Sept.

To my friend Dr. Ralph Schlaeger, expert radiologist and scholar in medicine and its history. In memory of many happy years at Columbia-Presbyterian.

With my compliments and best wishes

Mike [illegible]

DEATH OF THE CLINICIAN

Death of the Clinician

REQUIEM OR REVEILLE?

By

MICHAEL J. LEPORE, M.D.

Professor of Clinical Medicine
New York University School of Medicine
Attending Physician
Department of Medicine
St. Vincent's Hospital and Medical Center
University Hospital and Bellevue Hospital Center
New York, New York

CHARLES C THOMAS • PUBLISHER

Springfield • Illinois • U.S.A.

Published and Distributed Throughout the World by

CHARLES C THOMAS • PUBLISHER
2600 South First Street
Springfield. Illinois 62717 U.S.A.

ISBN 0-398 04591-7

Library of Congress Catalog Card Number: 81-9266

With THOMAS BOOKS *careful attention is given to all details of manufacturing and design. It is the Publisher's desire to present books that are satisfactory as to their physical qualities and artistic possibilities and appropriate for their particular use.* THOMAS BOOKS *will be true to those laws of quality that assure a good name and good will.*

Printed in the United States of America

AFG R-1

Library of Congress Cataloging in Publication Data

Lepore, Michael J.
Death of the clinician.

Bibliography: p.
Includes index.
1. Medical education–United States–History–20th century. 2. Medical colleges–United States–Faculty–History–20th century. I. Title.
R745.L52 610'.7'1173 81-9266
ISBN 0-398-04591-7 AACR2

To Ardean, my bride for over forty years, and to our son, Dr. Frederick Everett Lepore, whose love and understanding have made it possible for me to be neither full-time nor part-time but *over-time* in service to my institutions, my profession, and my patients.

PROLOGUE

The American doctor of today is the product of a highly competitive, gruelling, and demanding educational system designed to select and prepare the best candidates for the profession of medicine. It was not always thus. During the eighteenth and nineteenth centuries, almost any man in America could study medicine if he could afford the tuition fees or had family contacts for arranging service as an apprentice to an established practitioner. Too stupid to be a lawyer, too lazy to farm, and too immoral to be a minister were all too often the criteria for directing a son of the gentry into the profession of medicine. Not even a high school education was needed, and it was possible to become a doctor after only six months of study. Whatever its faults, and there were many, the system provided the public with ample numbers of doctors even though they were poorly educated, unscientific and semiliterate.

Efforts to improve standards of medical education were made almost from the beginning, but it was a slow and arduous process, and many years would pass before significant progress was made. According to Professor Lawrence J. Henderson, of Harvard Medical School, it was not until "somewhere between 1910 and 1912 in this country [that] a random patient with a random disease, consulting a doctor chosen at random, had, for the first time in the history of mankind, a better than fifty-fifty chance of profiting from the encounter."[1]

In 1910, with the publication by Abraham Flexner, a nonphysician and a relatively unknown high school teacher, of his now famous Bulletin Number Four of the Carnegie Foundation for the Advancement of Teaching, *Medical Education in the*

1. Strauss, Maurice B., Ed.: *Familiar Medical Quotations.* Boston, Little, Brown and Company, 1968, p. 302.

United States and Canada,[2] events were set in motion that would revolutionize American medical education. Emphasis would now be focussed on medicine as a science, while the practice of the art would be relegated to a secondary role.

The immediate impact of the Flexner report was to close many of the substandard medical schools of the day, leaving the field to those better equipped, staffed, and organized. Overproduction of poorly educated and ill-trained physicians was sharply curtailed and standards of medical licensure and practice improved.

Flush with his victory over the diploma mills, proprietary medical schools, and their proponents and armed with evidence accumulated from his inspection visits, Flexner saw the need for additional reforms and proceeded to fight for them. Closing wretched schools was not enough. Standards of education had to be raised in all the surviving ones, and new schools were to be built based on university criteria. A great believer in the university as the bastion of all educational progress, he pounced upon the proposal of Carl Ludwig, a famous German physiologist, to make of the chief clinical teachers in the medical schools university professors who would isolate themselves from "the distractions" of private practice and confine their activities within the walls of a hospital or medical school, be paid a salary for their "whole-time" or "full-time" work, and dedicate themselves entirely to teaching, training, and research in medicine. This was the reform that had already been instituted with great success in the so-called preclinical or basic science departments of anatomy, physiology, biochemistry, and pathology, and Flexner and his collaborators could hardly wait for similar reforms to be applied to the "practical" or clinical chairs.

Under Flexner's scheme, physicians and surgeons who were in private practice and responsible for most of the clinical teaching of the day would be assigned second-class status in the medical schools, the control of policy, curriculum, teaching assignments, as well as patient care being in the hands of full-time faculty.

So effective were Flexner's arguments and so cleverly and aggressively did he use the financial resources of the Rockefellers and those he recruited from other philanthropists to manipulate

2. Flexner, Abraham: *Medical Education in the United States and Canada.* A report to the Carnegie Foundation for the Advancement of Teaching. Bulletin No. 4 (1910). Washington, D. C., Science and Health Publications, 1960 reproduced.

university policy in support of his full-time plan, that most of the new schools of the twentieth century and many of the older schools selected to undergo reform were persuaded to commit themselves to his policy of strict full-time, at least for a time. During the 1920s and 1930s, there seemed to be little open dissent with Flexner's philosophy of medical education. Those who did protest, and there were a few powerful voices, were either squelched, suppressed, or ignored and bypassed in the stampede for philanthropic grants, scientific medicine, and Nobel prizes.

Since Flexnerian full-time was very expensive and few schools had the endowment and the resources to implement it, the initial experiment was, perforce, on a limited scale. Not until after World War II, when enormous sums of federal money became available for research and full-time staffing, would the movement expand to the degree that serious problems would arise, weaknesses become apparent, and complaints begin to fill the air.

Dissatisfaction and complaint, at first rather subdued, soon reached crescendo proportions, expressing the unhappiness of many individuals with what they perceived to be undesirable trends in medical education and health care delivery, attributable in part to the full-time system. Selected for special emphasis were defects in the education and selection of medical students, the overemphasis of science to the neglect of the art of medicine, the diminishing role of the practicing clinician in academic medicine, the subservience of the care of the individual to excessive dependence on technology, machines and tests and, in general, the dehumanization and depersonalization of patient care. This is not to imply that the revolution instigated by Flexner had failed in its entirety. There is no question that the full-time system brought some substantial benefits to the schools where it was installed, but, as with all innovations, it had its weaknesses as well as its strengths.

Blindness to these weaknesses on the part of Flexner and his disciples obstructed further reform and, in fact, served to polarize the medical profession into two armed camps, the "full-timers" or academicians versus the "part-timers" or practitioners. Fuel for the argument was provided by Flexner's intransigence, inflexibility, tactlessness and, on occasion, irrascibility. It was not the first time, nor would it be the last, that a revolutionary and an innovator might outlive his usefulness once his initial contribution had been made.

It is this topic, the full-time controversy, that forms a major theme of this book. An understanding of it is essential to judging the developments of the past half-century in the making of the American doctor, and I shall devote considerable space to presenting and commenting on the argument.

I shall present overwhelming evidence that Flexner's strict full-time concept for the clinical chairs was an unworkable and contrived scheme dreamed up by a small band of basic scientists without clinical expertise and a coterie of laymen led by Flexner, having access to large foundation grants, who sought to revolutionize American medical education by manipulating university policy through gifts of substantial sums of money. Should the most important key clinical teachers in our medical schools be as Flexner envisaged, an elitist group eschewing personal service to patients, delegating patient care to subordinates, insulated against twenty-four hour demands for service, isolated from contact with the community, and impervious to the requests of society for assistance in solving the problems of social reform so often associated with illness and disease? Would this not lead inevitably to the fulfillment of Sir William Osler's prophecy of 1911, in his famous letter to president Ira Remsen of Johns Hopkins University on full-time, in which he said, "The danger would be the evolution throughout the country of a set of clinical prigs the boundary of whose horizon would be the laboratory and whose only human interest was research, forgetful of the wider claims of a clinical professor as a trainer of the young, a leader in the multiform activities of the profession, an interpreter of science to his generation, and a counsellor in public and in private of the people, in whose interests after all the school exists."[3]

This warning by the greatest physician of modern times went unheeded and, in fact, was suppressed from view for fifty years. When the full-time system swept across the country, especially after World War II, many of Osler's predictions were fulfilled. Fortunately, before the system had taken over medical education

3. Chesney, Alan M.: *The Johns Hopkins Hospital and University Medical School,* vol. I. Balitmore, Johns Hopkins Press, 1963, pp. 180-81

in its entirety, voices of dissent were heard, and they gained in power and influence. The argument still goes on and, despite years of trial, study of the issue remains as divisive and controversial as it was in Osler's day.

THE VOICES OF DISSENT

Today, the voices of discontent with medicine and medical education are many and varied and come as a surprise to some who find it difficult to comprehend this dissatisfaction in an era when the health of the public has never been so good and medical technology and science have reached the highest levels ever. Who are those who complain and where do they come from? They can be divided into two main groups: those within the profession and those outside.

In a rapid and necessarily brief scanning of the area of conflict, I shall identify the main protagonists and indicate the sources of their unhappiness. Within the medical profession, we have the full-time *faculty,* unhappy with "routine" teaching assignments, inadequately rewarded financially and professionally for these activities, and bemoaning time lost from their laboratory investigations by ward and clinic teaching demands, committee work, and administrative duties. Next in line are the competent and seasoned *practioners* who like to teach but feel they have been shunted aside by the full-time staff who regard them as second-class citizens. The *medical students* are unhappy, their cries of irrelevance unduly influencing curriculum change and all too often indicating their failure and unwillingness to live up to the demands of scientific rigor and discipline. Undue emphasis on pass-fail, egalitarianism, and excessive commitment to electives of dubious value have contributed greatly to the decline of the medical school educational experience to the degree that students are now graduated who do not possess the basic skills needed to be a physician.

Admissions committees to the medical schools, charged to guard the gates and to admit only the best, confess freely their inadequacy for the assignment and complain that the criteria for admission become less and less reliable. "Dilution" of the undergraduate grades has progressed to the degree that an A is the equivalent of a B or even a C in the old days. The Medical

College Admissions Tests (MCATS) may tell us no more than does the grade in organic chemistry, and this merely tells us that the student with an A will almost certainly survive the first two years of medical school without giving us any prediction as to performance in the third and fourth years. The sheer volume of the applicants is overwhelming. Forty thousand applicants seek the 15,000 openings each year, and applications to as many as twenty or more medical schools are encouraged. In the present climate, I know of few faculty members who actually enjoy serving on an admission committee.

Finally, of the group within the profession, organized medicine, the *American Medical Association,* after a long period of leaving student affairs to the Association of American Medical Colleges (AAMC), is now so unhappy with the kind of physician being graduated from our medical schools that it plans, for the 1980s, to play a dominant role in the future direction of medical education, a role that may be fought tooth and nail by the deans of medical schools and the representatives of various specialty boards.

The voices of discontent outside of the house of medicine are even more strident and include *society,* which complains that the present system of medical education and training has unduly emphasized science and technology to the neglect of humanism; has overproduced specialists and subspecialists who fragment medical care; has failed to distribute doctors in ghetto, inner city, and rural areas; has failed to educate members of minorities for service to their people; has failed to stress service as a prime function of the doctor. Society criticizes doctors for being unavailable, too expensive, impersonal, spending too little time with their patients, being in a hurry, seldom listening, having undesirable personality traits and life-styles, and last, but not least, being not at all like the good old-fashioned family practitioner people have read about but seldom encountered.

Society believes that the present system of medical education is far too protective and solicitous of the doctor's comfort to the neglect of the needs of the patients. *Government,* many of whose leaders are noted for dissipating vast sums in pursuit of ill-defined and dubious social gains, asserts a proprietary interest in health care because "we are paying the bills." Is it not relevant to ask with whose money? The majority of well-informed citizens look upon politicization of American medicine, its socialization or what have you, as yet another step toward disaster and financial ruin to be avoided at almost all costs. *Costs* of medical care are responsible for many complaints as they skyrocket, although not nearly at the rate of our gasoline prices. We tend to forget that the quality of technology of medicine is getting better and better while a gallon of gasoline, like a good cigar, is still a gallon of gasoline, no more no less. When anger and fear are expressed at the finding that 10 percent of the gross national product is being spent for health care, the real question may be how effectively it was spent. Did it save lives and improve the quality of life? A society that spends more on its lawyers than its doctors and billions more on its automobiles than it does on its entire health care bill needs to reconsider its priorities.

THE PROFESSIONS UNDER SIEGE

Clearly, the profession of medicine is, to borrow a term from Professor Jacques Barzun of Columbia University, one of those "professions under siege." Siege is defined as "the encampment of an army about a fortified place to reduce and capture it by cutting off supplies, undermining, bringing guns to bear, and other offensive operations."[4]

In the preceding discussion, it is apparent that medicine is plagued and besieged by critics and well-meaning, but sometimes misguided, friends within the fortress as well as those outside. To categorically deny that anything is wrong with medical practice and medical education and to dismiss the complaints as the voices of troublemakers and malcontents without basis is, in fact, not only unscientific but patently untrue; it can lead to disaster. I, for one, believe that a good many things have gone wrong and cry out for their correction. In his elegant and perceptive essay, "The Professions Under Siege" Professor Barzun has put his finger on the quandary in which all of the professions find themselves, some more than others.[5]

The doctors, formerly worshiped as omniscient Good Samaritans,

4. *The Living Webster Encylopedic Dictionary*, Springfield, Massachusetts, G. & C. Merriam Company, 1971.

5. Barzun, Jacques: The professions under siege. *Harper's, 257/1541:* 61-68, Oct. 1978, p. 61.

> are now seen as profiteers, often of doubtful competence. Lawyers have never been popular, but they did seem the defenders of private and civil rights in time of need. Now they are thought neglectful and extortionate, when not actually dishonest. The poor academics, who won sudden prestige in the war years because they knew so much about so much that was useful, lost it all by their fecklessness in the troubles of 1965-68. As for the scientists, demigods since Darwin, they became objects of suspicion after Hiroshima. Their work was amoral; they dabbled in either treason or warmongering, and in any case their view of the universe was probably at the root of the modern malaise.

Barzun continues:

> The message for the professions today is that their one hope of survival with anything like their present freedoms is the recovery of mental and moral force . . . Policing, being negative, is not enough. It will not effect moral regeneration, which can come about only when the members of a group feel once more confident that ethical behavior *is* desirable, widely practiced, approved, and admired . . . . What all the professions need today is critics from inside, men who will know what the conditions are, and also the arguments and excuses, and in a full sweep over the field can offer their fellow practitioners a new vision of the profession as an institution.[6]

The Flexnerian revolution in American medical education was predicated upon the belief that university scientists, the key leaders, should be idealistic, of the highest integrity and character, and willing to make substantial financial sacrifices to advance the reformation. Flexner might turn over in his grave if he learned that the cream of the full-time academicians, the elite corps of research scientists, is now plagued with a highly publicized minority of miscreants in their ranks accused of cheating, dishonesty, plagiarism, and manipulation of data, the excuse being inordinate pressure to publish in order to advance careers and garner federal grants. Witness the resignation, under pressure, in August 1980, of the newly installed Bard Professor and Chief Physician at Columbia-Presbyterian Medical Center for "ethical insensitivity and other defects" in dealing with one of his former collaborators at Yale Medical School, who admitted falsifying research data and plagiarizing the work of other investigators.

Barzun concludes his essay on this note:

> When the problem is a failure of competence and morality, nothing will solve it but the work of an individual mind and conscience,

6. *Ibid.* p. 68.

> aided of course by the many scattered men of talent and good will who are only waiting for a lead. Without some such heroic efforts, we professionals shall all go down—appropriately—as nonheroes together.[7]

I take great comfort and considerable inspiration from Barzun's expression of faith and confidence in the individual to lead the way to reform. To paraphrase Professor Barzun, my desire is to function as a critic from inside, one who can be trusted by those who know what the true conditions are, and also the arguments and excuses, and in a full sweep over the field be able to offer fellow practitioners and academicians a new vision of the profession as an institution, the whole aim being to lift the critique from a set of complaints to a set of purposes—purposes no professional can gainsay because they are stated or restated by one who knows. Let this book, my *cri de coeur,* based on fifty years of personal observation and participation in the teaching and practice of medicine, serve not only as a critique but also as a catalyst and program for reform and improvement in the education, selection, training, and performance of the keen, dedicated, and remarkable young people who are destined to carry the torch, to meet the challenges and aspirations of the people we are privileged to serve.

M.J.L

7. *Ibid,* p. 68.

ACKNOWLEDGMENTS

In July 1975, little knowing what it would entail, I decided to speak out against some undesirable trends in medical education, training, and practice in the hope that my comments would stimulate reform and change. Some of the material was presented before committees of peers, teaching conferences, television, ward rounds, clinics, and various learned societies, but I wanted the message to reach the general public as well as my colleagues in medicine. This volume is dedicated to that end. The journey toward its publication has been exciting and rewarding for, in addition to renewing old friendships, it has led to many new ones. Access to fascinating correspondence, much of it unpublished and some of it held secret for fifty years or more, has added spice to the quest and led to all sorts of detours and unforeseen discoveries, the serendipitous experience of most research effort.

With considerable pleasure, indebtedness is acknowledged to Dr. J. William Hess of the Rockefeller Archive Center at Hillcrest, Pocantico Hills, North Tarrytown, New York, where many happy and busy hours were spent consulting original sources and correspondence assembled by the skilled and efficient staff in a scholarly, almost monastic setting.

To my revered professor of anatomy, Dr. George W. Corner, gratitude is expressed for granting access to the Flexner and Peabody correspondence in the library of the American Philosophical Society in Philadelphia. I owe much to Dr. Corner, including his active role in stimulating my interest in the history of medicine when I was a teenaged medical student at Rochester.

Miss Martha E. Swensson, my coworker and loyal associate of many years, has contributed substantially to the development of this book, not only in its preparation, organization, and research but as a source of steady encouragement and critical evaluation.

To Mr. Robert L. Volz, Head of the Department of Rare Books, Manuscripts and Archives of the University of Rochester, I acknowledge with pleasure assistance in making available the Eastman, Rhees, Whipple, and Flexner correspondence.

For Mr. Philip J. Weimerskirch, History of Medicine Librarian of the Edward G. Miner Library of the University of Rochester School of Medicine and Dentistry, I have sincere appreciation of his unfailing courtesy and helpfulness in locating some scarce items and for his cheerful encouragement.

Mr. Walter S. Ross of the *Reader's Digest* and the American Cancer Society, a seasoned and accomplished writer and a loyal friend, has helped to edit the book and has provided sound advice on numerous occasions.

My friend Mr. Sterling Lord has been gracious in his encouragement and generous in giving advice on this project.

To Mr. Payne E. L. Thomas, my publisher, I express sincere thanks for grasping the true message and thrust of the book and making it feasible to reach a wide audience.

For those who subscribe to my theme and to those who may differ, I quote this motto: *"AD PLACITUM PEREGI MEUM."*

CONTENTS

DEATH OF THE CLINICIAN

Chapter 1
DEATH OF THE CLINICIAN

Requiem or Reveille?

The major discoveries and scientific advances of the past half-century have served to expand the horizons of clinical medicine, diagnosis, and therapy almost beyond belief, giving the clinician of today a veritable arsenal of weapons for the battle against disease. Unfortunately, the price for these acquisitions has been the trend toward depersonalization and dehumanization of the care of the patient. Medicine as a science bids to displace medicine as an art. Medicine as a profession has edged toward a trade with regular business hours, no house calls, and excessive emphasis on material rewards. The personal contact of physician with patient, the intimate one-to-one approach, the laying on of the hands, is downgraded in our training and educational programs and is being delegated to nonphysicians. The art of history taking, physical diagnosis, and wise decision making has been relegated to the distant past rather than the present or future. Medicine by computer, Xray, nuclear scanning, and laboratory tests bids fair to take over, leading one observer to predict that in fifty years doctors will be obsolete.

I believe this prediction is totally in error, and I present the argument for the preservation and encouragement of an endangered species, the master of clinical medicine. My call is for reveille, not for requiem.

What is the definition of the word *clinician*? Our dictionaries tell us that the noun, clinician, is derived from the Greek *klinikos,* meaning bed. Animals do not usually sleep in beds, humans do. The clinician may then be defined as a physician who cares for humans in sickness and in health, at the bedside, in the clinic, in his office, or at home. What are the prime qualifications of a

Presented in part as the Cardinal Spellman Memorial Lecture, St. Vincent's Hospital and Medical Center of New York, October 26, 1979.

clinician and what does he do? Over one hundred years ago, John Brown (1810-1882) summed these up as: CAPAX, PERSPICAX, SAGAX, and EFFICAX and he defined these terms as follows.

> CAPAX–there must be room to receive, arrange, and keep knowledge;
> PERSPICAX–senses and perceptions keen, accurate, and immediate to bring in materials from all sensible things;
> SAGAX–a central power of knowing what is what and what is worth, of choosing and rejecting, of judging; and finally,
> EFFICAX–the will and the way–the power to turn all the other three–capacity, perspicacity, sagacity, to account in the performance of the thing in hand, and thus rendering back to the outer world, in a new and useful form, what you have received from it.[8]

I know of no computer capable of performing these functions.

In 1907, Sir William Osler, the greatest physician of modern times, defined the clinician's essential duties in the following terms.[9]

1. Acquire facility in the art of *diagnosis* to guide rational therapy.
2. Develop critical *judgement* to appreciate the relative value of symptoms, physical signs and laboratory data, and give the patient and his family a forecast and *prognosis*.
3. So conduct the *treatment* that the patient may be restored to health at the earliest possible period, or, failing that, be given the greatest possible measure of relief, whether by medications, by diet, by exercise, or by all the physical means available, and *often by the exercise of his own strong personality*.
4. Lastly, so to arrange sanitary and hygienic measures that wherever possible, disease may be *prevented*. (Italics added by Doctor Lepore.)

Here again, I know of no computer capable of performing these functions.

In 1932, in an address at the University College Medical School in London, Sir Wilfred Trotter had these wise comments on what he called "Aptitudes of the Doctor."[10]

---

8. Strauss, M. B. (Ed.): *Familiar Medical Quotations*. Boston, Little, Brown & Company, 1968, p. 401.
9. Osler, W. and McCrae, T.: *Modern Medicine*, vol. 1., Philadelphia, Lea Brothers & Co., 1907, p. xxxiv.
10. Trotter, Wilfred: *The Collected Papers of Wilfred Trotter (1872-1939)*. London, Oxford University Press, 1941, pp. 97-100.

> As long as medicine is an art, its chief and characteristic instrument must be *human faculty*. We come therefore to the very practical question of what aspects of human faculty is necessary for the good doctor to cultivate . . . .
>
> *The first to be named must always be the power of attention, of giving one's whole mind to the patient without the interposition of anything of oneself.* It sounds simple but only the very greatest doctors ever fully attain it. It is an active process and not either mere resigned listening or even politely waiting until you can interrupt. *Disease often tells its secrets in a casual parenthesis.* . . .
>
> *The second thing to be striven for is intuition.* This sounds an impossibility, for who can control that small quiet monitor. But intuition is only inference from experiences stored and not actively recalled. For that reason we should acquire experience and more experience . . . .
>
> *A humbler requirement but one not less necessary is the art of handling living flesh.* Here at any rate is something everyone can teach himself. Hands co-ordinated to smooth, firm, and gentle movement are to the sick body the complement of the attentive receptive mind. It yields its secrets to them but denies its secrets to the muttonfist as it does to the beefy mind . . . .
>
> The last aptitude I shall mention that must be attained by the good doctor is that of *handling the sick man's mind* . . . . In the exercise of this art he will have to convince the patient of his interest in the case, he will have to let him feel that something significant is being done all the time and he will have to teach him that his object must be health not comfort. When these purposes are clearly visualized they are easy enough to attain. *The most important is that the doctor should convince the patient of his personal interest.* The simplest way to do this is *to be interested*, and the effort will have its reward. *To the deep unreason with which all patients approach the medicine man, his interest is more potent than knowledge and skill, the latest development in science, or the utmost virtuosity in art.* (Italics added by Doctor Lepore.)

In contemporary terms, fifty years after Trotter, I present this list of the essential qualities of a good clinician.

Abilities

1. Competence: knowledge, thoroughness, accuracy.
2. Availability. What good is brilliance and skill if the doctor is not available?
3. Ability to listen: to hear what *is* told, what *is not* told, and what *cannot* be told.[11] To excel in nonverbal communication.

11. Henderson, J. L.: Physician and patient as a social system. *N Engl J Med, 212/18:* 819-23, May 2, 1935.

4. Ability to observe the obvious, and the not so obvious.
5. Ability to select and use diagnostic tests with wisdom, economy, and discretion.
6. Ability to collect information, sort it, and *make decisions*.
7. Ability to communicate: with the patient, his family, and the public.
8. Ability to adapt, to make changes: flexibility and versatility.
9. Ability to temper scientific practice with humanism.
10. Ability to work, the master word in medicine.
11. Ability to work solo.
12. Ability to work as a team member.
13. Ability to impart knowledge—to teach.
14. Ability to accept responsibility.

Character

1. Integrity—trustworthiness (worthy of confidence). Morality. Honesty.
2. Wisdom—sound judgement.
3. Loyalty.
4. Reverence for life.
5. Love for patients (*carita*).
6. Devotion to the welfare of patients.
7. Respectful of the individual and his rights.
8. Respected by his peers and his institutions.

Personality Characteristics

1. Affability, courteous manners, presents himself attractively. Observes appropriate dress code.
2. Reliability—predictability, dependability.
3. Compassion.
4. Capacity for giving—more than he takes. Generosity.
5. Courage.
6. Enthusiasm (inspired by God).
7. Optimism and a good sense of humor. The capacity "to quickly laugh for fear of crying."
8. Self-discipline.
9. Patience.
10. Durability—staying power.
11. Imperturbability, equanimity—steadfast under fire.
12. Resourcefulness.

13. A self-learner–a lifetime student.

I demand of our educational and medical school system, our society, our hospitals, doctors, and students the selection, development, nurture, and replication of men and women who have these important key traits.

One of my friends[12] has suggested that what we need in modern medicine is a society for the preservation of the use of the five senses (SPUFS). The members would be called young spufers and old spufers. These senses, as you know, are those of seeing, feeling, hearing, taste, and smell. One might add the sixth sense of cenesthesis (the sense of normal functioning of the organs of the body) and the seventh sense, or visceral sense, perhaps in contemporary terminology, *gut feeling.* Last, but not least, a sense of humor and an appreciation of laughter as a therapeutic tool.

Sir William Osler expressed it in these words: "The art of the practice of medicine is to be learned by experience; 'tis not an inheritance; it cannot be revealed. Learn to see, learn to hear, learn to feel, learn to smell, and know that by practice alone can you become expert."[13]

Having described some traits of the ideal clinician, let me pursue the question of what a clinician really does and present evidence that such physicians will never be replaced by a computer, CAT scanner, laboratory tests, or any technological or mechanical device.

How does a clinician, armed chiefly with his special senses, attempt to solve the problems brought to him? How does he make the diagnosis? How does he apply rational therapy? How does he prognosticate? Does he need all of those machines and laboratory tests, or can he and his patients survive with a minimum of these? Does he sometimes make the diagnosis in spite of the tests and machines rather than because of them?

I am in no sense trying to turn the clock back to the past. The advances of modern technology are here to stay and there are more to come. My plea is to harness them in the patient's best interests; utilize them effectively, efficiently, and wisely, with an

12. Richards, Dickinson W.: Are our medical school faculties qualified to teach medicine? *Resident and Staff Physician*, Oct. 1971, pp. 76-88.

13. Bean, William B. (Ed.): *Sir William Osler Aphorisms*, Springfield, Thomas, 1961, p. 129.

eye to their cost, not only in money but in patient discomfort and exposure to hazards. I plead for the application of the five God-given senses each one of us possesses in the problem solving that is the essence of good medical practice. No machine and no computer can ever displace these. These senses are part of us and they must never be neglected.

For the younger members of our profession, my hope is that what I have to say will serve as a stimulus to continue to develop their five senses and to have confidence in what the physician, as a person, is able to accomplish as a healer. Do not be overwhelmed by the burgeoning technology and machines surrounding us. Be their master; make them your servant. Remember that, unlike the scientific facts taught to you in medical school, half of which will be obsolete in five or ten years (your teachers unable to predict which half will survive), the art of history taking, physical examination, and decision making grows better with each year of experience and practice and should never leave you as long as you maintain control of your special senses.

Let me now turn to illustrations of how the clinician does his daily work and how he makes his reputation and his living. Rather than express the opinions and experiences of others, I shall present examples of patients from my own private, ward, and clinic practice.

The first patient was seen at Duke University Hospital in 1934. She was a forty-five-year-old woman with a history of diarrhea, weakness, extreme weight loss with emaciation, sore tongue, and a macrocytic hyperchromic anemia, with free HCl secreted in the gastric juice. She was presented at medical grand rounds as a patient with probable carcinomatosis, primary site unknown. As she was being wheeled out of the conference room, an intern rose to question the diagnosis, which he felt was undocumented. This was almost unheard of for an intern and led to a rather spirited debate. During the course of the discussion, Dr. Frederic M. Hanes, Chairman of the Department of Medicine, asked whether the intern had an alternative diagnosis. The intern proposed nontropical sprue, a wasting , diarrheal disease often associated with macrocytic anemia. When pressed for tests to substantiate this diagnosis, he suggested a glucose tolerance test, which had been reported by Danish investigators to be flat and interpreted as evidence of malabsorption of glucose. The test was done and turned out to be flat. The patient was treated with liver extract and responded dramatically, with weight gain, remission of anemia, and abatement of diarrhea. This was case number one of sprue at Duke Hospital and was forerunner of a large series that was collected over the years by Doctor Hanes who became a world authority on sprue. This disease is no longer rare. In the infant and child, it is known as celiac disease and may lead to stunted growth. Some of the best jockeys in England were afflicted with celiac disease. Now that we know that the disease can be effectively treated by a special gluten-free diet, the horse race enthusiasts of Great Britain have been known to complain that they have been deprived of the source of some of their best young jockeys.

The second patient I would like to discuss was a fifty-six-year-old French baker who was admitted in October 1952, to the Columbia-Presbyterian Medical Center with a ten-week story of diarrhea, weight loss, fever, chills, polyarthritis, weakness, and tan pigmentation of the skin. He was thoroughly studied during his stay in the ward and found to be anemic and to have malabsorption with a flat oral glucose tolerance curve, a markedly elevated ESR rate, and an abnormal small intestine study. The opinion of those who were in charge of his care was that he was suffering with nontropical sprue, and I was called to see him in consultation. Fever is not a manifestation of sprue and neither is an elevated red cell sedimentation rate, so I smelled a rat. To make a long story short, my diagnosis was not sprue but something called Whipple's disease. I had never seen a case, but I knew that my revered mentor and teacher, Dr. George Hoyt Whipple, founding Dean of the University of Rochester School of Medicine, had published the first example of the disease destined to bear his name while an instructor in pathology in 1907 at Johns Hopkins Hospital. I recommended that the patient undergo abdominal exploration to document the diagnosis for, in 1952, this was the only way it could be confirmed. The attending physician was the late Dr. Charles A. Ragan, who was sympathetic to the need for an exploratory operation, but the formidable and brilliant Dr. Robert F. Loeb, our department chairman and Bard Professor, quashed the suggestion in very strong terms saying he did not believe in exploring to settle a diagnosis. This was entirely in character for Doctor Loeb, who had five aphorisms for medicine: the first, to follow the Golden Rule and the last, and by no means least, to keep the patient out of the surgeon's hands. The patient was discharged but found his way back to the Vanderbilt Clinic where I was in charge of him. As is true in many academic centers, cooperation between the departments of surgery and medicine left something to be desired and, in fact, at times the atmosphere suggested two armed camps. My next move, admittedly fraught with danger, was to bypass the medical service by arranging the patient's direct admission to the surgical service for exploration which was performed on November 12, 1952. The findings were those of classical Whipple's disease. In those days, the diagnosis of Whipple's disease was the equivalent of a death certificate. Since then, we have learned that long-term antibiotic therapy is curative, and there is all the more reason to discover the disease and to institute rational therapy.

The third patient was a sixty-six-year-old woman with a bleeding gastric ulcer who was scheduled to have her stomach removed the following day in a New Jersey hospital. She happened to be the aunt of Dean Houston Merritt's secretary, who located me in the Vanderbilt Clinic where I was finishing a gruelling session at five o'clock. A good deal of pressure was put upon me to see the patient, who had already been examined by many consultants. I finally arrived at the hospital (in New Jersey) at about nine o'clock that evening. The patient's internist had been quite annoyed at the flood of consultants and failed to meet me at the hospital. This did not make me very happy. I reviewed the chart and immediately became suspicious. The record showed that this patient's blood count and hematocrit values had been stable for the preceding three days without requiring transfusion. The disturbing item was that the special nurses, assigned around the clock, were reporting black tarry stools despite repeated enemas. The assumption was that the patient was still actively bleeding. As I finished my examination, I asked for a glove and performed a rectal examination that revealed exactly what I suspected, a large black fecal impaction that had been untouched by the enemata. The black enema returns were due to old blood in the rectum. My diagnosis was that the bleeding had stopped at least three days before and that the patient did not need an operation. This really created quite a storm, especially with her physician, who rather pointedly asserted that I was out of line with all of the other consultants and asked if I would accept the responsibility if she bled again during the night. My answer was "Of course I will," and I gave him my home telephone number. The patient never bled again and lived another ten years, succumbing to hypertensive cardiovascular disease. Some time after her death, her husband made a gift to me that equipped the Borea Endoscopy Unit at St. Vincent's Hospital, a living memorial to a wonderful woman.

The fourth patient was a sixty-nine-year-old man who was seen by me in consultation in January 1963, in another hospital in New Jersey, because of recurrent gastrointestinal bleeding manifested by black, tarry stools and profound anemia. He had already been explored twice prior to my consultation and had undergone a partial gastreectomy with vagotomy. The presumptive diagnosis was bleeding duodenal ulcer, but no ulcer had been found on exploration, gastrostomy, or in the resected specimen. He continued to bleed, and this was why I was asked to see him. The diagnosis was let out of the bag when I looked into his mouth and saw on the left buccal mucosa a large blue bleb nevus. As I was examining him at the bedside, surrounded by residents and attending staff, I turned and asked whether anyone had noticed any other lesions of this type. The answer was in the negative, but having found one in the mouth that had been missed cold, I continued with my examination and, to everyone's chagrin but mine, found another similar blue bleb vascular malformation on the sole of the right foot. My diagnosis was bleeding from blue bleb vascular malformations that I thought I could see in the transverse duodenum on some x-ray films that had been taken. At operation, the diagnosis was confirmed and the transverse duodenum was resected, putting a stop to the bleeding for some years.

The fifth patient was referred to me for what I shall call a mortician-category consultation. By this, I mean she was sent to me by her highly competent personal physician who had diagnosed cancer of the stomach with metastases to the left hip and told the family it was hopeless, that she could be dead within three to six months. I was extremely reluctant to see the patient merely to reaffirm the death sentence, but I was prevailed upon to do this by the plea that if I agreed with the diagnosis, the family would be willing to accept it as the last word and would feel that everything had been done. The patient was in her forties, looked quite well, and complained of indigestion. The x-ray films showed a large ulcerated lesion on the lesser curvature of the stomach and a large solitary bone metastasis of cancer to the left hip. It all seemed to fit together until, as I proceeded with my usual complete physical examination, I felt a firm, golf-ball-sized mass in the left lobe of the thyroid gland, extending behind the sternum. This, I felt, was almost certainly a cancer of the thyroid gland. This physical finding led me to question whether the primary cancer was in the stomach. I admitted her to Harkness Pavilion where we established that the gastric ulcer was benign and healed quickly on medical therapy. Total thyroidectomy was done by Dr. Lawrence Sloan for what proved to be carcinoma of the thyroid. The bone metastasis was secondary to the thyroid cancer and was treated with radioiodine 131 with an excellent response that was sustained for several years.

The sixth patient was a beautiful and famous actress who was referred to me because of a right lower quadrant and pelvic mass for which a specialist at Memorial Hospital had recommended operation for an ovarian tumor. A professor of gynecology at Columbia-Presbyterian disagreed with this diagnosis, found no evidence of an ovarian tumor, and recommended consultation with me. She brought with her a list of physicians she had seen, among them some of the best in America and a few of the worst. She had been in Harkness Pavilion for over ten days some months before, at which time she had undergone considerable diagnostic testing under the supervision of one of our senior professors. Dr. Ross Golden, the great radiologist, did a gastrointestinal and small intestine study and raised the question of amebiasis of the cecum. He was told by the attending physician that he was overdiagnosing this condition. However, to accommodate Doctor Golden, two stool specimens were sent to the laboratory for examination for ova and protozoa including amebae, and they were reported as negative. When I examined the patient, I found a mass in the right lower quadrant that I suspected was an amebic granuloma of the cecum. I also knew that in a political or economy move, our chief parasitologist had been moved out of her quarters on the eighth floor of Presbyterian Hospital to a laboratory in the Board of Health Building on the corner of 168th Street and Broadway. It seemed never to have occurred to those responsible for this decision that it would be next to impossible to get a fresh, warm, purged stool to that laboratory on a freezing day in March all the way from Harkness Pavilion, one long city block away. Recognizing this possible flaw in the otherwise impregnable diagnostic workup in Harkness, I sent the patient to the late Dr. Howard Shookhoff for a warm purged stool examination in his laboratory. He reported promptly that the stool was loaded with Entameba Histolytica, the pathogen responsible for her illness. I cured her with appropriate antiamebic medication.

The last patient, a thirty-nine-year-old, single secretary, was admitted to St. Vincent's Hospital in September 1976 because of a weight loss of thirty pounds and recurrent indigestion with sharp midepigastric pain radiating through to the back, worse after eating. Complete diagnostic workup was essentially nonconclusive until the significance of a loud systolic epigastric bruit was appreciated. This led to abdominal arteriography that revealed severe narrowing and stenosis of the proximal celiac artery, and the diagnosis of celiac axis compression syndrome was made. An operation was performed at another medical center in New York where the diagnosis was confirmed at operation on September 27, 1976, at which time a constricting band obstructing the celiac axis was dissected away and the artery dilated. The patient failed to improve after operation and was followed by the surgeon who readmitted her to his hospital in April 1977, where many studies were performed, including a gastroscopy and abdominal arteriography, with what were interpreted as essentially normal findings. The patient was advised to seek psychiatric help. At this point, she returned to St. Vincent's Hospital where we disagreed with the previous opinions and felt that her problems were in her abdomen and not in her head and did not call for psychiatric help. Our diagnosis was that the first operation had been an incomplete one and had not solved her problem, which remained essentially that of celiac axis compression. Reoperation was performed and a most extraordinary lesion discovered—

encasement of the celiac axis by a dense, almost cartilaginous process that proved to be neurofibromatoses encasing the artery. Resection was performed, and the patient slowly but steadily improved, regaining the thirty pounds she had lost during the period of the followup. She remains well to date, three years after the operation.

I could narrate many more of these experiences, but I think the point has been made that the clinician, using his five senses, should be able to outgun the computer and the machines, making them his servants not his masters.

The *first* patient with sprue was diagnosed by being aware of the possibility and refusing to accept an undocumented diagnosis of cancer. The *second* (Whipple's disease) was a matter of alertness to the message that the laboratory data were trying to convey and the importance of having the courage to differ with higher authority even to the point of risking one's professional future to protect the patient's interests. The *third* (gastric ulcer with hemorrhage) illustrates the importance of Osler's aphorism that a specialist is a doctor who does a rectal examination. The *fourth* (blue bleb nevus) emphasizes the importance of seeing and believing. The *fifth* patient shows the value of a careful physical examination and viewing with skepticism any diagnosis of a fatal illness without searching carefully for alternatives—especially if the presenting diagnosis is not supported by tissue documentation. The *sixth* (amebiasis of the cecum) is the old, old story of trusting no one but yourself and taking nothing for granted. It serves also to illustrate the value of the consultant having his roots in the community and its institutions, privy to and familiar with its idiosyncracies and problems, knowing the weaknesses of institutions and personnel, and using this information effectively in the detective work needed to succeed in the art of clinical diagnosis. For this, there is no substitute for time, experience, persistence, perspicacity, and staying power. The lesson from the *seventh* patient is that when you know your patient and have confidence in her, do not acquiesce to a psychiatric diagnosis that may simply close the door to remedial therapy of a physical ailment.

The clinician is not dead, but he is an endangered species. My call is for reveille, not requiem.

Chapter 2
THE CLINICIAN

An Endangered Species

In his monograph, *The Post-Physician Era,*[14] Dr. Jerrold S. Maxmen, an Assistant Professor of Psychiatry at Albert Einstein College of Medicine, makes this claim: "We are entering into a new medical era—an era I believe will culminate in the total obsolescence of the physician, and in a radical transformation of our entire health care system." He goes on to predict that "in fifty years, doctors will be obsolete, replaced by computers and a new breed of health care professional called 'the medic' " whose training would take only twelve to eighteen months as compared to eight years required to train a doctor. My personal comment is "God forbid" that this should happen. Few physicians or medical educators would agree with these predictions, but they do raise serious questions.

Those of us who have been privileged to witness the rise and decline of the great practicing clinicians in our academic centers may be tempted to agree in principle but surely not in fact; however the trend is alarming. The clinician is not dead. He is in short supply, and his future is very much in jeopardy. Clearly, something has gone wrong. Despite major advances in the scientific and technological aspects of clinical practice and improved health of the public, complaints are filling the air. In Wildavsky's catchy phrase, medicine is "Doing Better and Feeling Worse."[15] Many explanations have been offered for this curious contradiction. I shall single out, as a major factor, the planned disappearance from academe of the practicing clinician, all too often bypassed in important policy decisions, relegated to minor tasks, and looked

14. Maxmen, Jerrold S.: *The Post-Physician Era.* New York, John Wiley and Sons, 1976, p. 15.
15. Wildavsky, A.: Doing better and feeling worse: the political pathology of health policy. In Knowles, John H. (Ed.): *Doing Better and Feeling Worse.* New York, W. W. Norton & Co., Inc., 1977, pp. 105-23.

upon by some academicians and full-time faculty as a second-class citizen. The broadly based master clinician or diagnostician has largely disappeared from our midst, and I submit that the current climate and restricted opportunity in academic centers are in a large measure responsible for his decline. How and why did this come about and what can be done to reverse the trend?

In the stampede to the specialities and subspecialities, general medicine has been grossly neglected for many years, especially since World War II. In academic centers, all too often only those who fail to make it as subspecialists gravitate to general medicine. Any medical student can see that the way to get ahead in academe is to latch on to an esoteric, narrow subspeciality and to stay with it and in the process lose contact with the patient as a whole. These trends have been encouraged by the proliferation of subspecialty boards and the emphasis on knowing more and more about less and less. Doctor Petersdorf, of the American Board of Internal Medicine, has commented that the number of those being certified as specialists in Infectious Diseases, for one, is so high that they may well end up spending "their time culturing each other."[16]

It is no exaggeration that on teaching services we tend to emphasize diseases most of the future doctors will seldom encounter and stress technology that may be unavailable to many of them after they go into practice. The focus on the laboratory has led to the worship of numbers, often a computer printout with little or no appreciation of the possibility for error or of the foibles and weaknesses of the machines.

Diagnostic techniques are stressed to the exclusion of thinking, communicating, taking good histories, and doing meticulous physical examinations. To top it off, the rewards for testing exceed, by far, those for thinking and time spent with the patient; and doctors, who are only human, tend to neglect thinking for testing.

When, for example, the performance of coronary arteriography, colonoscopy, or an ERCP (endoscopic retrograde cholangiopancreatography) is rewarded by fees that dwarf those allowed for a physical examination and careful history, it takes a very

16. Petersdorf, R. G.: The doctors' dilemma. *N Engl J Med, 299/12:*628-34, Sept. 21, 1978, p. 631.

dedicated clinician to continue to commit large segments of his time to the latter. Much of the blame for this should be assigned to insurance plans and third-party payers that reward testing and technology more generously than thinking. All of this and more has led to depersonalization and dehumanization of health care and discontent among some of our lay friends. Unless something is done to reverse this trend, the clinician, already in a weakened position, will remain increasingly vulnerable to attack. He is indeed an endangered species.

Too much of the education of medical students is based upon problems seldom seen outside of hospitals. Outpatient activity and primary care are given second-class status. Nonpracticing clinicians, serving as key teachers, are often short in clinical skills and sadly lacking in experience. Therapy for short-term illness may be well taught, but chronic illness is generally poorly handled. "Foot-of-the-bed" rounds and "chart" rounds have all too often replaced bedside teaching and the laying on of the hands, with the student seldom being brought into contact with the patient. The person as a whole is neglected, while his heart, his lungs, his kidneys, or his liver receive maximal attention, chiefly from strangers seen only in a crisis and seldom available for around-the-clock comprehensive care and followup. Decisions by committee supplant those that should be made by one's own personal physician. So-called intensive care may be noted more for its intensity than for its care! Personal care has plummeted in our teaching programs and needs reemphasis. The care of the sick can never be impersonal if it is to succeed. No capsule, no injections of medication, and no machine or test, no matter how sophisticated, can ever replace the committed personal physician. In any illness, real or imaginary, the physician himself becomes an important part of the treatment.

Seldom in our teaching and training programs are the joys and satisfactions that come from personal rendition of medical services to patients given proper emphasis. Enthusiasm for curing and healing people is all too often displaced by morbid preoccupation with disease processes or rare, exotic, and all-too-often incurable disorders. TLC, which used to stand for tending loving care, has been supplanted by thin layer chromatography for this generation of medical students.

Speaking of our medical students, what has the present system of medical education done to them and for them? At the college level, it has encouraged undue competition, grade grubbing, a narrowly based education with little or no exposure to the humanities. The study of modern languages has virtually disappeared. When you ask prospective medical students why this is so, the answer is that the medical schools have dropped the language requirement. Is it not time to change the entrance requirements to meet the needs of a modern physician to be a person of broad education and culture and not merely a technician? Multiple choice examinations have led to the emergence of a quasi-illiterate elite with ability to achieve high scores without the capacity to write acceptable English prose, or any other for that matter. Competition is of such a high order that it has made cheating a way of life rather than an occasional deviation. In medical school, similar trends prevail. Basic science education, instead of being expanded and given more space in the curriculum to cope with the enormous explosion in new scientific information, is steadily encroached upon and forced to yield ground. Medical students, not quite dry behind the ears, seek to escape the rigors of scientific discipline by crying out "irrelevant" if basic science courses seem demanding. There is nothing new about this. Medical students have always complained. The real difference is that in this era people in charge listen to them.

Similar escapes from responsible scholarliness are seen in permissiveness and the excessive trend toward electives that leave medical students chiefly to their own devices at a stage in their lives when they badly need supervised activity, discipline, and graded responsibility. Pass-fail is a disaster, as so many medical graduates have found when the time has come for application for internship and residency. Close supervision of history taking and physical examination by well-qualified instructors is as rare as hen's teeth. It is any wonder that discerning physicians complain that by the end of the fourth year in most medical schools the students graduate without ever having developed the basic tools needed for the care of the sick? So serious and flagrant are these deficiencies that the AMA, seeking to actively intervene in medical education to correct what it perceives to be major faults, is proposing a return to the long-discredited rotating internship, albeit a modified form. The AMA wants to ensure that every doctor is equipped with the fundamental techniques and clinical skills needed to function as a general physician no matter whether he is ultimately a dermatologist, a psychiatrist, a radiologist, or whatever. Shades of George Hoyt Whipple, founding dean of the University of Rochester's School of Medicine, whose educational creed was that four years in a good medical school should produce a doctor with the equivalent of a rotating internship as well as well-defined basic clinical skills in history taking, physical examination, and decision making. Perhaps we need to turn the clock back fifty years or so.

Many of these undesirable trends might have been avoided if the practicing clinician had not been bypassed in academic medicine and assigned minor and weaker roles in the teaching of the medical students and house staff. Most of the contribution of practitioners to medical teaching in the past was without salary or compensation other than the joy of fulfillment of the Hippocratic Oath. The money value alone of these teaching services was astronomical and reflected the altruism and generosity of the medical profession in very real terms. When in the history of any profession has so much been given with so little in the way of financial return? Why did we permit this tradition to decline? How can we restore the practicing clinician to one of his finest roles where he belongs as a stimulating influence in the teaching and training of each new generation of doctors?

Chapter 3
REFORM IN MEDICAL EDUCATION

I want to influence in some measure the life of my time in so far as that can be done through education.

–A. Flexner, Sept. 1904[17]

Granted that the diminished role of practicing clinicians in medical school teaching is a significant phenomenon of the past twenty-five years or more and conceding that it has led to many undesirable developments, we need to ask ourselves how this came about and how to change the trend.

Seventy years ago, most of the clinical teaching in our medical schools was by volunteer faculty who practiced in the surrounding community and taught medical students as a privilege and duty without financial reimbursement. There were, of course, exceptions to this, especially in the proprietary schools organized mainly for profit from fees paid by students whose chief qualification for admission was their ability to pay tuition. The basic sciences, anatomy, physiology, biochemistry, and therapeutics, at first taught by part-time practicing clinicians seeking to climb toward the clinical chairs, were soon to become staffed by salaried personnel who would devote their full time to teaching. With the passage of time, many of the latter would covet the financial rewards being reaped by their clinical colleagues and resent their affluence and prestige. In addition, some would accuse the clinical professors of neglecting their teaching assignments for lucrative private practice while enjoying the privilege of academic status and rank while contributing relatively little to the university.

Foremost among those who wished to place restraints and controls upon the clinical professors was Franklin P. Mall, professor of anatomy at Johns Hopkins. During postgraduate studies

17. Flexner, Abraham: *An Autobiography*. A revision of author's *I Remember, 1940*. New York, Simon and Schuster, 1960, p. 61.

in Leipzig, Germany, in 1885-1886, under the great physiologist, Carl Ludwig, Mall had often discussed medical education and had been imbued by his mentor with the concept that teachers of clinical medicine, like their preclinical colleagues, should be of university rank and caliber; be paid a salary; be forbidden the "distractions" of private practice; and required to confine their work to teaching, training, and research within the university and its clinics and hospitals. This proposal, which became known as the whole-time or full-time method of teaching, led to important repercussions in medical education in America. Professor Mall, described by some as an anatomist who did little or no teaching and by others as a genius (neither term being necessarily incompatible with the other), brought his revolutionary ideas to Johns Hopkins in 1893, where the clinical teaching was in the hands of renowned clinicians with large consulting practices, among them William Osler, professor of medicine, William Halsted, professor of surgery, and Howard Kelly, professor of gynecology, all serving on a part-time basis, earning most of their living from private practice.

Osler and Mall would soon clash on approaches to the teaching of medicine, but Mall knew better than to openly oppose the great clinical stars of Hopkins and risk incurring their wrath. He did, however, persuade one of his proteges, Lewellys F. Barker, then a member of his department, to embrace the concept of full time in the clinical chairs. Barker was professor of anatomy at the University of Chicago when, by his own admission, he acted as Mall's mouthpiece by delivering an address in 1902 before the Western Alumni of Johns Hopkins University on "Medicine and the Universities." It was in this talk that he openly espoused Mall's program of doing for the clinical chairs in medicine what had already been accomplished with the preclinical ones, i.e. to place the occupants of the major clinical chairs on a full-time salary, eschewing private practice and confining their activities to teaching, research, and training within the university, its clinics, and its hospitals.[18] The proposal was greeted with predictable responses, the preclinical scientists very much in its favor, while the clinicians gave it a cold shoulder. Besides, it was all hypothetical. There simply was not enough money to fund the con-

18. Barker, Lewellys F.: Medicine and the universities. *Am Med, IV:*143-47, July 26, 1902.

cept. In addition, what did Barker or Mall know about clinical medicine? They were both professors of anatomy with no experience in the practice of medicine. Nonetheless, the essay established Barker as the main proponent of full time in the clinical chairs.

The concept of full-time teaching in the clinical departments made little or no headway until a reformer named Abraham Flexner entered upon the scene and became its aggressive and vigorous champion. Flexner, born in 1866 in Louisville, Kentucky, the sixth of nine children in a family of impecunious circumstances, was destined to revolutionize American medical education. His ancestry and his background give little insight into the interesting career he was to pursue. His father, who had started as an itinerant peddler and amassed a modest fortune only to lose it in the panic of 1873, died in 1882 when Abraham was sixteen years old. In the great Jewish tradition of family loyalty, the oldest son, Jacob, a pharmacist, saved money for Abraham's education and, in 1884, gave him one thousand dollars to go to Johns Hopkins University to finish his education. Abraham knew he could not afford to remain in Baltimore longer than two years, and by dint of great energy, ability, and ingenuity, he was able to complete his course and obtain his degree in two years instead of the usual four. He returned to Louisville in 1886 to teach in the local high school and was addressed as "professor." Soon he started tutoring special pupils and, in 1890, was persuaded to open his own private school, "Mr. Flexner's School," which occupied his interests for the next fifteen years. The school prospered and he was able to help his younger brother, Simon, obtain a medical degree and, later, to direct him to Johns Hopkins where he became first assistant to Dr. William H. Welch, professor of pathology and founding dean of the medical school

The ties between Abraham and Simon remained very close and served to prepare the former for the important career he was to pursue in medical education. Years later (1920), Simon, who had risen to become head of the Rockefeller Institute and was the recipient of many well-earned honors, would pay this heartfelt tribute to his brother, Abe:

> But this fact in no way affects the great debt I owe you. To have sent me to The Hopkins and Doctor Welch in the far-away autumn

of 1890 has meant more for me than anyone except myself can know. It was not only that you made it possible with money that I should go that is so remarkable—great indeed as that event was—but that you should have possessed the insight that convinced you that Dr. Welch was the master in pathology that is almost miraculous. You also were a very young man then. This judgement merely preshadowed all the splendid things which you have done since then—many far beyond praise. But, I thought that I would like you to know where my thoughts have been roaming these two days and how deeply I feel my unredeemable debt to you, Abe.

In June 1905, dissatisfied with the routine work of his first-rate private school and burning with ambition to "influence in some measure the life of my time in so far as that can be done through education," Flexner closed his school and decided to go to the Graduate School at Harvard and then to Europe. "I was determined to make a career in education, and though my acquaintance with schools, school systems, and colleges was slight, and felt by me to be slight, I was fully, though vaguely, convinced that all were in need of thoroughgoing reform."[19]

When he returned from Europe three years later (1908), he was without a job and without money and was prepared to do "almost anything of a scholarly nature."[20] When Dr. Henry S. Pritchett of the Carnegie Foundation for the Advancement of Teaching offered him the assignment to make a study of medical schools, Flexner was certain he was confusing him with his brother, Simon, only to have Pritchett say, "I think these professional schools should be studied not from the point of view of the practitioner but from the standpoint of the educator. I know your brother, so that I am not laboring under any confusion. This is a layman's job, not a job for a medical man."[21] The offer of the "layman's job" to examine the medical schools had come about in a curious way.

THE ROLE OF THE AMERICAN MEDICAL ASSOCIATION IN REFORMING MEDICAL EDUCATION

It may come as somewhat of a surprise to the informed layman of today, and even to some physicians, that the initial thrust to improve medical education in America came from the AMA and several of its committees. Over the years there has been a

19. Flexner, *Autobiography*, pp. 60-61.
20. *Ibid.*, p. 71.
21. *Ibid.*, p. 11.

tendency to play down the role of the AMA in furthering standards of medical education and health care and, in fact, to regard it as a reactionary, mossbacked, politically active organization chiefly interested in maintaining the *status quo* and protecting a profitable monopoly. In the interest of scientific accuracy and fair play, credit must be given to the important efforts made by the AMA to close the poorer schools, to elevate the standards of medical education and practice, and to eliminate the proprietary for-profit medical schools and to replace them with university-type medical schools.

In 1846, Dr. Nathan Smith Davis, destined to become known as the father of the AMA, succeeded in persuading the New York State Medical Society to call for a national convention of physicians in Philadelphia where, in 1847, the AMA was organized and committed to the concepts "that young men received as students of medicine should have acquired a suitable preliminary education" and "that a uniform elevated standard of requirements for the degree of doctor of medicine should be adopted by all the medical schools in the United States."[22] One of the most important actions of this convention was the establishment of a committee on education that functioned for fifty-seven years before it was superseded by the Council on Medical Education when the AMA was reorganized.

As early as 1850, this committee complained in its annual report that medical education was defective because there were too many medical students and a scarcity of qualified teachers; that the quantity of medicine taught was too limited, the quality superficial, and the "mode of bestowal of honors of medicine too profuse and unrestricted." In 1858, James R. Wood, chairman of the Committee on Medical Education, arranged for the formation of the Association of American Medical Colleges to further efforts of the AMA to improve medical education. Hardly an annual meeting of the AMA would go by without comments deploring the conditions in medical education and offering resolutions for their correction, but little was accomplished, it seeming easier to show the defects of the system than to devise remedies. In addition, opposition to reform appeared, the influence of the

22. Fishbein, Morris: *The American Medical Association: 1847-1947*. Philadelphia, W.B. Saunders Co., 1947, p. 34.

medical college "professors" in the AMA being blamed for obstructing attempts to establish national standards for medical teaching and enforcing them upon their respective institutions. Many resolutions were passed and appeals made to the medical colleges of the day with little or no discernible effect.[23] Clearly, it was not enough to hold meetings and to pass resolutions favored by a minority of idealistic reformers. Something more was needed and it was not long in arriving.

In 1878, the Illinois State Board of Health, led by its secretary, Dr. J. H. Rauch, studied the number and character of the country's existing medical schools and adopted minimum requirements of medical schools as a necessary step toward the recognition of their diplomas by the State Board of Health of Illinois. This important regulatory step, accompanied by gradually increasing requirements over the years, forced medical schools to raise their standards if their graduates were to be licensed to practice in Illinois. Other states soon followed Illinois, and as a result the standards of medical education in America were substantially improved.[24]

A DOCTOR IN SIX MONTHS

When the AMA was established in 1847, admission requirements for medical school were virtually nonexistent; the M.D. degree was being awarded for less than six months attendance in addition to a period of apprenticeship, the degree admitting the holder to the practice of medicine in almost every state of the Union. By the end of the nineteenth century, a four-year course of at least six months each was required for the degree, which qualified the holder for licensure examination in almost every state but did not admit him directly into practice. Admission standards had also undergone some improvement, a high school diploma being required by many schools and, by a few, two years of college. Despite the evidence of progress, many members of the medical profession remained dissatisfied and frustrated by the failure of their efforts to produce more radical changes, and measures were undertaken to accelerate reform.

In 1901, a major reorganization of the AMA occurred, and in

23. Billings, Frank: Medical education in the United States. President's address, 54th Anual Session of the AMA. *JAMA, XL/19:*1271-76, May 9, 1903.

24. *Ibid.*

1902, Dr. John A. Wyeth, its president, took an important step toward the reformation of American medical education when he appointed a committee to survey medical education in America and to make recommendations concerning the role the AMA should play in the improvement of medical education. The choice of the membership of the committee was brilliant, especially in its chairman, Dr. Arthur Dean Bevan, of Chicago, who was to play a major role in improving medical education in America. The other members of the committee also bore distinguished credentials and represented a cross section of America. In 1904, the committee recommended the creation of the Council on Medical Education of the AMA, which was authorized to act as the agent of the AMA in its efforts to elevate medical education.

The first Council appointed by the AMA president, Dr. John H. Musser, had as its chairman Arthur Dean Bevan, who was to hold this position with great distinction for the next quarter of a century. Other members of the first council, all outstanding medical educators of the era, were Victor C. Vaughan, dean of the University of Michigan Medical School; Dr. William T. Councilman, professor of pathology, Medical School of Harvard University; Charles H. Frazier, professor of surgery, University of Pennsylvania School of Medicine; and J. S. Witherspoon, professor of medicine, Vanderbilt University School of Medicine.

In 1905, when the Council held its first conference, conditions in medical education in America were deemed unsatisfactory by comparison with those in England, Germany, and France, but there was evidence of substantial, albeit inadequate, improvement in the American medical schools during the preceding twenty years.

There were already in existence five medical schools requiring two or more years of college education before admission, the schools being: Johns Hopkins, effective in 1893, Harvard in 1900, Western Reserve in 1901, Rush University of Chicago in 1904, and the University of California in 1905.

The Council considered and indeed adopted what it called an "ideal standard" for the medical schools but decided, on further reflection, that it was impractical for the immediate future and settled for the following minimum requirements. Preliminary education of four years at high school, a four-year medical course, and the passing of a satisfactory examination before a state licensing board. Having established a standard of reference for medical education, the Council then moved on to the evaluation of existing conditions. Seeking some objective criteria, it found important data in the reports of the results of the state board examinations in medicine published in the *JAMA*. Tables were developed from these facts, dividing the medical schools into four classes based on the percentages of failures before the state boards. Class 1 were those schools with less than 10 percent of failures; Class 2 with from 10 to 20 percent failures; Class 3 with more than 20 percent of failures; and Class 4 "unclassified colleges in which there were less than ten graduates or most of whose graduates were licensed by their own home state board or in which we felt that the evidence was insufficient to permit conclusions."[25]

Admitting that failures of graduates on state board examination did not tell the whole story about a medical school, the Council felt that by publishing these data in the *JAMA* the medical schools would be prodded to improve themselves.

Doctor Bevan went on to say in 1928,

> I remember as well as though it were yesterday, although it was twenty-two years ago, that when I presented these tables, I said, "It is evident from a study of the medical schools of this country and their work that there are five especially rotten spots which are responsible for most of the bad medical instruction. They are: Illinois with fifteen medical schools, Missouri with fourteen medical schools, Maryland with eight medical schools, Kentucky with seven medical schools, and Tennessee with ten medical schools. That is fifty-four medical schools in these five states and not more than six of these can be considered acceptable." These startling figures led to an immediate and drastic reform.[26]

It was decided that the Council should make personal inspections of each of the 160 or more medical schools "to ascertain the character of their plants, of their work, and of their faculties, and in general their fitness to teach medicine, and to mark them as one might in giving a civil service examination." The assignment was a difficult one, but each school was visited by a member of the Council or by the secretary, Dr. N. P. Colwell, and most were examined by both the secretary and a member of the Coun-

25. Bevan, Arthur Dean: Cooperation in medical education and medical service. *JAMA, 90/15:*1173-77, Apr. 14, 1928.
26. *Ibid.*, p. 1174.

cil. The schools, examined on ten criteria rated at ten points each with a maximum possible score of 100, fell into three large groups. Class A, those marked above 70, the acceptable class; Class B, marked 50 to 70, the doubtful class; and Class C, marked below 50, the unacceptable.

Doctor Bevan continues.

> The ten points on which the schools were marked were the following:
>
> 1. Showing of graduates before state boards.
> 2. Requirements of preliminary education and its enforcement.
> 3. Character of the medical curriculum.
> 4. Medical school plant.
> 5. Laboratory facilities and instruction.
> 6. Dispensary facilities and instruction.
> 7. Hospital facilities and instruction. (These last three necessarily included the men giving this instruction.)
> 8. Extent to which the first two years are officered by men devoting entire time to teaching and also evidence of original research.
> 9. Extent to which the school is conducted for the profit of the faculty directly or indirectly, rather than for the teaching of medicine.
> 10. Libraries, museums, charts and teaching equipment.[27]

The Council's report of April 29, 1907, found that of the 160 schools examined, 82 were in Class A, 46 in Class B, and 32 in Class C.

> As a result of the report of this first inspection, a great wave of improvement in medical education swept over the country. Fifty schools agreed to require by 1910, or before, at least one year of university physics, chemistry and biology, and one modern language as a preliminary education before matriculating in medicine. Immediately a number of consolidations were arranged in many cities having several schools. A number of schools, as the result of state boards refusing examinations of their graduates, went out of business and it became evident that the 160 schools would be reduced within a short time to probably less than a hundred. By the time of the report of the second inspection, in 1910, the number of schools had been reduced from its high water mark of 166 to 126, a reduction of forty, almost 25 percent.[28]

I have gone into some detail in relating this story chiefly because I personally believe that Doctor Bevan, Doctor Colwell,

27. *Ibid.*, pp. 1174-75.
28. *Ibid.*, p. 1175.

and the AMA were given inadequate recognition for the major roles they played in reforming American medical education, the major credit going to Abraham Flexner and the Carnegie Foundation. This was not unplanned as we shall soon see. The AMA and its Council, rebuffed in their desire to proceed more vigorously with the crusade against unacceptable medical schools, faced with opposition and dissension in their rank and file and by the medical colleges, refused a modest grant of $5,000 by their own colleagues to pursue their investigation, decided to turn for help to the Carnegie Foundation for the Advancement of Teaching. The minutes of the meeting of the AMA Council on Medical Education held in New York in December 1908, contain these revealing passages.

> At one o'clock an informal conference was held with President Pritchett and Mr. Abraham Flexner of the Carnegie Foundation. Mr. Pritchett had already expressed by correspondence the willingness of the Foundation to cooperate with the Council in investigating the medical schools. He now explained that the Foundation was to investigate all the professions, law, medicine, and theology. He had found no efforts being made by law to better the conditions in legal education and met with some slight opposition in the efforts he was making. He had then received the letters from the Council on Medical Education and expressed himself as most agreeably surprised not only at the efforts being made to correct conditions surrounding medical education, but at the enormous amount of important data collected.
>
> He agreed with the opinion previously expressed by the members of the Council that while the *Foundation would be guided very largely by the Council's investigation, to avoid the usual claims of partiality no more mention should be made in the report of the Council than any other source of information.** The report would therefore be, and have the weight of an independent report of a disinterested body, which could then be published far and wide. It would do much to develop public opinion.

By turning over the facts to the Carnegie Foundation and asking Flexner to be the hatchet man, the AMA was avoiding rebellion within its ranks and ensuring wide publicity for the report by crediting it to a neutral and idealistic, newly organized foundation. The price it was paying for agreeing to soft-pedal the role of Bevan and Colwell and the AMA was a small one in return for the great benefits to medicine envisioned as resulting from the study. This

* Italics added by Doctor Lepore.

bargain was so well kept that although it is known that Doctor Colwell accompanied Flexner on most of his visits to the medical schools and that much of the material in the Flexner Report was derived from AMA sources, nowhere in this 326 page report is there any mention of Doctor Colwell, Doctor Bevan, or the AMA Council on Medical Education. Only in Pritchett's introduction to the report is some credit given to these individuals, but I hasten to add that Pritchett in later years freely acknowledged the enormous help derived from these sources. I am not complaining about this, I wish merely to state the facts and have indicated how this arrangement came about in the interest of medical education at large.

There is another reason for paying Doctor Bevan his due. Not only was he forthright, courageous, and honest in his judgements, he also had rather interesting views on medical education in general and expressed this caveat.

> Medical education cannot be left safely in the hands of the medical profession alone .... Medical education has been turned over by the great reorganization of the last twenty years largely to the university; and we all feel that this is the best solution. *But it is very evident that the medical school cannot be safely left in the hands of the universities alone; something more is needed. Uprooted from the medical profession, uprooted from the community, and transplanted to the scientifically prepared soil of the university campus, the medical school will lack those things which the medical profession and the community alone can give .... The great function of medicine can be developed in the best way only by the cooperation of all the factors involved, the community, the medical profession and the university.*[29] (Italics added by Doctor Lepore.)

The Flexner Report—Bulletin Number Four of the Carnegie Foundation for the Advancement of Teaching, published in 1910,[30] made its author famous overnight. With its publication, the campaign to improve the medical schools of our country was off to a great start. Standards of admission were raised so that more and more emphasis would be placed on a college education for admission to medical school. The medical schools themselves were on notice that they improve their facilities, faculty, and curricula

29. *Ibid.*, pp. 1176-77.
30. Flexner, Abraham: *Medical Education in the United States and Canada.* A Report to the Carnegie Foundation for the Advancement of Teaching. *Bulletin No. 4.* 1910. Reproduced Washington, D.C., Science and Health Publications, 1960.

and arrange solid relationships with hospitals to provide adequate practical experience for their enrolled students.

Early on, it was realized that the basic or preclinical sciences of the first two years of medical school, e.g. anatomy, physiology, biochemistry, pharmacology, and pathology, should be assigned time, laboratory space, and equipment and staffed by teachers who would devote their full time to teaching and research. No longer would it be possible for a "professor" of physiology to be a practicing physician or surgeon who was given the assignment as a stepping-stone to a clinical chair. No longer would the professor's high hat be used in lieu of a kymograph to illustrate physiological principles.

Anatomy was no longer the part-time activity of a busy practitioner, nor could pharmacology or biochemistry be taught by didactic lectures by peripatetic instructors. Learning from their colleagues in Europe, methods of research study were being introduced, and it was clear to any student of education that familiarity with and active participation in research were essential to the development and the future growth of teachers of the basic sciences. For these individuals there was agreement that endowment and full-time salaries were mandatory, and as quickly as they could the university-based schools made provision for them. Funds were limited and the salaries modest, but talented idealistic men were willing to make enormous sacrifices to further the science of medicine. Since patient care was not involved in their work, the M.D. degree was not a prerequisite; Ph.D.s were welcome and soon became the dominant group staffing the basic science departments. The establishment of full time in the preclinical and basic science departments was a major forward step in American medical education, but there were some undesirable features. Practicing clinicians no longer had the opportunity to teach medical students early in their training. The first two years of medical school were turned over to basic scientists, many of them without M.D. degrees. Some students chafed at the long delay before their exposure to clinicians and to patients and questioned the wisdom of postponing this phase of their education. The basic science faculty would soon dominate curriculum planning, admissions policy, and the direction of the program of their medical schools. As the basic scientists took over from practicing clinicians, the science of medicine was advanced, but to some observers it appeared that the art of medicine suffered. Nevertheless, the overall effect was to revolutionize American medical education, giving it the firm scientific base it had lacked and opening the door for the brilliant discoveries that lay ahead.

The Flexner Report's pitiless exposure of defective medical schools came at the right time, and with the support of the AMA and the state licensing boards the 160 medical schools of 1905 were reduced to ninety-five by 1915, eighty-five by 1920, and eighty by 1927. Fewer doctors were being graduated, but they were adequate for the country's needs and infinitely better prepared for practice than their forebears. Having won his great victory by eliminating the inferior medical schools, Flexner now sought bigger game. His next assignment was to study medical education in Europe; starting in 1910 he included medical schools in England, Scotland, France, Germany, and Austria. From this came, in 1912, Bulletin Number Six.[31] This did not make the impact that Bulletin Number Four had made. The European schools were not influenced very much by his recommendations or evaluations.

---

31. Flexner, Abraham: *Medical Education in Europe: Bulletin No. 6.* A Report to the Carnegie Foundation for the Advancement of Teaching. New York, Carnegie Foundation, 1912.

Chapter 4
FLEXNER CHAMPIONS FULL TIME IN THE CLINICAL CHAIRS

In the Spring of 1911, shortly after his return from Europe and while he was busily engaged in writing "Bulletin Number Six: Medical Education in Europe. A Report to the Carnegie Foundation for the Advancement of Teaching," Abraham Flexner received an invitation to have lunch with Frederick Taylor Gates, the chief Rockefeller almoner, whose enthusiasm for medical research had already persuaded John D. Rockefeller to establish the Rockefeller Institute. Mr. Gates lost no time in getting to the point. "I have read your Bulletin Number Four from beginning to end. It is not only a criticism, it is also a program."[32] Flexner replied that it was intended to be both and included two maps, one showing the existing schools and the other the schools and distribution he thought would be ideal. Gates then asked, "What would you do if you had a million dollars with which to make a start in the work of reorganizing medical education?" Flexner replied without a moment's hesitation that he would give the money to Dr. William A. Welch of the Johns Hopkins Medical School. When asked why, he replied,

> With an endowment of four hundred thousand dollars, Doctor Welch has created, insofar as it goes, the one ideal medical school in America. Think what he might do if he had a million more. Already the work Doctor Welch and his associates have done in Baltimore is having its effect in reorganizing the personnel of medical schools elsewhere, and we must not forget that but for the Johns Hopkins Medical School there would probably be no Rockefeller Institute for Medical Research in New York City today.[33]

Gates suggested that Flexner request permission of his chief to go to Baltimore to make a detailed study of the situation. Doctor Pritchett, pleased that Bulletin Number Four was attracting

32. Flexner, Abraham: *An Autobiography* (1940 revised). New York, Simon & Schuster, 1960, p. 109.
33. *Ibid.*, pp. 109-10.

the attention of the Rockefellers, gladly acquiesced, and Flexner arranged to spend three weeks in Baltimore on this assignment.

When Flexner made his visit to Johns Hopkins Medical School, he was invited by Dr. W. H. Welch to an elegant dinner at the Maryland Club where they were joined by Franklin P. Mall, professor of anatomy, and William S. Halsted, professor of surgery. At an appropriate moment, Doctor Welch asked his colleagues what they would do if the medical school were offered one million dollars in additional endowment. Flexner reports that Mall said, "If the school could get a sum of approximately a million dollars, in my judgement, there is only one thing that we might do with it—use every penny of its income for the purpose of placing upon a salary basis the heads and assistants in the leading clinical departments, doing for them what the school did for the underlying medical sciences when it was started. That is the great reform which needs now to be carried through."[34] Here for the first time, Mall after years of prodding others to carry the torch for full time in the clinical chairs, was out in the open, campaigning for the cause he had long espoused in private.

Mall was no stranger to Abraham Flexner, who had gotten to know him well during a stay in Munich in the summer of 1910. Years later, Flexner recalled this experience in these glowing terms.

> I had during the whole of my stay in Munich an extraordinary piece of good luck. Professor Mall of the Johns Hopkins was there with his family during the entire time. We visited laboratories and clinics together . . . . He was a shrewd and effective teacher, whether in his own laboratories in Baltimore or in the course of his wanderings with me. Lightly, almost unconsciously, he would ask the simple question which would call my attention to something which, as he thought, I ought to notice . . . . In the report which I subsequently wrote, the chapters dealing with medical education in Germany were profoundly influenced by Mall's apparently unconscious comments, criticisms, and suggestions.[35]

You may rest assured that Mall discussed other matters with his apt disciple, including the full-time concept, which had become an obsession. I have already alluded to the fact that Mall attrubuted the origin of the full-time concept in clinical medi-

34. *Ibid.*, pp. 110-11.
35. *Ibid.*, p. 103.

cine to his former mentor, the great physiologist, Carl Ludwig. Although both Ludwig and Mall had M.D. degrees, they had never practiced medicine and had no clinical experience or background. Ludwig felt that private practice by occupants of the clinical chairs and their assistants was undesirable, harmful to their teaching obligations, and should be forbidden. To make up for the loss of income, it was proposed that adequate salaries be paid so that the "distractions" of private practice would be avoided, leaving the individual free to devote his full time to the university pursuits of teaching and investigation.

This concept was being applied with spectacular success in the preclinical departments of anatomy, physiology, etc., and Ludwig and Mall and their disciples believed that extension of the concept to the clinical chairs was the logical next step; they could conceive of no valid objection to this proposal. This was a hypothesis. There was no full-time concept for the clinical chairs in Germany or anywhere else at the time. It was a dream of a highly idealistic brilliant laboratory scientist who had very little real concept of the world of medicine outside the walls of his university and who had limited contact with practitioners of medicine and their patients. Be that as it may, Mall drank all of this in, and it was to become one of the major themes of his life when he returned to the United States. Mall himself had a very limited grasp of what it takes to make a good clinician, and he failed to understand the effort, time, and skills needed to acquire clinical competence. He seemed to feel that money was the major factor in the clinician's life, and he frequently remarked that a man must choose which "G" he will worship—Gold or Glory. It is of interest and perhaps revealing that he did not mention God. Most of Mall's heavy work was done quietly and behind the scenes, others acting out the parts or making the speeches. Only occasionally is his fine, almost Machiavellian hand seen as it is in this excerpt from a letter to his friend, C. S. Minot, in 1911: "We are also thinking of reforms in medical education, but of the hospital side. The problem would be easy if the pork barrel were removed. Its removal would no doubt remove the exploiting medical professor and open the way for the real university professor of medicine. We are told that medical and surgical professors cannot take interest in medical problems and the sick unless they are paid for each move, that the sick man is not as conducive to real science as the dead or as a dog. It falls to us to demand of the last two years of medicine what they demanded (?) of the first two and I think that the day of reckoning is at hand."[36]

FLEXNER ATTACKS THE PRACTITIONER-TEACHERS

Let us now turn to Baltimore in 1911 where we join Abraham Flexner as he met with his close friend Franklin P. Mall, with Welch, and with Halsted. Flexner proceeded to examine the Johns Hopkins Medical School and immediately after the site inspection sent a very critical report regarding the clinical faculty to Mr. Frederick T. Gates of the Rockefeller General Education Board. This report was confidential and unpublished until 1963, more than fifty years later, when it was finally made public with Mr. Flexner's permission, in Chesney's history of the Johns Hopkins Hospital and Medical School.[33] In the section on the faculty, Flexner made these comments:

> As contrasted with the instructors on the laboratory side, the clinical staff has been on the whole less productive and less devoted. The instructors do not devote their time to science and education —indeed, only a few of them devote any considerable part. This is not in the first place their fault; for only one of them gets compensation enough to warrant the school and hospital in requiring a large share of his time and energy . . . . (T)he clinicians have with very few exceptions proved too easy victims to the encroachments of profitable practise. Not only has productive work been sacrificed to private professional engagements, routine teaching and hospital work go by the board when a large fee is in prospect. Classes are turned over to subordinates in order that the chief may leave town to see patients, not because they are scientifically interesting, but because they are pecuniarily worthwhile. The meagerness of original output and the conditions existing in the private wards, as above set forth, are not independent of each other, they are both traceable to one cause, namely, the displacement of science and education by business.[38]

Contrast this harsh appraisal with the statements made only sixteen months before by the very same examiner in his now fa-

36. Sabin, Florence R.: *Franklin Paine Mall: The Story of a Mind.* Baltimore, Johns Hopkins Press, 1934. p. 261.

37. Chesney, Alan M.: *The Johns Hopkins Hospital and University Medical School,* Vol. III. Baltimore, Johns Hopkins Press, 1963, pp. 287-309.

38. *Ibid.*, p. 299.

mous Bulletin Number Four.

> The Johns Hopkins Medical School, for which neither the State of Maryland, nor the City of Baltimore has ever done anything, is thus the only medical school in Maryland that either ought to or can live, and to its development greatly increased means should be freely devoted .... At this date [December 1909] the Johns Hopkins University is the only academic institution in the state capable of conducting a modern medical school. It would be safe, interesting and instructive to leave medical education in Maryland for a decade or two wholly in its hands.[39]

Elsewhere in this report, nothing but high praise was heaped upon Johns Hopkins Medical School, and it was held up as a virtual paragon for others to emulate.

What happened in the sixteen-month period between the two reports? What was going on? Was Flexner's original visit of several weeks in 1909 to Hopkins inadequate to reveal the failings of the school? Who was influencing him during the first visit? With whom did he consult? Was someone else feeding the information during the second visit? Had he already been very thoroughly briefed on the issue of full time by someone? Was he already committed to the full-time concept and persuaded that the only way to move ahead with it was to aggressively attack the existing system at Hopkins that others had found to be the best medical educational experience in America? How, in 1911, could he impugn the motives and the ideals of a group of clinicians described by others as among the best this country has ever seen? Who were these men? In the roster of the Department of Medicine, we find these names of illustrious teachers and clinicians: Lewellys F. Barker, William S. Thayer, Thomas B. Futcher, Thomas McCrae, Rufus Cole, Charles P. Emerson, Thomas R. Boggs, Louis Hamman, Paul W. Clough, Francis W. Peabody, Charles R. Austrian,and Ralph H. Major. Students of these outstanding men had only praise, reverence, and affection for them, and their influence spread across the country to other schools, elevating standards wherever the disciples went. The surgical staff was equally brilliant, including, besides its chief, William S. Halsted, John M. T. Finney, Joseph C. Bloodgood, Harvey Cushing, Hugh H. Young,

39. Flexner, Abraham: *Medical Education in the United States and Canada.* Bulletin No. 4 (1910). Washington, D.C., Science and Health Publications, 1960, p. 239.

and Richard H. Follis. In gynecology, the great Howard A. Kelly and his associate Thomas S. Cullen brought fame to the institution, as did J. Whitridge Williams and Karl Wilson did to obstetrics. The resident physicians and surgeons of this era were men with stars in their eyes, carefully chosen, rigorously trained, and devoted to the highest standards of patient care, research, and teaching. Many were destined to fill important posts in other institutions, bringing to Hopkins fame and glory, as well as comfort and solace to their patients.

The answer to some of these questions may be found in the close relationship that had developed between Mall and Flexner starting in 1910, well after the original site visit at Hopkins of December 1909 for the Carnegie Foundation's Bulletin Number Four.

Welch himself, in his June 11, 1911 critique of the Flexner Report to Mr. Gates of the Rockefeller Foundation, sought to soften its tone saying,

> Mr. Flexner's admirable report sets forth clearly and, in the main, accurately, the resources, working and needs of the Johns Hopkins Medical School and Hospital. The main lines of argument embodied in his interesting and valuable suggestions are not affected by a few minor errors, for which he is not responsible, such as the understatement of the hours devoted to teaching by some of the instructors, or the inadequate estimate of the productivity of some of the members of the staff based upon the often incomplete records of published papers in the School catalogue . . . .[40]

He goes on to state that later in this report he would touch upon the topic of the value to the Hospital and School of patients in the private wards and the value of the services of teachers engaged in outside practice. He indicates that he differs with Flexner on these matters seeing some benefits accruing to the hospital, the school, and the students from the active participation of practicing physicians in the teaching program.[41]

> Among the practitioners are some who love to teach and are really excellent teachers whose services it would be a great detriment to the school to lose. The opinion is entertained by some that under the plan by which the chief clinical professors are entirely withdrawn from outside practice, there may be the greater need of

40. Chesney, *The Johns Hopkins Hospital,* vol. III, p. 143.
41. *Ibid.*, p. 155.

teachers who have such practice to supplement the instruction.[42]

Flexner decried the access of private practitioners to the private beds in the hospital, inferring that they were being used to make a "financial fortune." He seemed very skeptical of any real idealism among the men in private practice and felt that as long as positions are "bartered for unpaid or poorly paid service, carrying with it large opportunities and some real necessity for money-making, few will reject the overtures of fortune."[43] The impression given to other observers by the men at Hopkins who practiced was that they enjoyed teaching and clinical investigation and were willing to subsidize these activities from their private practice income for the joy and satisfaction they derived. The teaching and scientific activities of this breed of man were simply not for sale. They were freely given, the private income providing financial support, the inner satisfaction from a professional life dedicated to the relief of human suffering being the ultimate reward.

Repeatedly in his correspondence, Flexner alludes to the money motive as the basic one influencing doctors' career decisions. He seems to believe that doctors' actions, work patterns, and services are ruled predominantly by money matters and feels that control of the financial aspects of their lives is the key to ensuring their full commitment to the life of the university professor. This concept is abhorrent to many and certainly, in the era under examination, no doctor worth his salt regarded his medical school pay as a major factor in determining the amount of time spent in research or teaching.

Flexner failed to understand the way of life and the idealistic motivation of many outstanding clinicians. This is the misconception that led to a bitter schism between practitioners of medicine and academicians. With Flexner there was no middle ground, it was "either/or" with little or no provision in his scheme for talented men and women who liked to teach, perform research, and still render superb personal care to their patients.

Unfortunately, there were two major exceptions in the clinical faculty at Hopkins at the time of the Flexner inspection. Barker and Kelly were so committed to making money that their teaching and research suffered. Many observers on the scene believed

42. *Ibid.*, p. 155.
43. *Ibid.*, p. 300.

that it was largely because of the heavy involvement in private practice of these two professors that Mall, Welch, and Flexner were pressed into action to impose full time in the clinical chairs. For some, the remedy seemed worse than the disease.

The report by Flexner was supposed to be confidential, but there were many leaks. From this point on, Flexner, who had made friends of the mighty and whose only enemies in medicine had been people of small consequence, was now taking on some real giants, and he was heading for trouble. Foremost among these was the brilliant professor of surgery at Harvard, Harvey Cushing, who strongly opposed the full-time concept and said of the Flexner Bulletin Number Four:

> This sensational publication served to call public attention to the deplorable conditions that prevailed and had a profoundly beneficial effect not only in accelerating the elimination of many poorly equipped and conducted medical schools, but at the same time in raising the standards of the survivors. While in this monumental report, the Johns Hopkins was singled out and held up to view as approaching the ideal, only two years elapsed before the clinical departments of this particular school came privately, by the same virile pen, to be severely criticized. To correct what were regarded as abuses of their academic positions a full-time service for chiefs of the clinics was proposed.[44]

Cushing went on to express his vehement opposition to full time and advocated in its stead what has become known as geographic full time.

Even before Cushing's outcry, Osler himself had taken the offensive and was clearly out in the open leading the battle against full time. As was pointed out previously, Osler disliked Mall's teaching methods and did not hesitate to say so, accusing him of neglecting the students by leaving them to their own devices. He also differed with him sharply on the full-time issue, and Welch, who greatly admired Osler, had reason to be very cautious in yielding too soon or too readily to Mall's viewpoint.[45]

The controversy over full time in the clinical departments was now common knowledge and medical teachers were soon split into two diametrically opposed factions. Strong emotional reac-

---

44. Fulton, John F.: *Harvey Cushing: A Biography*. Springfield, Thomas, 1946, pp. 382-83.
45. Fleming, Donald: *William H. Welch and the Rise of Modern Medicine*. Boston, Little, Brown & Company, 1954, p. 171.

tions and considerable bitterness were engendered. Good friends became enemies and ceased to speak to one another. The battle was in part one of town versus gown but it was also one which pitted clinicians who took care of the sick against laboratory-oriented scientists who dealt with cats, frogs and dogs and diseases rather than with human beings. This struggle is not ancient history, for the issue remains as important in medicine to this day as it was at the turn of the century. Should scientists whose work is confined to the laboratory set the conditions under which clinical faculty should work and be rewarded? Are the work hours of the laboratory scientists, nine to five, without night or weekend duty, realistic or in keeping with the Hippocratic oath for practicing clinicians whose major commitment should be around-the-clock service? Is the care of the sick ever to be a mere "distraction" rather than the *raison d'être* of the dedicated clinician? These are a few of the questions raised by the full-time issue that merit further discussion.

To assist the reader in understanding this controversy and its importance to American medicine, it is essential that certain terms be clearly defined. "Full time" or "whole time" for teachers of clinical medicine, as advocated by Flexner, is the contractual agreement of the medical school and hospital to provide full salary for the clinical staff on the condition that they confine their professional activities to the medical school and the hospital; focus on teaching, training, and research; ignore the community outside the university citadel; have no outside office or practice; and accept no fees for professional services to any patients. Geographic full time is defined as having physicians on the premises, some without salary, others on a base stipend, all with permission to engage in private practice on a fee-for-service basis, with or without a ceiling on income. Part time is usually interpreted as volunteer faculty engaged in private practice in the community outside the hospital and contributing teaching services to the hospital and medical school without salary. Many variations on these themes have been developed over the years, but the essential and most controversial was, from the very beginning, Flexner's insistence that his version of strict full time be the key mechanism for staffing the major clinical departments of our medical schools. Any deviation was regarded as heresy by Flexner and grounds for rescinding gifts made by the Rockefeller funds.

Since he was not a physician, Flexner failed to appreciate that the full-time system he was championing was replete with major weaknesses and out of touch with the realities of medical practice. He missed the message that teachers of clinical medicine should function primarily as role models for their students, most of whom would end up practicing medicine and not as research scientists. He failed to understand that the truly committed clinician does not regard the personal practice of medicine as a "distraction"; it is the prime reason for his existence. Without continuing personal practice, clinical skills cannot be developed, nor can they be maintained and improved. The surgeon who does not operate soon loses his skills and dexterity. The physician who does not practice may soon lose his skills in diagnosis, history taking, and decision making. The full-time clinical professor, isolated from the community and his patients; confined to his laboratory; devoting much of his time and energy to myriads of committee meetings, national meetings, site visits and fund raising mainly from government sources, emerges primarily as an administrator and medical politician rather than the role model envisioned by Flexner as the idealistic, cloistered scientist-teacher. Flexner envisioned commitment to science rather than dedication to service as the major theme of the physician-teacher's way of life. Flexner found little idealism in those committed to the personal practice of medicine, and he saw only their alleged venality, avarice and greed. He failed to appreciate that the art of medicine is every bit as important to the care of the sick as is its science.

Flexner's full-time concept for the clinical chairs must be viewed in context of the period for which it was proposed as a panacea for medical education. Most of the medical education of the era was didactic and conducted in lecture halls and amphitheatres by volunteers whose outside activities in the private practice of medicine would not infrequently conflict with their teaching obligations. Students were seldom involved in the care of patients and had little or no personal experience with them. Preceptorship was on the wane.

Osler's great innovation in medical education, which he introduced in 1894 at Johns Hopkins by bringing medical students to the wards and teaching them at the bedside, was still in its infancy and a rarity in most medical schools. Witness that, in 1910, Roosevelt Hospital in New York City turned down a magnificent gift with the promise of more to come from Edward S. Harkness because the grant was conditioned on the acceptance of medical students as clinical clerks on the wards. The excuse given by the Roosevelt Board was that the use of "the sick poor for teaching purposes would be in contravention of the terms and spirit of [founder] James Roosevelt's will."[46]

The patients available for teaching purposes were, in the main, indigents who accepted the rather primitive hospital accomodations of the day without complaint, the conditions oftentimes being much better than those in their own homes. Private rooms were virtually nonexistent, large open wards being the custom. The general public feared hospitals as sources of contagion and spread of disease and tended to avoid them at all costs. When middle-class people were sick, they preferred to be examined and treated in their own homes by their personal physicians, and even when operations were necessary they elected to have them performed in their homes.

In an era without C.A.T. scanners, elaborate radiology units, ultrasound, diagnostic laboratories and electronic monitoring systems, there was really very little to be gained from being in a hospital except perhaps an opportunity to be exposed to cross infection, impersonal care, loss of privacy, and separation from one's family. Medical therapy of the day was empiric and unscientific and almost as apt to harm the patient as to help. There were only a handful of drugs of known efficacy, and many of the great physicians, including Osler, were therapeutic nihilists.

House calls were the order of the day, and there were ample numbers of general practitioners to make them. Consultants frequently visited patients in their homes. Servants and household help were abundant, and families were large, supportive, and willing to help each other. Instead of being exiles to a hospital where strangers assumed their care, the substantial assets of love,

---

46. Roosevelt Hospital, Special Committee on History of, Drs. C. W. Cutler, Jr., A. T. Martin, and T. C. Peightal: *History of Roosevelt Hospital, 1871-1957.* New York, Roosevelt Hospital, 1957, p. 54.

(TITLE PAGE)

WHOLE-TIME
CLINICAL PROFESSORS

A LETTER TO PRESIDENT REMSEN
JOHNS HOPKINS UNIVERSITY

FROM
WILLIAM OSLER

NOT FOR PUBLICATION

Figure 1.* Source: Chesney, Alan M.: *The Johns Hopkins Hospital and University Medical School,* vol. III. Baltimore, Johns Hopkins Press, 1963, p. 176.

sympathy, personal loyalty, and devotion lavished by one's family were put to work in supporting and comforting those who were ill, a far cry from the conditions of the current era. As a result of these trends, private patients stayed out of hospitals and clinics, and hospital teaching was usually conducted on indigent, nonpaying patients. Since clinical teachers were either unpaid or given only a pittance for their efforts, they had to develop outside practice in order to pay their bills and provide for their families. To insist that clinical teachers stop all private practice and accept inadequate salaries on full time was asking them and

* This is a family letter, strictly confidential and not for publication. It is sent only to the President and the Trustees of the University, the President and Trustees of the Hospital, to Mr. Abraham Flexner, to Dr. Hurd, Dr. Winford Smith and Dr. Norton of the Hospital, and to the Professors in the Medical School. Other copies are not to be had.

their families to submit to bankruptcy or penury. Under Flexner's full-time system, those patients who wished to see the physician of their choice and who were able and willing to pay for his services would be told that they could not do this because their doctor was on a full-time salary and forbidden to take private patients. The adverse effects of such a policy on relationships between doctors and their communities beggar description. Such a policy is not in the patient's best interests, not the physician's and, even more significantly, not in the best interests of the community or the hospital itself. The trend would serve to isolate the key leaders in medicine from the problems outside of the ivory tower, a policy strongly advocated by Flexner but clearly inconsistent with emerging modern concepts of responsibility of the university toward society as a whole. Above all, there was the full-time system's weakness in denying to the physician the opportunity to establish meaningful and warm personal relationships with his patients and their families and to experience the personal fulfillment and joy of the physician as a healer. Clearly, Flexner's full-time concept was an idea whose time had not come.

Chapter 5
OSLER ATTACKS FLEXNER

But, lastly and chiefly, divert the ardent souls who wish to be whole-time clinical professors from the medical school in which they are not at home to the Research Institutes to which they properly belong and in which they can do their best work.[47]

–Sir William Osler, 1911.

When Flexner visited Hopkins in 1911, Osler was no longer on the staff, having assumed the Regius Professorship of Medicine at Oxford in 1905, but he remained deeply interested in Hopkins and was kept fully informed of any major developments. On July 6, 1911, he received a letter from Ira Remsen, President of Johns Hopkins University, informing him of the latest decision on the full-time matter and including copies of Mr. Flexner's captious report of the Hopkins site visit and Welch's response in his letter and memorandum of June 11, to Mr. Gates of the General Education Board. Osler had obtained a copy of Flexner's report some time before from his protégé, Dr. Howard A. Kelly, who was strongly opposed to full time, but he had not had a chance to read it until August 1911. On August 25, 1911, he wrote to Kelly saying that he was sending an open letter to Remsen on the subject, commenting as follows: "It is a great pity Flexner's report was issued so full of errors and misconceptions and I am stating it frankly."[48]

The letter to Remsen was sent off on September 1, 1911, from Oxford, and it proved to be a bombshell on the full-time issue. In this famous letter that was suppressed from public view for fifty years, Osler attacks Flexner with considerable vigor saying:

---

47. McGovern, J. P. and Roland, C. G.: *William Osler: The Continuing Education.* Springfield, Thomas, 1969.

48. *Ibid.*

> The Report as a whole shows the advantage of approaching a problem with an unbiased mind, but there are many mistakes from which a man who knows the profession from the outside only could not possibly escape. It is a pity the Report was allowed to go out in its present form, as his remarks show a very feeble grasp of the clinical situation at the Johns Hopkins Hospital; but this is not surprising, and perhaps is not his fault, since he has not had the necessary training, nor, from the outside, could he get the knowledge to understand it. To say, for example, p. 14, as contrasted with the instructors in the Laboratory side the clinical staff has been on the whole less productive and less devoted is simply not true. I deny the statement in toto—they have been more productive and quite as devoted. It is singularly unfortunate that he should not have been able to appreciate the work of the very men who have done as much, or more, than any others to build up the reputation of the school and to advance the best interests of the profession. To mention, out of many, only five names—the most stable on the staff!—Finney, Thayer, Bloodgood, Cushing, and Cullen . . . . It is hard to say which is the more prevalent on pp. 14 and 15 of the Report—unfairness or ignorance; but in either case gross injustice is done to the men who have made the Johns Hopkins Clinical School.[49]

Needless to say, Kelly wrote Osler on September 24, 1911, expressing his satisfaction with the letter and hoping it would give the *coup de grâce* to the full-time movement.[50]

The comments on the laboratory scientists were not taken lying down. W. H. Howell, the professor of physiology, came to their defense in a strong letter to Osler dated October 5, 1911. "I am afraid that I do not wholly agree with your point of view and I am exceedingly sorry that you cannot advocate the view that the majority of us believe in, namely, that it could be a great advantage to the science of medicine if the clinical teachers were relieved of the distractions of an outside practice."[51]

Flexner's comments on the stagnation of the clinical staff at Hopkins as opposed to the fluidity of the laboratory staff reveals with startling clarity his basic misconceptions of the role of the clinical teacher and his ignorance at the time of the state of affairs for practicing clinicians in Baltimore. He points with pride to the mobility of the junior staff in the preclinical sciences

---

49. Chesney, *The Johns Hopkins Hospital,* vol. III, pp. 177-78.
50. *Ibid.,* p. 183.
51. *Ibid.,* p. 184.

and stresses that they remain at Hopkins for only a short period before taking off for new fields. Where else would a laboratory scientist go with all opportunities for promotion blocked to him in his present insititution? What other options were there? For the clinician, the opportunities were abundant and close by to apply his skills and knowledge to the care of the ill of the community and to contribute his teaching service to the hospital without reimbursement. This he could do without demanding a salary, office space, secretarial help, or other kinds of support from the hospital. Such a man with his roots in the local area, would be dependable, available, and committed to his hospital for his entire career seeking little in return but a sympathetic and stimulating climate to carry on his professional work and to teach students and house staff. His rewards would come, not from his academic rank but from the joy and satisfaction of maintaining high standards of practice and teaching and setting an example for others to emulate. Flexner spoke with scorn of those physicians who remained for years at levels below the rank of professor, saying, "The top men on the junior clinical staff remain because they have long since ceased to be scientifically significant, and hence outside institutions do not desire them; at the same time, these men have developed in Baltimore lucrative private practices which they would not abandon to accept an academic call elsewhither. Their high positions in the Hopkins assist their professional prosperity and demand no great sacrifice of time."[52]

Again, we see envy and the inordinate emphasis on money, which I do not feel is the prime motivating factor in the career decision making of most good physicians. Again, we witness Flexner's inability, or unwillingness, to comprehend the true role of the physician-practitioner in the function of a hospital and its medical school. The stability and "lack of mobility" of the clinical staff are as much an asset to the true goals of the medical school and hospital as are mobility and brief tenure in the careers of the junior preclinical scientists who of necessity must go elsewhere to perform their life work. The role model of the clinical teacher is enhanced by his commitment to people and to the community about him. Students are sensitive to these

52. *Ibid.*, p. 300.

aspects of the clinician's life and many seek to emulate him in their career choices, placing dedicated service to people above service in the laboratory. Finally, Flexner seemed unaware that, denied academic promotion and admitting privileges at Hopkins, many of their ablest clinicians were diverted to the community hospitals of Baltimore where they developed and directed outstanding services. Some of the most brilliant stars of the Hopkins faculty never had admitting privileges to the Johns Hopkins Hospital and were forced to use other hospitals in order to minister to their patients. Hopkins' loss was to the advantage of the Baltimore community hospitals, which developed into what has been called "Baltimore's Secondary Medical Centre."[53]

Osler continues in his letter to Remsen saying that the chief of a university clinic stands for many things besides research.

> In life, in work, in word, and in deed he is an exemplar to the young men about him, students and assistants. "Cabined, cribbed, confined" within the four walls of a hospital practising the fugitive and cloistered virtues of a clinical monk, how shall he, forsooth, train men for a race the dust and heat of which he knows nothing and—this is a possibility!—cares less? I cannot imagine anything more subversive to the highest ideal of a clinical school than to hand over young men who are to be our best practitioners to a group of teachers who are ex officio out of touch with the conditions under which these young men will live. The clinical teachers belong to the fighting line of the profession, whose ambitions and activities they should share and direct. Do you imagine for a moment that men whose interests are mainly in the research aspects of medicine, and who have no touch with the rank and file—the men behind the guns—do you suppose they would get into the arena and share the struggle of their brethren? A few with Welch's broad spirit would—a majority would live lives apart, with other thoughts and other ways.[54]

Osler continues, his words more prophetic, as relevant today as the day they were written.

> As students of the wider problems of social reform so closely associated with disease, the clinical men should come into contact with the public, whose foibles they should know, and whose advisers they should be. To seclude the ablest men in their respective departments from this contact would not be possible in the United States,

53. Bernheim, Bertram M.: *The Story of Johns Hopkins: Four Great Doctors and the Medical School they Created.* Kingswood, The World's Work. Ltd., 1949, p. 178.
54. *Ibid.*, p. 179.

> where the profession lives so much in the "open": and the attempt would, I believe, defeat itself. Those best fitted as teachers in the medical schools, the men with larger outlook, would soon kick over the traces and leave the positions to the quiet student-recluses, keen at research, but as little fitted to train medical students for the hurly-burly of life as I would be to direct your laboratory.
>
> I cannot bear to think that any successor of mine should grow up deprived of those delightful associations which I enjoyed with the profession and the public. How barren would I feel my life without these memories! And a great gap would be left in the education of a clinical teacher who had not known that inner life of the public which we meet in our ministry of health. To some extent seen in hospital work but not in the same way, it helps to develop the side of a teacher's character very precious in his influence upon young men.[55]

And then he goes on to the often-quoted—

> . . . The Trustees of the Hospital will do well to hesitate before handing over their magnificent "plant" to a group of men to "run" on the narrow lines of a Research Institute, and risk the termination of that close affiliation with the profession and the public which has made their clinical school the most potent distributor of scientific medicine in the United States.[56]

Next he turns to the question of fees and private practice saying,

> To the enormous value of the outside work in one's personal and professional development I can bear strong testimony. In looking over my writings for this specific purpose I am surprised to see how much of my very best material came from this source. The difficulty is to keep practice within bounds, but it should not be impossible to frame regulations to ensure that the major part of the time of the clinical professors is given to the clinics.[57]

These statements I can attest to with conviction as will many others who practice medicine as well as teach it. Private patients are challenging, exciting, often unusual, and always stimulating. They can be followed for long periods and form the basis of careful and personal evaluation of the course of disease, the prognosis, and the response to therapeutic measures. This experience is difficult, if not impossible, to match in the full-time hospital setting. Osler continues,

> Against the sin of prosperity, which looms large in Mr. Flexner's Report (p. 17), the clinical professor must battle hard. I was myself believed to be addicted to it; but you will be interested to know, and I would like the Trustees of the Hospital to know, that

55. *Ibid.*, pp. 179-80.
56. *Ibid.*, pp. 180-81.
57. *Ibid.*, pp. 180-81.

> I took out of Baltimore not one cent of all the fees–none of which came from hospital patients–I received in the sixteen years of my work. The truth is, there is much misunderstanding in the minds, and not a little nonsense on the tongues, of the people about the large fortunes made by members of the clinical staff.[58]

Osler then criticizes Flexner's Alternative Scheme I, which offers a full-time salary of $7,500 to the clinical professors, and he says with some sarcasm:

> We are all for sale, dear Remsen. You and I have been in the market for years, and have loved to buy and sell our wares in brains and books–it has been our life. So with institutions. It is always pleasant to be bought, when the purchase price does not involve the sacrifice of an essential–as was the case in that happy purchase of us by the Women's Educational Association–but in Alternative Scheme I we chance the sacrifice of something that is really vital, the existence of a great clinical school organically united with the profession and with the public. These are some of the reasons why I am opposed to the plan as likely to spell ruin to the type of school I have always felt the Hospital should be and which we tried to make it–a place of refuge for the sick poor of the city–a place where the best that is known is taught to a group of the best students–a place where new thought is materialized in research–a school where men are encouraged to base the art upon the science of medicine–a fountain to which teachers in every subject would come for inspiration –a place with a hearty welcome to every practitioner who seeks help–a consulting centre for the whole country in cases of obscurity. And it may be said, all these are possible with whole-time clinical professors. I doubt it. The ideals would change, and I fear lest the broad open spirit which has characterized the school should narrow, as teacher and student chased each other down the fascinating road of research, forgetful of those wider interests to which a great hospital must minister.[59]

Sir William closes with this famous paragraph:

> But, lastly and chiefly, divert the ardent souls who wish to be whole-time clinical professors from the medical school in which they are not at home to the Research Institutes to which they properly belong, and in which they can do their best work.
>
> Believe me, my dear Remsen,
>
> Sincerely yours,
> (signed) William Osler.
>
> Oxford,
> September 1, 1911.[60]

58. *Ibid.*, p. 181.
59. Chesney, *The Johns Hopkins Hospital*, vol. III, p. 182.
60. *Ibid.*, p. 183.

Chapter 6
WELCH AND HALSTED AND FULL TIME

Welch was now faced with a serious problem that threatened to break up the happy family he had so carefully nurtured at Hopkins. He himself, a laboratory scientist and research investigator, felt that the full-time plan that had succeeded so brilliantly in the preclinical sciences could also improve the clinical departments and that this was the obvious next step. His protégé, Mall, was pressing him hard on this issue, as was Abraham Flexner, the brother of Welch's disciple, Simon. But Welch was always his own man and understood better than many of his close advisors what it really meant to be a physician. His brief experience in practice in New York, his family background in medicine, and his close association with Osler were all factors enabling him to appraise the full-time concept with a balanced viewpoint and comprehension denied the preclinical basic scientist. As the leading light in his great medical school, his responsibility was heavy, and he was very sensitive to the human and personal implications of the controversy. No matter what the pressure, he was not about to be stampeded into premature or poorly conceived action. He was by nature a very deliberate and gentle man of the highest character and integrity.

William H. Howell, the distinguished professor of physiology at Johns Hopkins, had quite predictably already come out in open support of the full-time concept in an address given at Yale University in 1909, "The Medical School as part of the University."[61] Here he said that the clinical chairs should either be placed on full-time, or so-called university basis, practice being limited to the hospital and dispensary and the laboratories attached to them, or that limitations be placed on the time given

61. Howell, W. H.: The medical school as part of the university. *Science, 30/761:* 129-40, July 30, 1909.

to outside practice so that definite allocation of time and energy be devoted to teaching and research.

Support of the whole-time concept by the preclinical scientists could be taken for granted, but what of the clinicians at Hopkins? On the clinical side, Welch was concerned over Howard Kelly's opposition, for he was a great star in gynecology and had attracted renown to Hopkins by his enormous surgical skills and innovative operations.[62] Kelly, dubbed by his sponsor, Osler, "the Kensington colt," at the tender age of thirty-one was brought to Hopkins in 1889 from Philadelphia by Osler to head the department of obstetrics and gynecology. He "came nearer to being a genius than any other man on the medical faculty," in the opinion of G. Canby Robinson,[63] whose appraisal was disputed by George H. Whipple and by Donald Fleming who said Kelly was the only "common-place intellect among the Big Four" at Hopkins. He was an extremely devout man (an Evangelical Christian) who detested drink, vice, and graft and who regularly conducted prayers for surgeons, nurses, and observers before he operated. Osler said of him,

> When in the full swing of his practice Doctor Kelly had probably the largest professional income of any surgeon in the United States. He charged very large fees, $10,000 and $12,000 for some of his more important operations. He seemed conscienceless in the matter, and, yet, men have told me that after conversation with him, they were glad to get away without making an assignment of their estates. He was exceedingly liberal and gave with great freedom both to the hospital, to his assistants, and to general charities.[64]

He had very little to do with the medical students and, as a teacher, his fame rests with the residents he trained, among them Cullen, Robb, and Hunner, as well as a host of others who became leaders in American gynecology.

Kelly led the battle against full time at Hopkins and sided with Osler as Halsted did with Welch. In May 1911, he wrote a series of six letters to Osler on the full-time proposal and indicated his disapproval. As the conflict became more and more intense,

---

62. Robinson, G. Canby: *Adventures in Medical Education.* Cambridge, Harvard University Press, 1957, p. 54.
63. Fleming, Donald: *William H. Welch and the Rise of Modern Medicine.* Boston, Little, Brown & Company, 1954, p. 90.
64. Bates, D. G. (Ed.): Inner history of Johns Hopkins Hospital. *Hopkins Med J, 125:* 184-94, Oct. 1969, p. 191.

Kelly became disaffected with the policies and decisions being made at Hopkins, and in 1916 requested a leave of absence. In February 1919, he resigned from the staff to devote more time to the Kelly Clinic where he continued to pioneer in gynecologic surgery and radium therapy for cancer. Years later, on the occasion of Kelly's 75th birthday, Welch wrote, "I have always felt, as did Osler, that you did more than any of us to extend the fame of the Johns Hopkins University to distant parts; and the hospital afforded no greater attraction than the opportunity to see you and your work, and the new methods which you were so rapidly developing."[65]

J. Whitridge Williams, professor of obstetrics, was strongly in favor of full time and on one occasion had written, "There is no doubt that Mr. Flexner's criticism of the clinical branches is amply justified, and that the remedy he proposes is substantially correct"[66] In this, he was clearly at opposite poles from Kelly, head of the department of gynecology. He also strongly favored a combined department of gynecology and obstetrics that was anathema to Kelly and to Osler.

Halsted was of another type. He, too, was Welch's protégé and had been the recipient of substantial encouragement and faithful support despite his known tragic addiction to narcotics. Welch reported to Gates in 1911 that Halsted was enthusiastic about full time and was backing it. How true was this? Does the record bear this out? Here again, letters once secret and confidential tell us more than Welch himself may have known. Halsted is felt by many to have been the prototype of the full-time academic surgeon. His record indicates that this was not entirely true, for he had a lucrative private practice that provided him with substantial income, the fees for individual patients reaching, at times, five figures. He preferred to operate in Johns Hopkins Hospital but, on request and for an extra fee, would operate in the patient's home in Baltimore.[67]

Osler, in his *Inner History of the Hopkins*—the little black book that held its secrets until 1968 when arrangements for its

65. Chesney, *The Johns Hopkins Hospital*, vol. III, pp. 139-40.
66. Turner, Thomas B.: *Heritage of Excellence: Johns Hopkins Medicial Institutions 1914-1947.* Baltimore, Johns Hopkins Press, 1974, p. 117.
67. Olch, P. D.: William S. Halsted and private practice: a re-examination. *Surg/72/5:* 804-11, Nov. 1972.

publication were approved—had this to say of Halsted.

> Mixing but little with the local profession he never acquired a large consultation practice, in fact, he cared so little for it that he did not keep office hours. He received a very good income from a very few patients as his fees were enormous—at least they were so regarded. He was not popular with the trustees, at first partly on this account, as they heard so many comments on his high charges. The natives were simply aghast at them—in fact, I used to think them high but I never "went back on him," though he often got me into trouble. He charged a patient of mine $10,500 for a gall-stone operation—a most serious and protracted case, with two operations but the woman got well. The people were wealthy and I stood by him and told the artist story to the old man, who at the last felt thankful that the fee was so small. He really had not much conscience in [the] matter of charges, but he had the feeling of a high class artist about the value of his work . . . . When we recommended him as full surgeon to the Hospital in 1890, I believed, and Welch did too, that he was no longer addicted to morphia. He had worked so well and so energetically that it did not seem possible that he could take the drug and do so much. About six months after the full position had been given, I saw him in a severe chill, and this was the first intimation I had that he was still taking morphia. Subsequently, I had many talks about it and gained his full confidence. He had never been able to reduce the amount to less than three grains daily, on this he could do his work comfortably and maintain his excellent physical vigor (for he was a very muscular fellow). I do not think that any one suspected him—not even Welch.[68]

In a later notation in the black book, Osler added, "Subsequently, 1-10-98, he got the amount down to 1½ grains, and of later years (1912) has possibly got on without it."[69]

Welch was not fooled, but he kept the secret well. While a patient in Johns Hopkins Hospital for the fourteen months preceding his death, on April 30, 1934, Welch was treated by Dr. David Sprong, a member of the house staff in Urology. In a letter, dated May 29, 1968, to Dr. Emile Holman, Sprong quotes Welch as having said,

> Although it has been widely reported that Halsted conquered his addiction, this was not entirely true. As long as he lived he would

68. Osler, W., Bates, D. G., and Bensley, E. H. (Eds.): The inner history of Johns Hopkins Hospital. *Hopkins Med J, 125:*184-94, Oct. 1969.
69. Penfield, W.: Halsted of Johns Hopkins. Osler Commemorative Issue. *JAMA, 210/12:*2214-18, 12-22-69.

> occasionally have a relapse and go back on the drug. He would always go out of town for this and when he returned, he would come to me, very contrite and apologetic, to confess. He had an idea that I could tell what he had done. I couldn't, but I let him go on thinking so because I felt it was good for him to have someone to talk it over with.[70]

Wilder Penfield, commenting on Halsted's addiction says,

> Let us leave the matter there! This surgeon might have dropped out and disappeared, a martyr in the cause of science. Others did. Not he. During the long years of struggle against the dreadful discomfort of drug hunger, he grew in stature. He became a man of imperishable memory among surgeons, a hero in the story of American medicine—Halsted of Johns Hopkins.[71]

Getting back to Halsted and full time, what were his personal views? Was he really in favor of it? What is the evidence? This question was reexamined in 1972 by Olch who uncovered two undated handwritten manuscripts captioned "Barker and Barkerisms," listed as items 10051, 10052, 13329-13338 in Halsted papers, Welch Medical Library, Johns Hopkins University, Baltimore. These were apparently written in reply to Barker's address of 1902, in which he publicly espoused the whole-time concept. They indicate quite clearly *that at that time* Halsted was strongly in favor of private practice on a geographic full-time basis, and he advanced cogent arguments in support of this concept. In his Annual Address in Medicine delivered at Yale University, June 27, 1904, on "The Training of the Surgeon," he *expands upon the items mentioned* in the published memoranda saying,

> To be an impressive teacher of surgery, to attract important cases in large numbers, to exert an influence far and wide as a surgeon, to know his subject thoroughly, the surgeon must operate every day and always. A very considerable part of the surgeon's time must be spent in the operating room; more and more, it would seem, as time advances, for the number and variety of operations which a general surgeon performs each year is prodigiously increasing . . . . With a fixed salary the surgeon may devote himself to the work of his choice, whatever that may be. If his tendencies are in the direction of research, he will neglect his operative work, if he is a natural operator, he will chafe under the restrictions which prohibit the acceptance of fees so easily within his reach.[72]

70. Holman, Emile: *Pharos*, Oct. 1971, p. 139.
71. Penfield, W., *JAMA*, p. 2217.
72. Olch, *Surg.*

> I should like to see the plan which Doctor Barker advocates carried out to the letter, and if it should succeed no one would rejoice more than I. But I would not advocate giving the surgeon or physician a larger salary than the others. The salaries of all must eventually be increased at least two- or three-fold. *There is, however, a compromise which even at present is altogether feasible. Let the surgeon be permitted to accept remuneration for services to certain patients operated upon in the hospital which the university provides or controls. His consultations and operations should all take place at the hospital.*[73] (Italics added by Doctor Lepore.)

By 1914, Halsted had changed his mind about geographic full time and accepted pure full time with a salary of ten thousand dollars a year. In document 12107, we find this statement,

> I am free from prejudice in trying to take position in this matter, because it would now make, so far as my income is concerned, very little difference, to me whether it (my income) was limited to a $10,000 salary or not. The assurance of such an income, which is perhaps a few thousand dollars less than what I am at present making, would quite compensate for the uncertainty of making so much in the future.[74]

Why did he change and what factors influenced his decision? Olch surmises that Halsted may have made so much money by 1914, in those income-tax-free years, that he had amassed ample funds for his old age. That this was not true appears in a letter written to Welch, February 28, 1929, by Miss M. Carey Thomas, president of Bryn Mawr College, and sister of Dr. Henry M. Thomas of the Hopkins staff, in which she eloquently championed the cause of higher salaries for the full-time staff. Miss Thomas said,

> Dr. Halsted told me that when he went on the full-time Hopkins salary of $10,000, he had to economize in many unaccustomed ways. He had no children and owing to Mrs. Halsted's ill health, as you know, they entertained not at all. I tried to persuade him to employ a college-bred stenographer, but he said he could not afford it. As you perhaps do not know (Mrs. Halsted told Zoe after his death) he left her barely enough to live on, and if she had not died within a year or two she would have had to face real poverty.[75]

---

73. Halsted, William S.: *Surgical Papers Vol. II. The Training of the Surgeon.* Baltimore, Johns Hopkins Press, 1924, pp. 512-31. Paper delivered June 27, 1904.
74. Chesney, Alan M.: The coming of full time to the Hopkins and Halsted's attitude toward the plan. *Surg., 32/3:*482-84, Sept. 1952.
75. Turner, Thomas B.: *Heritage of Excellence: Johns Hopkins Medical Institutions 1914-1947.* Baltimore, Johns Hopkins Press, 1974, p. 580.

The theory that Halsted had hoarded a large sum of money during his earlier years as a surgeon seems untenable.

Halsted was now sixty-two and as he was growing older he was becoming rather irregular about his teaching and operating activities, and more and more distant from his private patients. He was also ill with gallstones, cholangitis, and common duct stones and, as we know, remained addicted to morphine. He may have realized that his operating days were numbered and grown to regard the full-time salary as security for his late years, much more attractive than it would have been in his youth. By his own statement, despite an occasional enormous fee, his income averaged not much more than the full-time salary being offered. Last but not least, he had been Mall's closest friend, and Olch surmises that this was the crucial factor that swung him over to full time. My own evaluation is that Welch, more than anyone else, was responsible for Halsted's acceptance of full time. Halsted knew that Welch, his mentor and protector, wanted the change and sooner or later he would acquiesce.

Getting back to the meeting at the Maryland Club in 1911, when Welch assembled Mall, Halsted, and Flexner to discuss full time, the date is of some importance with regard to Halsted's position. In 1904, he was in favor of *geographic* full time, allowing the surgeon to collect his own fees, and by 1914, tired and ill, he accepted so-called salaried full time without private practice fees. Welch said after the meeting of 1911, that Halsted was committed to full time and would support it, and I have no reason to doubt this statement. My question is whether Halsted's decision to go full time was because it was indeed the best choice for medical education or whether it merely reflected his fatigue, illness and age, and personal considerations that may have unduly influenced him. Would Halsted have accepted salaried full time at age forty? These are questions for which we have no clear answers, for all of the players in the scene have long since departed, leaving relatively few clues and much room for speculation.

Chapter 7
BARKER SUCCEEDS OSLER

When Osler, in 1905, attended his last faculty meeting at Hopkins prior to leaving for the Regius Professorship at Oxford, he turned to Mall and said, "Now I go, and you have your way." The disagreement between the two professors had by now become quite open. Osler made no effort to conceal his disdain for Mall's so-called inductive method of teaching, and he criticized both Mall and Halsted for their remoteness from the medical students.

> A man who is not fond of students, and who does not suffer their foibles gladly, misses the greatest zest in life, and the teacher who wraps himself in the cloak of his researches, and lives apart from the bright spirits of the coming generation, is very apt to find his garment the shirt of Nessus.*[76]

True to form, even before Osler's final faculty meeting, Mall had already begun to make his move to have "his way" by championing behind the scenes, the cause of his protégé, Lewellys F. Barker, as Osler's successor in the chair of medicine at Hopkins. At first there had been some discussion that Welch might succeed Osler with Thayer as his associate, but this drive was shortlived, for Welch would have no part of it. Barker was at this time Professor of Anatomy at the University of Chicago and woefully weak in clinical experience, a fact which he candidly admitted in his autobiography.

> It was to the surprise of nearly everybody that the position was offered to me. For though I had been well trained in the preclinical sciences of anatomy, histology, pathology, and chemistry, I had as yet meager experience in the teaching and practice of internal medicine . . . . The only way that I can account for the decision arrived at is by assuming that those in authority (and especially Welch and Mall) were sympathetic with the ideals of internal medi-

---

76. Fleming, *William H. Welch*, p. 163.

> cine that I had promulgated in my address entitled, "Medicine and the Universities," and though the funds available were insufficient to establish a so-called "whole-time" position, they hoped that I would approach those ideals as closely as I could in the circumstances even though some private practice would be necessary to supplement salary.[77]

Of course, Barker, who by his own admission had been Mall's mouthpiece in the famous lecture on full time of 1902, had more information than he professed regarding Mall's role in securing the position for him. Mall had been working indefatigably for Barker's return to Hopkins, and he regarded Barker's training as ideally suited for the preparation of a university professor of medicine along the lines he (Mall) had envisioned and championed for many years. When Barker expressed some fear that his years in anatomy, histology, and neurology and his inadequate clinical experience might be a drawback, Mall encouraged him by writing,

> Ludwig took undesirable positions until he was fifty—Professor of Anatomy, Professor of Zoology, and Professor in der Kriegsakademie—before he got to Leipzig. You are fifteen years ahead of him. Now you will have the opportunity to fill a university chair of medicine and do what no man has done in America, found a research department. The place for you is here, and you may rest assured that I will try to pay my debt to you by supporting Medicine as you did Anatomy when we fought together. Please forgive me for writing but I cannot hold in longer.[78]

But Mall seems to have overlooked the fact that Ludwig was not a clinician and never occupied a clinical chair, making the first portion of his letter to Barker clearly a *non sequitur*. This oversight has been carried over into more recent times. I recall a story told about the late Dr. David Rittenberg, Professor of Biochemistry at Columbia University College of Physicians and Surgeons, when he sat on the search committee for a new Bard Professor of Medicine to succeed the great Dr. Robert F. Loeb. As I recall the tale, the committee labored mightily to establish criteria for the position and considered all sorts of qualifications, among them that this person be of the "right age," neither too young nor too old, with research publications, excellent scientific training, competence in original research, etc. Above all, this particular committee decided that no individual would be con-

77. Barker, Lewellys F.: *Time and the Physician.* New York, G. P. Putnam's Sons, 1942, pp. 151-52.

78. *Ibid.*, p. 151.

sidered for the Bard professorship if he had at any time been in the personal private practice of medicine. When the criteria were hammered out and passed around for review, it was Rittenberg who commented that he thought they were really very good, but there was one basic defect: "According to these criteria, I could qualify as the Bard Professor of Medicine, but I don't have an M.D. degree." Shades of Mall and company, the weakness persists even to this day! Clinical experience and the actual care of the sick have for some years been relegated to a minor role in the halls of academe. It has been assumed that competence in clinical medicine is easily acquired as a sort of side line. Any scientificially trained M.D. can become an expert clinician almost overnight! Nothing could be further from the truth, and there is ample evidence to the contrary. The making of a clinician, given good basic qualities, requires hard work, experience, years of effort, and a sincere and overwhelming commitment to the care of human beings, sick and well.

Mall's error in selecting Barker becomes evident as we pursue Barker's performance in the chair at Hopkins. To top it off, and much to Mall's astonishment, a startling about-face was to occur in Barker's personal commitment to the full-time concept.

Barker's appointment in March 1905 to Osler's chair was viewed by some as a direct affront to Osler; a laboratory scientist and a nonclinician had been appointed to succeed the outstanding clinician of modern times. Some were to regard this as a blow against the tradition of clinical medicine so beautifully exemplified by Osler and his associates, and there was some bitterness expressed at the passing over of William S. Thayer, the distinguished clinician and teacher who had been Osler's right-hand man. To placate the Oslerians and also to protect its gamble with the clinical reputation of Hopkins by appointing a laboratory man to the position, William S. Thayer was promoted to Professor of Clinical Medicine and Associate Physician. This concession led to an erroneous report in *The Sun* of Baltimore on April 4, 1905, under the heading, "Osler's work divided."[79] "The trustees of the Johns Hopkins University yesterday divided the chair of medicine, occupied by Dr. William Osler, into the chairs of medicine and clinical medicine." Actually this was not true,

79. Barker *Ibid.*, p. 152.

Barker was at the helm and completely in charge of medicine at Hopkins.[80]

How did Barker perform as Professor of Medicine and Physician-in-Chief to the Johns Hopkins Hospital? His competence in the basic sciences and preclinical fields of the day was not in question, but how good a clinician was he? To answer this, we need to hear from one of his former students of this era. This student who was to have a great career in medicine himself was Thomas M. Rivers whose *Oral Biography* by Saul Benison has a number of gems presented in his own inimitable, completely candid fashion. When asked about Barker as a clinician, Rivers said,

> Lewellys Barker was an extremely intelligent man, but I don't think that he was a great clinician. Prior to coming to the Hopkins to replace Osler, who had resigned to become the Regius Professor at Oxford, Barker had been a professor of anatomy at the University of Chicago. He was appointed professor of medicine but that didn't make him a clinician. I watched Barker when I was an interne, and when he walked on the ward to make rounds he would always choose a patient who had been previously well worked up. If the patient were well worked up and Barker had the histories or notes from excellent diagnosticians like Thayer, Futcher, or Hamman, he would take the case. To listen to him discuss the history and the nature of a given disease was beautiful. Barker was a master at that. And his rounds and his clinics were not a complete bust, because he did add something. But he never liked to show a patient at a clinic unless he'd been previously well worked up. The reason I know this is because, every now and then when a patient was going to be shown in the clinic the next day, Barker would have me look up the literature and fetch the necessary books to his office. So I know that on certain occasions Barker knew what the diagnosis was on a patient for the next day, and he had a chance to cram up on the literature.
>
> Theodore Janeway, on the other hand, was just the opposite. He did not want to know what the patient had and he did not want to have the patient worked up before he saw him on the ward or even in the clinic. He wanted to take a crack at it cold. Now, that was the difference between Barker and Janeway. Barker I don't think would have gotten to first base if he'd taken a crack at a case cold. Janeway knocked a double, frequently a triple, and occasionally a home run, on the patient that he saw.[81]

80. Chesney *The Johns Hopkins Hospital,* vol. II, pp. 438-39.
81. Benison, Saul: *Tom Rivers: Reflections on a Life in Medicine and Science.* Cambridge, M.I.T. Press, 1967, p. 25.

So much for Barker as a clinician! Later in the same interview, Rivers had this to add.

> Janeway was full of surprises, Barker was never a surprise. Most of us young fellows who had been around the hospital any length of time knew his limitations. Later Barker was offered the full-time professorship in medicine and turned it down to go into private practice. Just let me say that Barker was one of the few practitioners of his day that actually made a million dollars from the practice of medicine and the investment of what he made at the practice of medicine. But even in private practice, his success depended upon two people, Dr. Thomas Sprunt and young Dr. Walter Baetjer, who were two of the best diagnosticians in Baltimore.[82]

By the time of Flexner's visit to Baltimore in 1911, Barker, who had assumed Osler's chair in 1905, was obviously committed to private practice much to the displeasure and chagrin of Mall whose protégé he had been. It is therefore quite comprehensible that the Professor of Medicine at Hopkins was not privy to the special meetings being held with Abraham Flexner to deal with the full-time issue in the clinical chairs.

---

82. *Ibid.*, p. 27.

Chapter 8
GATES SUPPORTS FLEXNER

Flexner's high critical "confidential" report on the clinical faculty at Hopkins and his proposal to place the clinical division heads on full time reached Gates shortly after the site inspection visit of the spring of 1911. Gates, in characteristic fashion, reacted promptly and vigorously, advising Flexner to draw up a letter offering Hopkins one and one-half million dollars to carry out the recommendations of the report. Flexner, for once, thought this was moving too rapidly and suggested that it would be more tactful if he submitted the report to Welch and his associates and through them to the medical faculty and the university trustees for appropriate action, while indicating informally to Doctor Welch that a request for assistance would be viewed with favor by the General Education Board. Flexner states that "In the course of our discussion, Mr. Gates talked with his usual incisiveness of commercialism in the practice of medicine."

> Why [so a letter of Gates' asked] do you object to it or resent it? Isn't it because we feel that where commercial methods are fair the two parties must both know the value of the article or service? If you want to buy potatoes, an agreed price is fair because you and the grocer both know about potatoes. But as to the value of skill of a doctor's services, one of the two parties knows nothing. He has to take it at the word of the other. And that other, the doctor, makes more of his services or his individual skill than they would be worth if they could be appraised competitively.[83]

This is a rather surprising comment coming from a man who was apparently quite ruthless in dealing with Rockefeller competitors in the business world, to the point that he was accused at one time of being a wolf in minister's clothing and that "on occasion he could even outdeal Mr. Rockefeller himself." Was he perhaps seeking to achieve through medicine, idealistic and altruistic goals

83. Flexner, *Autobiography*, p. 113.

that had long eluded him in the highly competitive and ruthless world of business of that day? Was his commitment to the ministry finally surfacing after years of preoccupation with worldly affairs? Did he have guilt feelings regarding his business activities and was he seeking to redeem himself through his philanthropic endeavors as the chief almoner of the Rockefellers? Gates had a very low opinion of practitioners of medicine of the day and had no hesitation to express it.

That Gates was incompletely informed about the state of the art of medicine in America is made quite clear by Dr. George W. Corner, who suggests that Gates' professional contacts were in a relatively poor city parish and in rural areas. The doctors of America were not so ignorant and ill-informed as Gates would make them. There were substantial numbers of excellent clinicians and teachers in America, but Gates was not in touch with them.[84] Even his employer, Mr. John D. Rockefeller, used a rather inept homeopath, Dr. H. F. Biggar, as his personal physician. Raymond B. Fosdick has said, "There was a quaint streak in the elder Rockefeller. He would support modern scientific medicine with millions of dollars but for himself, he preferred the old methods that had the authority of tradition." This "quaint streak" appeared again in the person of a grandson, Nelson, whose physician was an osteopath.[85]

Gates can then be faulted on his lack of knowledge of the truly great members of the medical profession but, as Corner brings out, perhaps it was just as well for had he been better informed, he might not have been as upset about the conditions in medicine of that period and he might not have been impelled to seek drastic action.

As I review this aspect of Gates' life, I find it difficult to comprehend why he did not communicate with Sir William Osler on the subject of full time. If he did, there is no record of it.

Given that Osler was now at Oxford, surely the mail could have served for communication. In any event, why didn't Gates follow his previous life-style by making a personal visit to Hopkins? His reputation had been established in the past by dint of visits

84. Corner, G. W.: *History of Rockefeller Inst., 1901-1953.* Rockefeller Institute Press, 1964, pp. 21,41.

85. Fosdick, Raymond B.: *John D. Rockefeller, Jr., A Patriot.* Harper & Bros., 1956, p. 116.

to the scene of the action with personal evaluation of the participants and the problem. Was he too old for this? At fifty-eight, I hardly think so. Was he now leaning too heavily upon subordinates and emissaries and in the process falling into the same errors that his employer had made in the past? Were the ever-present Simon Flexner, the easily available Abraham, and the gung-ho concept of the Rockefeller Institute influencing him unduly to the side of the scientist to the detriment of his understanding of the practicing physician? Since it was a medical student, Elon Huntington, who had aroused his interest in medicine, why didn't Gates go down to Baltimore and talk to the medical students? Wouldn't it have been appropriate to go to Baltimore to interview in person some of the outstanding faculty whose motives had been so badly maligned in Flexner's report? After all, the problems being discussed were not laboratory matters. They had to do with the staffing and conduct of clinical departments, the care of the sick, and the education of students to become practitioners of medicine. Or was Flexner reporting matters in a light he knew would upset Gates, goading him into action?

Chapter 9
WELCH PROCRASTINATES

Why doesn't Doctor Welch either shoot or give up the gun?[86]

—Abraham Flexner, 1912.

According to the plan of action he had suggested to Gates, Flexner met with Welch and a group of Hopkins trustees in Baltimore at the end of March 1911 to answer their questions regarding his report. Proposition number one of the report, which stressed the full-time concept received considerable attention, and Flexner reported that Welch was more outspoken than he had ever been in support of the issue and indicated that any doubts or fears he may have had were now gone. Later that night, Flexner took the sleeper to New York, leaving the next move to the Johns Hopkins officials.[87]

While the Flexner report was supposed to be confidential, as we have already seen, there were many leaks, a copy reaching Sir William Osler who, on May 23, 1911, wrote to Welch,

> What a time you must be having over the question of whole-time clinical men! Cushing tells me I am quoted on both sides. It is difficult to give an opinion, not having heard the proposal. If, as Kelly mentioned in a letter, the salaries would be fixed at 7,500 dollars, it would spell ruin to the Hospital. You could, perhaps, get the good men for a few years for that, but they would flit off inevitably.[88]

Welch, personally committed to the full-time concept, realized that any precipitate action might destroy much of the harmony he had worked so hard to create at Hopkins among the staff and its trustees. He chose to go very slowly and in letters to Gates on May 10, 1911 and June 2, 1911 sought to reassure Gates that his delay was not because of any personal lack of commitment to the full-time concept. He indicated that the issue was controversial and "The questions involved are more complicated and

---

86. Flexner, *Autobiography*, p. 115.
87. *Ibid.*, pp. 113-114.
88. Chesney, *The Johns Hopkins Hospital*, vol. III, p. 138.

difficult than might at first appear, and there are considerable differences of opinion on essential points."[89]

> While the proposition to place the heads of certain clinical departments on the salaried, full-time basis seems relatively simple, it would mark a most revolutionary change in existing conditions of medical education, if adopted. I know that you must have become impatient over the delay in hearing from me, but I have encountered great difficulties in obtaining from our Trustees such an expression of their views as would enable me to report definitely what they are willing to do in this matter .... I am sorry to say that Doctor Osler is strongly opposed to the plan, going so far in a letter received today (June 2, 1911) as to say that it will wreck the hospital if we attempt it, at least on the basis of $7,500 salaries for the chief physicians and surgeons. I am myself equally strong on the other side of the question, and I expect to be able to report to you favorably.[90]

Gates now knew Osler's position and apparently made no effort to pursue the matter and to find out why the greatest physician of his time felt so strongly opposed to full time.

Welch continued to deliberate and finally on June 11, 1911 he sent Gates a "Report on the Endowment of University Medical Education," describing the needs of the medical school and how he planned to use the endowment that would be supplied by the General Education Board for the support of full-time university professors.[91] A copy of this report was sent to Osler, July 6, 1911, by President Ira Remsen of Hopkins, who commented, "I have heard that you do not look favorably upon the plan. I am sorry for this and I believe that if you had been able to discuss the problem with us you would have come out about where we have."

It looked like clear sledding at this juncture for Welch and Flexner and Mall, but a bombshell burst in their midst in September 1911 in the form of the now-famous Osler letter to Remsen on "Whole Time Clinical Professors," which we have discussed at some length in Chapter 5. The immediate effect was to stall forward progress of the plan and to delay its implementation until October 1913, nearly two and one-half years later. The delay was so irritating to Flexner that he wrote to his friend Mall saying, "Why doesn't Doctor Welch either shoot or give up the

89. Chesney, *The Johns Hopkins Hospital*, vol. III, p. 140.
90. *Ibid.*, p. 141.
91. *Ibid.*, pp. 142-58.

gun?" Mall, without authorization, showed the letter to Welch, seeking to goad him into action but failed to get the desired response. In fact, Simon Flexner, some time later, asked his brother, Abraham, what he had said to upset Welch, and the story of the divulging of a confidence by Mall was laid bare.[92]

At 5 P.M. on Monday, October 13, 1913, the Advisory Board of Johns Hopkins was called into a special meeting at which Welch finally made the long-awaited announcement stating that the General Education Board had suggested that Hopkins make formal application "for funds to enable us to place certain departments of the Medical School upon the full-time basis, provided that it was felt that we are able and willing to do so."[93] The necessary protocol was followed in securing approval of the various committees of faculty and trustees. On October 21, 1913, Welch, in his capacity as Chairman of the Administrative Committee of the Johns Hopkins University, with the approval of the Trustees of Johns Hopkins University and the Johns Hopkins Hospital, wrote to the General Education Board requesting endowment for the full-time plan as well as additional endowment for the departments of Medicine, Surgery, and Pediatrics. A milestone had been reached after years of struggle, but the road ahead was by no means smooth; the controversy would continue to rage, and persists to this day.

92. Flexner, *Autobiography*, p. 115.
93. Chesney, *The Johns Hopkins Hospital*, vol. III, p. 245.

Chapter 10
IMPLEMENTATION OF FULL TIME AT HOPKINS

On October 23, 1913, The General Education Board, meeting in New York under the chairmanship of Gates, agreed to appropriate the funds needed for the full-time proposal at Hopkins. Furthermore, it was recommended that in view of Doctor Welch's great services to the cause of medical education in America, the fund appropriated be called "The William H. Welch Endowment for Clinical Education and Research."[94] Welch who was waiting in an adjoining room while the meeting was going on was called in and congratulated by the trustees. "It was one of the great moments in my life," he was to say years later.

The die was cast and the call was for action. The chair in surgery and the one in pediatrics were no problems; the chair in medicine could be sticky. When Lewellys F. Barker was offered the chair in medicine at Hopkins in 1905, he asked Welch whether or not a "whole-time chair" was available, but Welch indicated that there were no funds for this and that the position would be on the same basis as Osler's, i.e. part-time salary with private practice as desired. Barker commented that it was the hope of Welch, Halsted, Mall, and himself "that the time was not far distant when some philanthropist might offer an endowment that would enable the University to plan the clinical departments on a 'full-time basis,' or what we regarded as a 'true university basis.' " Lacking this, Barker compromised by organizing his work so that the major portion of his time was devoted to "the clinic" and by limiting his private practice to definite hours on certain afternoons of the week. As his private practice grew, he secured able assistants who saw his patients when he was not available.[95]

94. Flexner, Simon and Flexner, J. T.: *William H. Welch and the Heroic Age of American Medicine.* New York, Viking Press, 1941, p. 321.

95. Barker, *Time and the Physician,* p. 185.

One of Barker's first official moves as a chairman of medicine was to organize three new laboratories or divisions—biological, chemical, and physiological—in the department of medicine to focus on research and clinical investigation into the phenomena of disease. Men destined to make their mark in American medicine headed each one: Rufus Cole, the biological; Arthur D. Hirshfelder, the physiological; and Carl Voegtlin, the chemical. The establishment of the chemical laboratory was made possible by Osler (now at Oxford) who asked the trustees of the University to allocate for this purpose a gift of $1,000 he had made to the University during a fund-raising campaign. An additional $1,000 was contributed by Barker's brother-in-law, Mr. R. T. H. Halsey, of New York.[96]

Barker felt that "this extension of research facilities in the laboratories of the Medical Clinic was certainly one of the most important advances made during the nine years that I held the professorship,"[97] and Chesney agreed that "it was his most enduring contribution to the Hopkins medical institutions."[98]

We have already learned of Barker's weakness as a clinician, but his qualities as an administrator were apparently of a high order, and he was skillful in selecting good assistants. He was able to enlist the continuing support and dedication of the nonsalaried clinicians on his staff, the chief being William S. Thayer, and because of this the clinical teaching at Hopkins did not suffer but continued to maintain the high standards set by Osler. Perhaps surprisingly, Barker's private practice grew rapidly and to such a point as to embarrass some of his best friends including Mall who saw his protege becoming the very sort of clinical practitioner-teacher he abhorred. Barker was well aware of this and in a talk in 1911 at McGill University, gave expression to his changing views on this topic, from the perspective of six years in Osler's chair and increasing involvement in private practice. He discussed his initial paper of 1902, "Medicine and the University," and indicated that he still adhered to his views but expressed doubt that they could be applied in precisely the manner he then suggested.

96. Chesney, *The Johns Hopkins Hospital*, vol. III, pp. 4-10.
97. Barker, p. 176.
98. Chesney, *The Johns Hopkins Hospital*, vol. III, p. 10.

> Though the clinic then seemed complex, I know, today even more of its intricacies and difficulties, and the problem looks less simple in solution at close range than it did at a distance . . . . In our reorganized medical schools it does not seem to me probable that it will be desirable soon, if ever, to have all the men of the faculty composed of nonpractitioners. It would seem distinctly advantageous to have at least some of the teachers of undergraduates and some of the men who care for the patients in the hospital also engaged in private practice, at least in consultative or operative work.[99]

As if in explanation of his original position as Mall's mouthpiece on full time, he goes on to say,

> It is among the inconveniences attending all important reforms that the disciple overstates the teacher, exaggerates some features of his doctrine and is oblivious to, or insufficiently appreciative of others. There is always danger of confusing novelty with originality and alteration with progress. Because we desire research is no reason for doing away with teaching and practice in the clinic. Nor would, in my opinion, the limitation of every professor in a university to the material rewards of an insufficiently salaried position prove a panacea or a magic "open sesame" to the medical millenium.[100]

Earlier in the same address he said,

> The struggle to live, financial worries, inability to educate the children of the family, too great personal hardship, and the social penalties of too small an income are sure more or less to inhibit a man in his work. Society ought not financially so to penalize the professorial class that the occupancy of chairs by the stronger personalities will be limited to bachelors, to childless men, to men enriched through the accidents of inheritance or marriage, or to married men who consent to doom their wives and children to the mitigated happiness which poverty affords.[101]

And finally, a shaft probably directed at his mentors, Mall and Flexner,

> Above all, all honest, earnest, hard-working men should be protected from the zeal and overstatements of headlong advocates who insinuate the absence of ideals among clinical men, or talk of graft, rascality, commercialism, and the exploitation of the clinical chairs for profit.[102]

A rereading of Barker's paper of 1902 on the full-time proposal

---

99. Barker, L. F.: Some tendencies in medical education in the United States. *JAMA, LVII/8:*613-21, Aug. 19, 1911.
100. *Ibid.*, p. 620.
101. Barker, *JAMA*, p. 615.
102. Barker, *JAMA*, p. 620.

for the clinical faculties reveals very little semblance of concern for the restraints imposed upon the whole-time staff by financial pressures. Quite obviously, in nine years time or less, Barker had come to grips with the hard facts of life and was now recognizing weaknesses in his idealistic or utopian scheme as it applied to his personal requirements.

In November 1913, soon after the announcement of the gift from the General Education Board, the Advisory Board of the Medical Faculty recommended to the Hopkins trustees that Doctors Barker, Halsted, and Howland "be offered the posts of Professor of Medicine, Surgery, and Pediatrics, respectively, upon the full-time basis made possible by the gift."[103] On January 13, 1914, Barker received a letter from Welch offering him the full-time chair in medicine with an annual salary of $10,000, the same proposal going to Halsted and Howland.[104]

The acceptances of Halsted and Howland were foregone conclusions, but the offer to Barker was clearly a charade, for in 1911, when the possibility of funds for full time was being actively discussed, Barker had written to Remsen offering to resign if the faculty were reorganized. Barker, confronted in 1913 by the actuality of the offer to occupy the chair on a full-time basis underwent a period of travail and soul-searching. In his autobiography, he speaks in considerable detail of his dilemma.

> The whole-time chair of medicine was offered to me, and Doctor Welch and other friends urged me to accept it if I could see my way clear to do so. I would have liked very much to take it, particularly as it was to be placed on the basis that I had so strongly pleaded for some twelve years earlier. It was embarrassing to find myself in a situation in which I had to decline the offer. How I should have welcomed it in 1905! But in 1914, I found myself in a familial and financial situation that had greatly changed.[105]

Barker had established that life is hard, facts already experienced by many of his colleagues who had opposed the full-time concept that he had championed so actively in 1902. They were not venal men, they too had aspirations and high ideals in medicine. But they also had to provide for their families and to meet the obligations imposed upon them by a society that expected

103. Chesney, *The Johns Hopkins Hospital,* vol. III, p. 254.
104. Barker: *Time & the Physician,* p. 199.
105. *Ibid.,* p. 190.

individuals to care for their own and to maintain strong family ties. Why espouse a cause that imposed considerable financial restraints upon the cream of American physicians? Was it not in truth utopian and unrealistic? Was it not too much to expect the clinical professors to turn their backs on the needs of their parents, their wives, their children and their close relatives? Were only the inheritors of wealth or the husbands of heiresses or those who for one reason or another embraced a monastic life and existence be able to afford the luxury of being university professors? Would these men and women be the best leaders for new generations of youth being prepared to provide for the health needs of our people and their communities? Should the professorships be awarded on merit or by default? In his 1911 lecture at McGill, Barker had already shown how his thinking had changed, and he seemed more in touch with the reality of life than he was in 1902. However, it was already too late. He was clearly on the defensive because of his expanded life-style and exhibition of worldliness. He had lost the real support of Mall and Welch no matter what was said in the open. His only chance was to turn his back on his profitable private practice and return to the fold. Failing this, it would be merely a matter of time before he would have to step down.

The Baltimore newspapers entered the fray, a cartoon, in the *Baltimore American* depicting the lot of the "Hopkins Physician" in a derogatory manner as an antiquarian, bearded infant being weaned from his bottle, "private practice," by the Rockefeller Fund. For some, the cartoon might be redone to show that rather than to wean them, the full-timers were to be placed smack onto the teat of the hospital's endowment! As the controversy raged, Barker received some interesting mail from his friends and colleagues across the nation and from overseas. Of especial importance was a letter, dated December 18, 1913, from Dr. Frank Billings, the dean of Chicago internists, who espoused a practical compromise on full time which he had developed and had found acceptable. In a few years, still another compromise, so-called geographic full time would be championed by Harvey Cushing at Harvard.[107]

106. Barker, *Time & the Physician*, p. 196.
107. Barker: *Time & the Physician*, pp. 197-98.

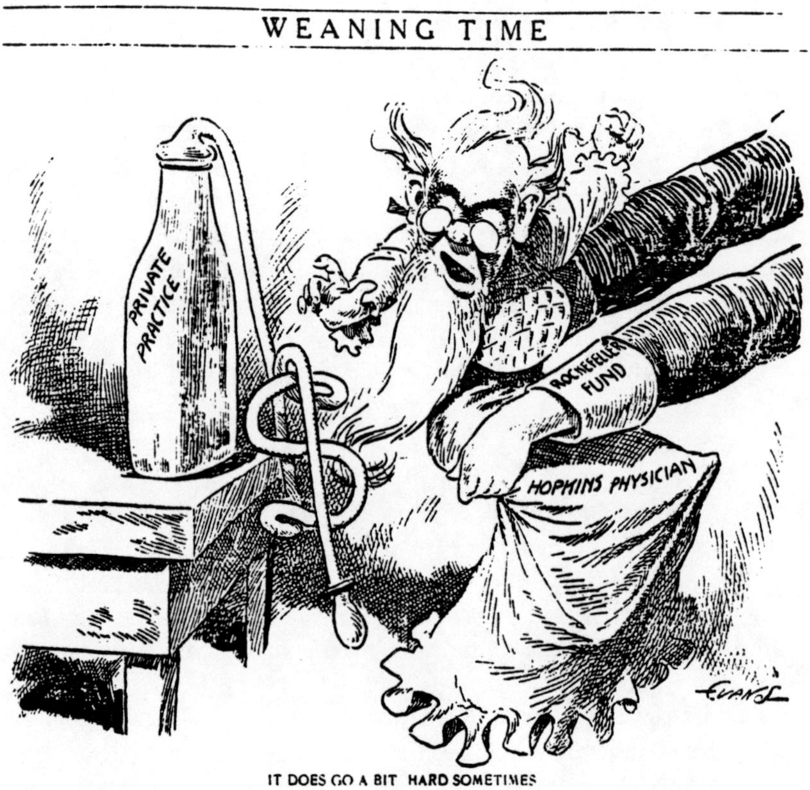

Figure 2.

On January 17, 1914, Barker refused the full-time chair and stepped down as of September to make room for the new incumbent and accepted appointment as Professor of Clinical Medicine.

On February 13, 1914, Cushing wrote from Boston,

> I have anxiously waited for your decision and I do not see how you could have made any other. I think you are entirely right and I doubt not that. I shall have to take a similar stand when the matter comes to a head here. I shall be in Baltimore soon and shall hope to have a long session with you. I hope that when my time comes to withdraw, I shall be able to formulate as graceful and eminently satisfactory a letter as you have done.[108]

108. Barker: *Time & the Physician*, p. 201.

Perhaps the retreat was too "graceful," for Barker was safeguarding his private practice and was aware that life could be more rewarding and much more comfortable if he chose to go along with the new system rather than to buck it. The argument against "pure" full time could have been eloquent and persuasive, but its champion had to be beyond criticism and fully as idealistic as the proponents of the scheme. For Barker to completely reverse his position of 1902 would have been well nigh impossible for his friends and enemies to comprehend and accept. He was clearly flawed by his rapid conversion to material rewards and his unwillingness, or inability, to give them up. Barker was not the person to challenge full time. The challenge would be in the person of Harvey Cushing, and we shall see later on that he was more than equal to the task.

Chapter 11
JANEWAY TO HOPKINS

With Barker displaced from the chair and demoted to Professor of Clinical Medicine, the next step by Welch and Mall would have to be very carefully taken. First, it was obvious they had erred in their choice of Barker with his weaknesses as a clinician as a replacement for Osler. To preserve the clinical reputation of the hospital, Welch knew that he could no longer be guided by Mall. He would simply have to appoint an outstanding clinician who would embrace the full-time concept and serve as a bridge to the not-distant future when the bright young men in training might be ready for the clinical chairs. Welch's first move was to offer the position to William S. Thayer, Osler's very able protégé, who had been passed over in 1905 for Lewellys F. Barker. Years later, when this decision was reviewed, a senior observer commented that Thayer was not as good in 1905 as he was in 1911. At any rate, Thayer turned down the full-time chair and Welch began to look elsewhere.

"Elsewhere" turned out to be New York City, more specifically, Welch's alma mater, the College of Physicians and Surgeons of Columbia University. There an outstanding clinician, Theodore C. Janeway, Bard Professor of Medicine and Visiting Physician to the Presbyterian Hospital, was carrying heavy teaching and patient-care responsibilities while coping with a large private practice as well. He was known as a brilliant clinician and had published in 1904 a monograph, *The Clinical Study of Blood Pressure.* His father, Edward G. Janeway, with whom he practiced, was well known to Welch, who admired him as New York's outstanding internist and clinical teacher of the day. Theodore Janeway is credited with having influenced Mrs. Russell Sage to found the Russell Sage Institute of Pathology in New York. He was also a member of the Board of Scientific Directors of

The Rockefeller Institute for Medical Research. He obviously had the proper credentials, but would he abandon a large practice and his friends and associates in New York, at age forty-two, to accept the challenge of a full-time position at Hopkins? Welch, apprehensive lest he lose Janeway, knowing that great pressures would be exerted to keep him in New York, applied every legitimate measure, including a request to Barker that he urge Janeway to accept the position. This Barker did in a telegram of congratulations in which he promised to cooperate fully with the new chairman.[109]

The challenge of the new position with its opportunities for advancing medical education in America was extremely attractive to Janeway's altruism and idealism. The load of his private practice in New York plus his teaching activities was so heavy that he looked forward to the full-time position at Hopkins, where most of his energy would be applied to the science and teaching of clinical medicine. Janeway accepted the offer and on July 1, 1914, became the first full-time Professor of Medicine at Johns Hopkins and the first in America. His appointment was greeted with enthusiasm by the staff, which welcomed the arrival of a superb and experienced clinician with educational and scientific attainments needed to restore luster to the chair once held by Sir William Osler. Snaring Janeway was not only a coup for Welch, it was also a triumph for full time, one line of reasoning being that the concept had to be sound if such an outstanding clinician would be willing to make such substantial sacrifices to accept it.

Janeway embarked upon his new assignment with vigor and élan, and it was not long before the wards of Hopkins were ringing with his praise. The adulation of his house staff, including Tom Rivers, was infectious. He was indeed an outstanding teacher for residents as well as medical students, and his attending staff learned quickly to respect the new professor from New York. Six months after the three major clinical departments had been placed on a full-time basis at Hopkins, the three department heads reported on their experience. Halsted, quite predictably, commented favorably that "a keen and wholesome rivalry has been aroused and the range of my clinical experience seems not

109. Chesney, *The Johns Hopkins Hospital,* vol. III, pp. 258-60.

to have been affected,"[110] and that he had found much more time to devote to his research. Howland felt that full time had increased his clinical opportunities, since "it allows more time to devote to the observation of patients." Janeway's reply was also in favor of the plan, his detailed letter on the subject sent to the General Education Board, stating,

> So far as the teaching of the medical student goes, I can only say that a year has convinced me that our students, under this plan, gain more effective, practical bedside instruction, a wider outlook on the whole fields of medicine and surgery from their constant contact with their teachers, and a greater stimulus to the investigation of many unsolved problems than any students I have come in contact with before. For the student I can see no disadvantage.[111]

Unfortunately for Janeway, despite freedom from the previous demands of his large practice in New York, many other responsibilities descended upon him, the heaviest being service in Washington in World War I as a senior consultant to the Surgeon General. The time which he felt might be free for research and teaching was being encroached upon by administrative demands and military requirements. Other problems were also cropping up, chief among these being his gradual disaffection with the full-time system, which had lost its appeal and he found at close sight less attractive than he had originally envisioned. The disillusionment progressed and finally in November 1917 it had reached the point that he resigned from the chair at Hopkins with the intention of returning to his private practice and part-time teaching in New York. In a letter to Welch, dated November 4, 1917, he indicated that his decision to return to New York and private practice, was, in part, based upon financial obligations to his family and also because he had lost sympathy with the full-time scheme. This was a serious blow to Welch and the proponents of full time, and it was not loudly publicized at the time. This was not a Barker turning on the system. This was a seasoned, brilliant clinician who had been excited about the concept and had found it to be wanting after he had given it a fair trial. As if the letter of resignation were not enough, Janeway expressed his views with clarity and eloquence in an address given before the Association of American Universities in Iowa City,

---

110. Flexner, S. and Flexner, J. T., *William H. Welch*, p. 326, note 94.
111. General Education Board: Report of the Secretary, 1914-1915, Chap. 2, p. 20.

November 10, 1917 and published in an obscure journal (*The Educational Review,* March 1918, p. 207) under the title, "Outside Engagements by Members of the Professional Faculties." The essay was lost to most medical readers until Henry Christian arranged for it to be reprinted in the *Journal of the American Medical Association* in April 1928, ensuring its belated exposure to a wider audience.[112]

In this essay, Janeway turns his keen analytical mind upon the full-time concept as it applies to clinical medicine, dissects it, diagnoses its weakness and its strengths, and then clearly indicates his own position on this issue and why and how he arrived at it. The comments seem as appropriate today as the day they were written sixty years ago and warrant careful scrutiny.

When Turner in *Heritage of Excellence* speaks of Janeway's brief tenure as chairman of the department of medicine at Hopkins, he says,

> By 1917, he had decided to resign his Hopkins post to return to private practice in New York City, a decision probably prompted by "some disenchantment" with the full-time system coupled with sheer physical and mental exhaustion. Before his resignation could be acted upon, he developed lobar pneumonia and died on December 27, at the age of forty-five, only three years after assuming the professorship.[113]

I would take issue with the interpretation that physical and mental exhaustion were important factors in Janeway's defection from full time. The detailed and brilliant analysis in his discourse of November 10, 1917 shows no evidence of a tired mind. It is acute, critical, constructive, and carefully thought through. Janeway, a mature and seasoned physician, had tried the system, seen its weakness, and had openly rejected it.

In today's language, what is Janeway's message? First, let us call a spade a spade; by "outside engagements" he was not talking about lectures or visiting professorships. He was clearly and unequivocally talking about personal private practice on a fee-for-service basis, the anathema of all pure full-timers. His position was that the things which made him an outstanding teacher were

---

112. Janeway, T. C.: Outside professional engagements by members of professional faculties. *JAMA, 90/16:*1315-18, Apr. 21, 1928.

113. Turner, Thomas B.: *Heritage of Excellence: Johns Hopkins Medical Institutions, 1914-1947.* Baltimore, Johns Hopkins Press, 1974, p. 105.

derived from this sort of experience that he had undergone while teaching and practicing in New York City. His feeling was that all physicians should be exposed to private practice at some stage in their lives. True, it is that he hedges somewhat when he advises that young men be sheltered from private practice early so that their capabilities and work habits in productive research may be formed. In practical terms, such an individual who finds his niche in research, seldom seeks the additional experience of private practice. He is already committed to a way of life that bars the "intrusions and distractions" of patients who are sick and asking for help for minor as well as serious matters. Another point Janeway might have stressed is that not all clinicians in practice are so attracted and committed to their private patients that as they grow older they do less teaching. I know for certain that once the right men in practice have developed income adequate for moderate family needs, the best ones seek to contribute more of their time to public service, some to teaching without reimbursement, and others to community and national activities. These are the ones to spot early. These are the ones to encourage and for whom the university should leave the options open, giving them recognition, encouragement, and the opportunity to participate actively and with dignity in the teaching and training of students and house staff as well as attending staff. This sort of man or woman brings lustre to his institution and serves as a bridge between the world outside and the ivory tower of academicians within the walls of the university.

This I believe to be the essence of Janeway's message in contemporary terms. We must also remember that in Janeway's day, in contrast to the surgeon whose main work was in the hospital, the physician's main activities were in his office and in the homes of his patients. In 1915, relatively little could be done for medical disorders. We had few if any specific drugs. Therapy was largely symptomatic and empiric, and the best men, including Osler, were therapeutic nihilists. There was little or nothing the physician could do for his patient in the hospital that he could not do just as well or better in his home.

For that period, the imposition of full time upon the clinical professor of medicine was indeed premature and untimely. It could constrict his experience in his contacts and handicap him seriously in the teaching and training of young people for the practice of medicine. The time was simply not ripe or appropriate for this drastic change in medical education. The troops were not available for the change, and neither staff nor public nor students were ready to embrace the plan. The reformers behind the scheme were not a whit dissuaded. They sincerely felt that it was the ONLY way and that no compromise was indicated. The motives of the practitioner-teachers were under constant attack: in the press, in foundation headquarters, and among the preclinical teachers. The schism between the practitioners and the academicians was becoming wider and wider, and the exchanges were at times rather vicious. The Council on Medical Education was claiming that the Rockefeller money and Flexner, an unexperienced layman and nonphysician, were trying to impose a revolution upon American medical education without adequate consultation with the profession at large. The practitioner-teachers were being accused of venality, greed, and avarice. Cartoons in the newspaper were presenting the practitioner-teacher in a very bad light.[114]

Of Flexner, Hans Zinsser, in his autobiography, *As I Remember Him*, had this to say:

> Oh, Abraham Flexner! We have fought with you on minor points, have alternately admired and disliked you, have applauded you for wisdom and detested you for opinionatedness. But in just retrospect—layman as you are—we hail you as the father—or better, the uncle—of modern medical education in America. You did, on occasion, hit below the belt, yet in the spirit in which Christian Knights slashed off the infidels' heads while shouting "Kyrie Eleison!" It was your report—uncomprising, cruelly objective, courageous and incisive—which opened the eyes of the medical profession to the state of their training schools, aroused public opinion to the need of better education of the guardians of health, and set the floodgates of the golden streams of philanthropy in medical directions.[115]

The cauldron was boiling and events were set in motion having great impact upon the education of every physician in America. There were bound to be areas of disagreement among honest and good men and women. The full-time controversy was dividing medicine into two armed camps. Statesmen would be needed to

114. See cartoon, "Weaning Time," *Baltimore American* (1913), in Chapter 10.

115. Zinsser, Hans: *As I Remember Him: The Biography of R. S.* Boston, Little, Brown & Co., 1940, p. 313.

reconcile the opposing views, seeking common ground for all in this struggle to improve the care of the sick and the well.

Chapter 12
HOPKINS AND P & S PLAY MUSICAL CHAIRS IN MEDICINE

In March 1922, Warfield Theobald Longcope was offered the chair in medicine at Johns Hopkins and accepted it, effective July 1, 1922. Longcope, born in Baltimore, March 29, 1877, came from a long line of physicians, a direct descendant of Nathan Smith, the great pioneer in medical education, and of Nathan Ryno Smith, leader and outstanding teacher of surgery in the University of Maryland.[116] Alan P. Smith, Longcope's great-uncle, had been the last physician to Mr. Johns Hopkins, who had appointed him one of the original trustees of the Johns Hopkins Hospital. Longcope received his B.A. degree from Hopkins in 1897 and his M.D. in 1901, having been a student of the Big Four, including Osler. Among those in his class destined to reach high positions in medicine, there were besides Longcope, Frederick H. Baetjer, Thomas R. Boggs, Frederick P. Gay, and Louis V. Hamman, to mention a few.[117]

Following his graduation in 1901, Longcope was appointed Resident Pathologist under Dr. Simon Flexner at the Pennsylvania Hospital where he served for three years until he succeeded his chief in 1904 as director of the Ayer Clinical Laboratory of the Pennslyvania Hospital. In 1909, he was given an additional appointment as assistant professor of applied medicine at the University of Pennsylvania, an assignment that provided access to clinical material and clinical teaching. During this era, his clinician friends regarded him as rather odd for his emphasis on the laboratory and the study of bacteria rather than "practical" clinical medicine and they soon dubbed him "Bugs" Longcope.

In 1911, Theodore Janeway, Bard Professor of Medicine at P & S called Longcope, now age thirty-four, to New York where he was his first assistant for three years and Associate Professor

116. Robinson, *Adventures in Medical Education.* p. 66.
117. Turner, *Heritage of Excellence.* p. 109.

of Medicine. When Janeway left New York in 1914 for the chair at Hopkins, Longcope succeeded him as Medical Director and Bard Professor of the Practice of Medicine at P & S. World War I influenced the next move when, in July 1917, Longcope was called to the Surgeon General's office and for overseas duty, where he undertook studies of influenza and streptococcal infections. During his absence from New York, Dr. Walter W. Palmer, who had been brought in from the Rockefeller Institute, was appointed Acting Director of the Medical Service at Presbyterian Hospital and ran the division with skill until Longcope returned in February 1919. Palmer then left to accept an associate professorship in medicine at Johns Hopkins. Here he remained until 1921, when in what might be characterized (except for its deadly seriousness) another round of musical chairs, Palmer returned to P & S to occupy the chair relinquished by Longcope who rather unexpectedly had resigned in 1921 because of repeated disagreements with Dean William Darrach of P & S. The experience was so frustrating to Longcope that he sought to escape from it by going into private practice, mainly as a consultant. Shortly thereafter, he received an offer to head the department of medicine at Yale University Medical School but declined. When, in March 1922, the offer reached him of the chair in medicine in his native Baltimore and in the university where he was educated, it proved irresistible and he accepted it, going on to serve with distinction, developing one of the strongest medical units in the world during his twenty-five years of tenure. His Presbyterian friends were "delighted at the happy outcome of an unpleasant conflict," and his good friend, Dr. A. R. Lamb, opined that Longcope in Baltimore "worked more contentedly than he probably could have in the hurly-burly of New York."[118]

When Longcope took over as director of the Department of Medicine at Hopkins, he moved vigorously to implement the full-time system. This had remained in abeyance during World War I and during the interregnum occasioned by Janeway's death, Hamman's interim appointment as chief during Thayer's World War I service, and Thayer's and Robinson's short terms of office. There was considerable animosity between the full-time men and

118. Lamb, Albert R.: *Presbyterian Hospital and Columbia-Presbyterian Medical Center: 1868-1943.* New York, Columbia University Press, 1955, p. 167.

the part-time faculty, especially apparent on the ward services but also evident in the outpatient department, where a number of part-time associate consultants were listed but rarely appeared in apparent protest of the full-time system.

> Longcope, wishing fully to implement the full-time system in spirit as well as in theory, initially made his principal full-time associate professors primarily responsible for clinical care and teaching on the wards. Thus, in addition to himself, the main burden fell upon Carter, Amoss and Harrop with Chesney playing a more minor role. While Longcope was a highly skilled physician who had a good background in pathology, and had served as head of medicine at Columbia, the same could not be said for his titular principal associates. Carter was a good clinician but tended to be a dilettante and to take his ward duties somewhat lightly. Amoss learned fast, but was relatively inexperienced as a clinician during the early years of his service at Hopkins, and Harrop, although sincere and well-meaning, was not a born clinician, to say the least, and his attention was focussed largely on problems of metabolism, especially diabetes. Each of these senior associate professors had one or more younger men working with them, some of whom were very good clinicians, and they too assisted in the ward teaching. But the senior members of the part-time faculty were for all practical purposes excluded from ward teaching in the 1920s which caused considerable dissatisfaction among that group and gave rise to questioning on the part of the fourth-year students.[119]

Above and beyond the concept of full time and its effects on the careers of graduate and postgraduate physicians is the unfortunate separation of the men in practice from the students in training. Some Hopkins students, appreciating that part-time teachers had much to contrubute, expressed their dissatisfaction with the system. The clinical weaknesses in their full-time teachers were all too apparent, and the students knew that stellar clinicians in practice in Baltimore were not asked to participate in their instruction. Other students, seeing their role models as primarily scientists and not clinicians, reacted by emulating them and selected careers that tended to place less emphasis on patients than on their diseases, often to the detriment of the patient. Polarization of the two groups of physicians was bad for the student, harmful for patient care, and unwise for American medicine. Some sort of compromise was needed, but it would be some years before the situation would improve at Hopkins.

119. Turner, *Heritage of Excellence*, p. 153.

Chapter 13
HARVEY CUSHING AND FLEXNER COLLIDE

I quote others only the better to express myself.

Michel de Montaigne
(1533-1592)[120]

By 1912, Abraham Flexner had been appointed to the General Education Board as a member and assistant secretary. His next move was to attempt to do in Boston what he had finally accomplished in Baltimore. The bait was an offer by the General Education Board in October 1913, of one and one-half million dollars to Harvard Medical School, "provided the chiefs-of-clinic at the Brigham Hospital would agree to serve as full-time officers on the same financial basis as that about to be instituted in Baltimore."[121]

Here, Flexner met with more than his match. Harvey Cushing, Brigham's surgeon-in-chief, had rather strong feelings about full time and had the courage and energy and eloquence to speak very frankly. A head-on collision was inevitable.

On March 30, 1914, Cushing wrote to President Lowell:

> It is my impression that the reasons for the adoption in Baltimore of the proposal from the General Education Board were based upon the feeling, chiefly on the part of the heads of the preclinical departments, that the school was getting into a rut, from which it should be extricated no matter how seriously the method adopted might temporarily wrench their machine. Unquestionably this feeling would not have arisen had the heads of the clinical departments been given the opportunity some years ago voluntarily to place themselves on a whole-service basis similar to that on which my colleague and myself now serve at the Brigham Hospital.
>
> It seems to me that the clinical departments of the Harvard Medical school, on the other hand, by their own initiative give promise

120. Montaigne, Michel: *Complete Works of Michel de Montaigne.* Translated by Donald M. Frame. Stanford, Stanford Univerity Press, 1957.

121. Fulton, *Harvey Cushing,* p. 384.

> of getting out of the rut into which they had fallen, and the injection at this time of a new element into the situation might seriously complicate it. Were we at a standstill or in financial straits, we might have to ask others to help pull our load, and to accept their terms no matter how experimental they might appear to be. On the other hand, were our engine running more smoothly than it is, we might otherwise be justified in venturing to test it on an unbroken road.
>
> Not without various difficulties we are slowly working out our own problems at the Brigham Hospital—problems which concern the continuous whole-time service of the clinical chiefs—problems therefore which are somewhat idealistic and which moreover are novel to those who are concerned with the hospital administration. The difficulties are gradually being smoothed out, but the experiment, from all points of view, cannot as yet be deemed a complete success. Before we have quite found ourselves, on this basis, it is proposed that we make a still more radical experiment in so far as our relation to the institution is concerned.[122]

The solution that Cushing and Henry Christian were developing at the Brigham was so-called geographic full-time, the professors being permanently based in the hospital and receiving a modest salary with most of their income being derived from private practice within the hospital.

To clinch the argument, Cushing in the final paragraph offers to resign his position if the Flexnerian full-time scheme is to be put in effect. Lowell replies on April 4, 1914,

> I understand your position perfectly. It is, substantially, that we have made a real innovation, which promises to be a great improvement in clinical teaching, in connection with the Brigham Hospital; and that it is unwise, at present to complicate this with further experiment, the results of which must necessarily be uncertain. Your position seems to me perfectly reasonable; and while it will prevent our applying to the General Education Board now for a gift for full-time clinical professors, it may not prevent our doing so at some future time, in case the experiment as now tried at Johns Hopkins proves successful.[123]

For the moment, this seems to have disposed of the full-time issue at Harvard but not for very long. Flexner raised the issue with Lowell once more in July 1914, and letters were exchanged by Cushing, Christian, and Lowell. Again, Cushing offered to give up his position and so did Christian. Flexner and the General

122. *Ibid.*, pp. 379-80.
123. *Ibid.*, p. 380.

Education Board continued to negotiate with Lowell and on March 7, 1915, Cushing, in reply to another letter from Lowell, offered to step aside for a full-time man if this was what the Brigham trustees desired. This letter, described by John F. Fulton, Cushing's biographer, as one of "disarming grace which under the circumstances could scarcely have been expected," might be viewed as a clever maneuver in the power struggle between Cushing and the General Education Board and his adversary, Abraham Flexner. Cushing probably had no real intention of resigning at that time. He fully realized how important he had become to the Brigham and the world of medicine and knew that the threat of resignation would throw the Brigham trustees into a tizzy. He was their great man and they were not about to lose him, especially since it was not going to cost the hospital anything if things remained as they were.

Why was Cushing so strongly opposed to Flexner's full-time scheme? The answer to this is presented with eloquence in Harvey Cushing's next to his last Annual Report of the Surgical Department of the Peter Bent Brigham Hospital. After discussing the initiation of clinical full time at Hopkins in January, 1914, he goes on to say that he and Christian had developed a geographic full-time system that he felt was superior to full time as defined by Flexner.[124]

Against Flexner's full-time scheme, he offered these cogent arguments. "On my part, a term of service limited to twenty years with an academic salary on which a family of children were to be educated and no pension in sight in case of accident or ill health seemed a dubious proposition."[125]

How prescient this was when in retrospect, we know that Cushing had three beautiful and talented daughters, each of whom would marry well. Any father can tell you that these are not inexpensive matters to encourage and facilitate. Cushing also expressed doubt that the full-time arrangement would in any way activate him to work harder and, in fact, he feared it might encourage indolence.

> If the purpose of the plan was to prevent the attendants in university hospitals from exploiting their position for their personal

---

124. *Ibid.*, pp. 382-84.
125. *Ibid.*, p. 384.

> ends, there was just as much reason to fear, human nature being what it is, that hospital superintendents and trustees might be tempted in a pinch to exploit their salaried professional attendants.

Finally, he said:

> Coming of a race of general practitioners, the intimate and confidential relation between doctor and patient—one of the most precious things in medicine—was in my blood and I could not look upon the cold institutional program with any great enthusiasm, much less with any expectation that it would serve to make something out of me that I was not already.[126]

On April 15, 1915, during Cushing's absence on war duty in France, Alexander Cochrane, President of the Brigham trustees, wrote a gracious and perceptive letter to President Lowell on the full-time issue and recommended rejection of the offer of the Rockefeller General Education Board. When Cushing returned from Europe three months later, the issue had been settled. Harvard had turned down the General Education Board's offer of 1.5 million dollars and had again rejected the full-time scheme. Cushing's vigorous stand against strict full time and the rational basis for his position had won the day. Harvard would never accept strict full time. In spite of heavy pressures, Harvard would stay with the modification initiated by Cushing and Christian, adapting it to meet changing circumstances.

After the Brigham had acted adversely on full time, David L. Edsall who had come to the Massachusetts General Hospital as Jackson Professor in Medicine in 1912, chafing at the loss of 1.5 million dollars for the medical school, wrote to President Lowell suggesting that the Massachusetts General Hospital be used in place of the Brigham. Edsall had already been "ambushed" once before at the University of Pennsylvania where he tried to introduce a mild form of full time (so-called half time), and he had witnessed some problems with it at Washington University, St. Louis, where he was for a short period Professor of Preventive Medicine. He was, therefore, very careful in his espousal of the cause and proposed a modification rather than the pure concept, a position not unlike that taken by Cushing and Christian at the Brigham. Flexner, representing the General Education Board, was opposed to the MGH as the hospital for the full-time trial because it was too far away from the medical school, was con-

126. *Ibid.*, p. 384.

trolled by an independent board of trustees without an administrative link to the school and, in his opinion, did not have the proper tradition. "And the situation in Boston was impossible anyway, the relations between the school and its many hospitals being too tenuous, complicated and impermanent."[127]

Despite these objections, Edsall persisted in his efforts and was able to persuade Flexner to consider the Massachusetts General Hospital for a trial of full time and proposals were prepared for presentation to the staff of the MGH prior to submission to the General Education Board. The MGH surgical staff met in November 1914 and turned down the entire plan, leading to a prolonged stalemate.

In June 1916, the matter was taken up again by a committee consisting of President Emeritus Charles Eliot, Walter Cannon, David Edsall, Reid Hunt, and W. S. Thayer. In December 1916, the committee proposed a trial of a modification of the full-time concept at Harvard to include several clinical units: two in clinical medicine; two in clinical surgery; and one each in pediatrics, obstetrics, and diseases of the nervous system. Dr. Wallace Buttrick of the General Education Board rejected this proposal saying in part:

> The full-time scheme was, in a word, meant to end one order of things and to instal a new order of things. Dr. Eliot's proposition continues the old order and adds the new order, in so far as medicine, surgery and pediatrics are concerned . . . . Thus Dr. Eliot's plan would not transform the general character of the medical school, as the institutions previously reorganized on the full-time plan have been transformed.[128]

Eliot replied:

> While the Harvard Medical School desires to put full-time professors at the head of all its clinical teaching, it expects to continue to employ a large number of part-time teachers, in order to utilize its extensive clinical and laboratory facilities, and give amply individual instruction in the great variety of subjects with which it deals. . . . There are more than three hundred lecturers, instructors, and assistants, most of whom are private practitioners as well as hospital practitioners . . . . The existence of this useful body of instruction given by part-time teachers, who are familiar with practice

127. Aub, J. C. and Hapgood, R. K.: *Pioneer in Modern Medicine: David L. Edsall.* Harvard Medical Alumni Association, 1970. p. 173.

128. *Ibid.*, pp. 176-78.

in homes as well as in hospitals, does not interfere in any way with the control of all the principal clinics by full-time professors. . . .

In closing, Dr. Eliot reaffirmed his university's independent tradition with the comment:

No "transformation" of the Harvard Medical School and no suppression of any of its parts or departments are needed or desired. Its history is honorable, and its present condition effective. It now asks from the General Education Board (1) aid in establishing that great improvement in medical education, the full-time professorship without private practice, and (2) in building up and maintaining a well-equipped Department of Preventive Medicine and Public Health.[129]

Again, Harvard had asserted its position clearly and indicated that it was not going to permit the General Education Board and its money to dictate its policies, The Board was equally adamant and when it became apparent that it would reject the Harvard proposal, it was withdrawn in May 1917 to await a more propitious opportunity.

In June 1918, David Edsall was appointed Dean of Harvard Medical School, and it was not long before he corresponded with Abraham Flexner again regarding full time, the latter adhering tenaciously to the pure concept while Edsall argued for a modified form, saying (August 3, 1919),

I am thoroughly convinced that we can not grow successive crops of good clinical teachers and investigators without actually seeing to it that they do, as they develop, get contact with the differing types of disorders and the methods of therapeutics that are used with the nonhospital class of the community. I think this more and more forcibly as I grow more convinced of the need of a full-time plan. In fact I know from personal experience that fine hospital internes and young instructors who have had only hospital experience with ward cases have so very distorted an idea of what good medical service to the community is that were I to choose between continuing the present conditions everywhere on the one hand or on the other hand having medical education entirely dominated by a group of men who had been brought up strictly in hospital wards, I know I should enjoy the latter more in my own work but I think I should feel that the other was right for the public.[130]

Flexner's reply in defense of pure full time was:

I should like to see the scheme, in its most rigid form, tried out

129. *Ibid.*

130. *Ibid.*, p. 276.

during the next ten or fifteen years in a half dozen institutions and then ascertain whether it needs modification . . . . I suspect that, if the funds are adequate to give decent salaries to men working whether as chiefs or as assistants on the full-time plan, the outcome will be favorable to the more rigid conception. (Aug. 14, 1919)[131]

Edsall's rebuttal of Flexner was well taken. "In all the experimental work that I have had to do and have observed, one of the most important elements is always flexibility rather than absolute rigidity."[132] Obviously, Flexner was meeting with a worthy adversary and getting a substantial education in the process.

By 1924, when Edsall addressed the Massachusetts Medical Society, he was confident that the modified full-time system had established itself.

Acceptance of complete personal responsibility in the usual and natural way with a few private patients in a hospital is much more effective in achieving the academic purpose in seeing such patients, than is the method that makes it purely a part of the duties to an institutional organization . . . . Skill in practise . . . is retained not by practise only, but by undivided and keen responsibility in practise . . . . Circumstances, not regulations, have led me through all stages of experience in this. I for some time did general practise, then for a long time only consulting practise, then a distinctly restricted consulting practise, then none. I believe, I trust with reason that I became better as a consultant as I went on, but I am sure I became coincidentally less and less skillful in the duties of family practise. Then in the several years in which other duties grew so pressing that consulting work, though continued, became in considerable degree a task rather than a highly interesting and alluring thing, I could clearly see that my skill such as it was, decreased, not simply as a consultant, but even in teaching and research. I imagine that this is usual.[133]

Edsall, having suffered from his two previous experiences at Pennsylvania and Washington Universities, saw the advantages of full time and at the same time fully realized its disadvantages and proceeded to bring about gradual change rather than a third revolution that might have ended in his being removed from office. What he finally developed is the Harvard Plan of full time, which has been a strong force in maintaining Harvard's reputa-

131. *Ibid.*, p. 277.
132. *Ibid.*, pp. 277-78.
133. Edsall, David L.: The product of medical education. *Boston Med & Surg Jnl, 191:*283-94, Aug. 14, 1924.

tion as an outstanding medical school and has served as a model for other institutions.

> By the spring of 1928, looking back on the accomplishments of ten years, Edsall permitted himself a cautious optimism on this achievement, and wrote:
>
> "A great deal of the betterment in the tone of the School and in the interest of the students in their work has been due to the extensive establishment of our system of modified full time in a large group of the clinical chairs." He was careful to point out, however, that the Harvard Medical School had "always maintained in each department a group of clinicians in active practice, as an essential part of the proper training of students."[134]

The financial support for these changes came largely from the Rockefeller Boards despite Harvard's refusal to comply with any rigid conditions imposed by them. The appointment in 1920 of Richard W. Pearce, a warm friend and former colleague of Edsall, as head of the division of medical education of the Rockefeller Foundation, opened a new era in the relationship between Harvard and the Rockefeller Foundation and unquestionably played an important role in the support given to Harvard for its educational programs in medicine. No longer would a Harvard president complain that his university was being neglected by the Rockefeller Boards!

134. Aub and Hapgood, *Pioneer in Modern Medicine*, p. 279.

Chapter 14
FLEXNER HYPNOTIZES MR. EASTMAN

I am not interested in education.

—*George Eastman, 1898*[135]

Flexner's crusade to reform medical education in America was pursued relentlessly following his appointment to the General Education Board[136] in 1912 and given added impetus by his appointment as its secretary, and in effect, its chief executive officer in 1917. The reformation was to be accomplished by persuading and enticing selected medical schools to accept full time for the clinical chairs in exchange for substantial gifts for endowment and construction. Strict full time was Flexner's prescription for curing the ills of medical education and he would never deviate from his support of the concept. If already established medical schools rejected the scheme, he would see that new schools were built and staffed by faculty agreeing to accept full time. Since enormous sums of money were involved, he could, of course, apply his concepts to only a small number of institutions. His hope was that they might serve as pilot ventures and stimulate others to follow their example. In addition, he had learned the lesson from Gates of supplying seed money for projects and never paying the whole bill, depending upon local and other sources to match the Rockefeller gifts. Both concepts were original and pioneering and were to set the pattern for major philanthropy for years to come. Between 1917 and 1928, the General Education Board disbursed $50,000,000 to medical schools and generated another $600,000,000 from other sources

135. Slater, John R.: *Rhees of Rochester.* New York, Harper and Brothers, 1946, p. 159.

136. Founded in 1902 by John D. Rockefeller "to promote education in the United States of America without distinction of race, sex or creed." From foreword of General Education Board Review and Final Report, 1902-1964.

in matching funds, a truly amazing performance.[137]

We have discussed the problems encountered by Flexner and the General Education Board when they attempted to reform or modernize several existing medical schools to fit their model at Johns Hopkins. While Flexner clearly enjoyed a good fight, the battles at Hopkins, Harvard, Washington University, and Vanderbilt, to name a few, were, at times, rather bloody and consuming of energy and time and left scars that persisted for many years. Undaunted, he dreamed of starting a medical school in New York City in the Johns Hopkins mold. With the encouragement of his superiors, he investigated the possibilities at Cornell and Columbia University, College of Physicians and Surgeons. Flexner reported that after a long and encouraging conversation with President Nicholas Murray Butler of Columbia at the Century Club, during which he "tried to explain the impossibility of carrying on a modern medical school that did its laboratory teaching at Fifty-ninth Street and Ninth Avenue and its clinical teaching with practicing consultants in the Presbyterian Hospital at Seventieth Street and Madison Avenue," he was referred to Dr. Samuel Lambert, Dean of the Medical School.

> But neither of them was half as much interested in scientific medicine as in the persons who held posts from which they would have to be dislodged. At Cornell the situation was not fundamentally dissimilar. The underlying subjects were properly equipped, taught, and inspired in a building on First Avenue. The clinical subjects were in the hands of practitioners and consultants at the New York and Bellevue Hospitals. So for the moment New York seemed impossible.[138]

That is the story as Flexner tells it, but another version of it reached me some years ago at lunch in the faculty dining room at Columbia Presbyterian Medical Center from Dr. David C. Bull, Attending Surgeon. According to Doctor Bull's version, Flexner fell in New York in the winter of 1917, fracturing his left ankle, and went to the accident room of a New York hospital where the fracture was set by Dr. Adrian V. S. Lambert. "The surgeon made a complete mess of his work. He put on a huge cast reaching

137. Flexner, Abraham: *Funds and Foundations.* New York, Harper and Row, 1952, p. 132.

138. Flexner, Abraham: *An Autobiography.* New York, Simon and Schuster, 1960, p. 180.

from foot to hip without using any pad," said Flexner.[139] As a result, Flexner suffered tortures. The cast should have been removed as soon as pain set in. It was not removed for three weeks, during which time he was kept under the influence of opiates. When finally it was taken off, there was no feeling in the foot, and the upper surface of the foot was necrotic. The surgeon was puzzled, but did nothing more than put on a fresh bandage. Flexner was sent home on crutches, but went every day or two to the surgeon's office where the bandage was changed. One day his wife went with him and amazed the surgeon by saying, "Dr. _______, do you know what you are about?" He stammered and admitted he did not. She said, "Very well, replace the bandage, and we will go down to Baltimore and see Doctor Halsted."[140] Flexner was admitted to Hopkins in November and remained there until February under the care of Halsted who took personal charge and meticulously changed the dressings himself and saw the patient twice daily. The problem seemed to be to restore "the vitality of necrotic tendons." On January 27, 1919, Abraham Flexner wrote to his brother, Simon, exasperated by the length of time he had to remain in the hospital and added, "Doctor Halsted's plan contemplated an ideal result but took no account of time or other circumstances. A line of treatment may be one thing in the case of a monkey or a guinea pig and ought to be another in the case of a busy person."[141] In a letter to Doctor Blalock, thirty-six years later in 1953, Flexner's account was somewhat different, for he had mellowed and now praised Halsted to the skies for his superb care and boasted that Alexis Carrel had come down from New York City to see the excellent end result and had said, "This is a magnificent surgical stunt."

So much for the Hopkins end of the story. Columbia came off second best. Dr. Adrian V. S. Lambert, Director of Surgery at Presbyterian Hospital, and his brother, Samuel Lambert, the Dean of the Medical School, were powerful figures in New York medicine. Doctor Bull told me that because of his adverse experience, Flexner swore he would never recommend a grant from the General Education Board for any medical school having a

---

139. Crowe, S. J.: *Halsted of Johns Hopkins.* Springfield, Thomas, 1957, pp. 238-40.
140. *Ibid.*, pp. 238-40.
141. Olch, P. D.: Personal letter to author, September 16, 1975.

Lambert on its staff! I tell this story not to discredit Dr. Adrian Lambert but to indicate that many large decisions may be influenced by very small personal reactions that may not have idealism or altruism as their basis and may lack objectivity. No matter what the true basis for his decision, Flexner's next move in medical education was to illustrate once more his cleverness and his innate capacity for infighting to achieve his goals.

Rebuffed in New York City in his attempts to remodel the two leading medical schools in the Hopkins pattern, he decided to start from scratch in Western New York State with a brand new medical school committed from the very beginning to the full-time principle. This would prove to be the only school created *de novo* by Flexner's efforts. Here the full-time concept would be put to the test without any old guard to interfere with the trial. For the first time, he would be able to conduct his experiment without opposition, for the staff had agreed to full time as a condition for appointment. Because this experiment was so unique, with many lessons to be derived, I shall describe what happened in Rochester, New York, in some detail.

Since a frontal assault on the entrenched power structure of Cornell and Columbia schools of medicine had failed to budge either institution in the direction desired by Flexner and the General Education Board, Flexner decided to take the situation by the flank. One day when he was riding home from a Southern trip in a Pullman car with Doctor Buttrick, the head of the General Education Board, Flexner, according to his own account, said quite casually, "The University of Rochester is a modest but good institution, isn't it?" Buttrick replied, as Flexner knew he almost certainly would:

> "Yes," he replied. "I know it well. Gates and I are graduates of the Rochester Theological Seminary. I know Rhees well—a fine college head. Why do you ask?"
>
> "It has occured to me that if we could help to plant a first-rate medical school there, perhaps New York City would wake up."
>
> "Why Rochester?" he asked.
>
> "There are medical schools at Buffalo, Syracuse, Albany; it won't be easy to find money or men to reorganize them. Rochester has a clean slate; and besides there is Mr. Eastman."
>
> "Do you know him?"
>
> "No, but I do know that he has endowed a dental clinic. Perhaps

that would prove a step toward medicine."[142]

Quite fortuitously, when Buttrick reached New York, he found on his desk, of all things, a letter from President Rhees saying he would be in New York the following week. The opportunity was seized and in Flexner's short interview with Rhees, he asked, "President Rhees, there is no medical school in Rochester; would you like to have one?" "Only if we could have a first-rate one." "We are not interested in any other kind. Do you know Mr. George Eastman?" "Oh yes, intimately." "Can you arrange a meeting between us in Rochester?" "I think so."[143]

Rhees' friendship with George Eastman had not come easily. For years he had undertaken a low-key, soft-sell approach to the bachelor businessman to inform him of the needs of the University of Rochester, and of its importance to the City of Rochester and its 250,000 inhabitants, and also, not incidentally, to the Eastman Kodak Company. Initially, Eastman had been cool toward education, for he himself was essentially self-taught. In fact, on one occasion, after giving Rhees a significant but relatively modest gift, he warned him that there would be no more and said he was not generally interested in formal education. Offended by the rebuff, Rhees managed to keep his "cool" for the time being, but resolved to never again solicit Mr. Eastman without some really major specific project in mind. As the years went on, Eastman had occasion to modify his original stance. He quickly realized that the key people in his organization were university trained and that his research chemists were at the heart of the entire future of Eastman Kodak. Without research, it would simply fade away as its competitors passed them with new concepts and innovative techniques. By 1920, Mr. Eastman had given tangible evidence of his change of heart in philanthropy. In Rochester, this was demonstrated by his establishment of the Eastman Dental Clinic and by major gifts for the Eastman School of Music of the University of Rochester. The climate for giving was good, cultivated as it had been by Rush Rhees, and the time was ripe for the major solicitation Rhees had been waiting for. The money was there; Mr. Eastman was single and had few, if any, dependents. Andrew Carnegie and John D. Rockefeller had set

142. Flexner, *Autobiography*, pp. 180-81.
143. *Ibid.*, p. 181.

the pattern for American philanthropy during their lifetimes, and George Eastman was keenly aware that his turn had come to commit his resources to the public weal.

Within forty-eight hours of his interview with Rhees, Flexner received a telegram inviting him to have breakfast with Eastman in his mansion on East Avenue in Rochester, New York. The description of the initial meeting conveys something of the character of the man being courted for his bounty. Organ music was being played and it continued through breakfast, stopping promptly at 10:00 A.M., at which time Eastman and Flexner adjourned to the study where they sat on a sofa before a wood fire, its ashes snow-white. Flexner, with his host's approval began by describing the history of medical education in America, some of the problems involved, and the struggle to create higher standards waged by the Council on Medical Education, the Carnegie Foundation, and Mr. Rockefeller's General Education Board. Specifically, he indicated that Rochester had been proposed as the site for a new medical school of the "university type" where the integration of the medical school with other components of the university could be ideally developed under the aegis of a sound administrator, President Rush Rhees. The new school was to be of the highest possible calibre, starting from scratch, unfettered by any preexisting commitments and destined to be a model for other institutions to emulate. Mr. Eastman asked Flexner to remain for lunch, a good omen. Following luncheon, the discussion was resumed and terminated at 4:00 P.M. because Eastman had to go to his office—or so he said. But, he invited Flexner to dine with him and President Rhees at 6:30. After an excellent dinner, the trio went to the study and Eastman, wasting no time on small talk, came directly to the issue.

> "I am interested in your project, but in these recent years I have given away thirty-one million dollars. What will the new school cost?" "Eight to ten million." "Let us figure on ten. I have spoken to my associate .... He tells me that I can spare two and one-half million." "Where is the rest to come from?" I asked. "From Mr. Rockefeller's Fund." "In that event, it would be our school, not yours; it must be yours." "That is the best I can do now." "There's no hurry. Wait till you sell more Kodaks."[144]

Flexner left only to be summoned back to Rochester by tele-

144. Flexner, *Autobiography*. pp. 182-83.

gram a few days later at which time he was offered three and one-half million dollars, which he again turned down. Flexner returned to New York empty-handed, wondering whether he had gone too far. Eastman let him stew for a few weeks and then sent him a handwritten note inviting him to lunch in his office in Kodak Park.

> "I can see him now as he rose behind his desk, smiling and pointing his finger at me," reminisced Flexner some years later. "I shall make you one more offer and then I never want to see your face again." . . . "I'll give you five million dollars, including the dental clinic valued at one million, if the Board will give five million." "Very well," I said, "that offer I will accept. But," I added, "beware; with one gift, we have finished, but you have just begun." "You are mistaken," he replied; "I, too, have finished." "We shall see."[145]

Flexner recalls that Eastman concluded the interview saying he was the best salesman he had ever seen and he would be glad to give him a job in the Kodak business with the highest salary ever. Eastman's own description of this episode was rather different. In a letter to a friend, he said,

> He [Flexner] is the worst highwayman that ever flitted into and out of Rochester. He put up a job on me and cleaned me out of a thundering lot of my hard-earned savings. I have just heard that he is coming up here June 2nd to speak at the graduating exercises of the allied hospitals. I have been asked to sit on the stage with him, but instead of that I shall probably flee the town for fear he will hypnotize me again.[146]

The morning following his key visit with Mr. Eastman, Flexner was back in his office in New York and he told Doctor Buttrick and Mr. Gates what he had done. "But," said Mr. Gates, "you had no authority." "I know that; but if the Board refuses, I'll make good on our understanding." Fortunately, the General Education Board approved and Flexner was vindicated. On June 12, 1920, Eastman wrote to John D. Rockefeller, Sr.:

> I venture to take this occasion to say that I am proud to have my name associated with yours in a philanthropic enterprise. For many years I have considered you the foremost philanthropist of the age and have admired the wisdom with which your vast wealth is being distributed. In this case it is not only the money contribution that this community appreciates, but the cooperation of your

145. *Ibid.*, p. 183.
146. *Ibid.*, p. 185.

> organization, without the skilled services of which the mere money would be impotent to obtain success.[147]

Flexner's boldness and his courage in getting the medical school at Rochester is in character. He exceeded his authority, was ruthless in getting the money he needed and was, in his own way, a Robin Hood among fund-raisers, using his intellegence, cunning, and quick wits to achieve his goals rather than a bow and arrow or a gun. He had a genius for sizing up the potential for giving of the millionaires on his list, and he was very skillful in manipulating others to comply with his wishes.

Not all of Flexner's mail on the Rochester venture was complimentary. One letter from his former mentor, Henry S. Pritchett, from Santa Barbara, California, dated July 28, 1920, read–

> This is excellent, I am delighted that so promising a venture in medicine is to be started in Rochester. At the same time, I feel a certain regret that the General Education Board should be giving so large a sum for a new medical school in a region already well populated by medical schools likely to survive, when there is such great need for bringing up the situation of medicine in the South.[148]

On February 7, 1921, in a letter to Buttrick of the General Education Board, Pritchett again criticized the Rochester project, saying–

> I had an interesting talk with Rhees at San Francisco the other day; he is a very good man and is going at his problem carefully and thoughtfully. I was a little disturbed that he should take Whipple from his present work of research. There is some question in my mind whether Whipple will contribute as much as Dean of a school in Rochester, as he will as head of the Research Department of an already strong medical school.
>
> I have never quite understood the theory upon which you invested five million dollars in starting a new medical school in Rochester, N.Y. It looks to me like going against all the things for which the General Education Board has stood. I asked Abraham about it and he explained it by saying that you got five millions out of Eastman, but the reply to that is, it seems to me, that Eastman got five millions out of you.[149]

The letters were out of character for Pritchett. As Mayor Fiorello La Guardia of New York once said, "When I make a mistake,

147. G. Eastman to J. D. Rockefeller, Sr., June 12, 1920, Rockefeller Archives.

148. H. S. Pritchett to A. Flexner, July 28, 1920, Rockefeller Archives.

149. H. S. Pritchett to Wallace Buttrick, February 7, 1921, Rockefeller Archives.

it is a beaut!"[150]

On commencement day, June 11, 1920, at Rochester, the two major gifts were announced to the general public amidst great enthusiasm. Rush Rhees now sought advice on the staffing of the medical school, going to Baltimore to see Welch; to New York to William Darrach, Dean of P & S; L. Emmett Holt; and Simon and Abraham Flexner. His advisors were unanimous in recommending that he choose a pathologist to head the school. Welch and Simon Flexner nominated George Hoyt Whipple. Abraham Flexner suggested Alonzo E. Taylor of the University of Pennsylvania, and Winford H. Smith, Director of Johns Hopkins Hospital, placed Milton C. Winternitz of Yale at the head of his list. The latter earned a caveat from his mentor, Welch, who told Rhees he was "brilliant but needed restraint"—perhaps the understatement of that year.

Fortunately for Rochester, Rhees was so impressed by all that he was told about Whipple that he made no overtures to the others and quickly sought to offer him the deanship.

Who was George Hoyt Whipple and why was he so highly recommended for the deanship of a new medical school with a full-time faculty destined to rival Johns Hopkins and to shake up the medical establishment in New York City?

150. Manners, William: *Patience and Fortitude: Fiorello La Guardia.* New York, Harcourt Brace Jovanovich, 1976, p. 219, line 11.

Chapter 15
GEORGE HOYT WHIPPLE (1878-1976)

Discipuli victoria magistri est gloria*

George Hoyt Whipple was a brilliant graduate of the Johns Hopkins University School of Medicine Class of 1905—the class that "graduated with" Osler, who left that year for Oxford to become Regius Professor of Medicine. Whipple received his training as a pathologist at Hopkins and rose to become Welch's first assistant. A superb teacher, topflight and imaginative investigator, and an excellent administrator, he was sought after by a number of medical schools whose offers he rejected until one he could not refuse arrived from California to direct the Hooper Foundation for research medicine at the University of California with the rank of university professor. He remained in San Francisco for seven years and in 1920 became the dean of the medical school. Here he gained administrative experience and organized and initiated important research investigations dealing with hemoglobin regeneration that would ultimately lead to a Nobel prize. The split aspect of medical teaching in a school with basic science being taught on one campus in Berkeley and the clinical subjects in San Francisco was observed by Whipple as extremely undesirable and unacceptable in a first-rate institution.

In October 1920, he received a letter from a stranger, President Rush Rhees of the University of Rochester, telling him that a new medical school was to be organized in Rochester and inviting him to "come east at once to look into the project with a view of heading it." On November 8, 1920, after consulting with President Barrows of the University of California, he wrote President Rhees a pleasant but firm letter in which he expressed his pleasure at being invited but declined on the grounds that he was reluctant to leave his post in San Francisco. Rhees, upset

* Motto of the George Hoyt Whipple Society.

over the refusal, talked again with Abraham Flexner, who had urged him from the very beginning to go to California in person to get his dean, and was advised by both Flexner and George Eastman to quit writing letters and go to California to make a personal presentation to George Whipple. Rhees made an appointment with Whipple in San Francisco in mid-January 1921, and told the Rochester University treasurer, "I don't know when I shall get back. I am not returning until George Whipple says 'yes'!"[151]

Convinced by now of the great importance of the Rochester project and attracted by its promise of ample endowment, no commitments to the past, and a great opportunity to start a new medical school on the Hopkins plan from absolute scratch, George Whipple knew he had to reconsider his earlier decision.

When he met Rhees, he took an instant liking to him and this was reciprocated. The conversations that followed explored many aspects of the Rochester plans. Whipple, having learned from bitter experience, laid down a number of conditions regarding his role and the demands to be made upon him. Among these, based upon unpleasant experiences in California, were freedom from the distractions of community service and outside medical affairs. Other stipulations were "that the medical school be physically part of the university with adequate hospital facilities under its own control; that the buildings and grounds were to be paid for out of income already accumulating from endowment. For himself he stipulated that as dean he would have executive control of the school's affairs and that facilities for his own research would be provided as soon as possible."[152]

All of the conditions were acceptable to Rhees and the Trustees, and on February 25, 1921, the Trustees unanimously appointed George H. Whipple Dean of the University of Rochester School of Medicine and Dentistry and Professor of Pathology, effective July 1, 1921.

WHIPPLE AT ROCHESTER

Rush Rhees, perhaps at the suggestion of Abraham Flexner, offered Whipple the opportunity to go to Europe for several

---

151. Corner, George W.: *George Hoyt Whipple and His Friends: The Life-Story of a Nobel Prize Pathologist.* Philadelphia, J. B. Lippincott Company, 1963, p. 113.
152. *Ibid.*, pp. 115-16.

months of study and observation of trends in medical education in England and on the continent prior to entering upon his duties at Rochester. This generous offer was quickly turned down by Whipple who felt that the challenge of his new position was so great that the sooner he could get to work the better. Arrangements were made for Rochester to assume the expenses for the anemia research in California until the dog colony could be moved to Rochester. Whipple set out in mid-August 1921 from San Francisco for the east coast with a detour to Charleston where Mrs. Whipple and the two children, Hoyt aged four and Barbara aged four months, remained for a visit with their family while Whipple went on to Rochester, arriving September 20, 1921. Here he stayed for a while in Rush Rhees' home, beginning a friendship destined to last for the rest of their lives.

Here again, I must pause to stress the importance of individuals and their personal relationships in advancing medical and social progress. Had Rhees and Whipple failed to become good friends, much of the progress at Rochester would have been delayed and, indeed, might never have occurred. It would have been very easy for the University president to envy the medical school its wealth and its status in academic medicine. A lesser man than Rhees might have sought for the undergraduate school the funds and endowment attracted by the medical school and have played one against the other. Instead, Rhees encouraged Eastman and others to continue to contribute generously to the medical school and at the same time to elevate the standards, equipment, and faculty of the undergraduate school, seeking to raise them to the levels of its school of medicine. Graduate instruction, at first leading only to the master's degree, was slowly and steadily advanced and, in the twenties, the departments, thought to be adequately equipped and staffed, gave instruction leading to the doctorate.

The undergraduate school expanded its sights and sought to keep pace with the school of medicine and the school of music. By 1924, it was clear that the College of Arts and Science had to embark upon a major expansion in order to keep up with the demands of the people and their expectations. George W. Todd, a Rochester businessman with no previous connection with the affairs of the college, spearheaded a campaign to raise $10,000,000 for the College of Men and succeeded in reaching his goal, attracting 13,651 subscribers, among them George Eastman with his usual generosity. An added dividend was Eastman's gift of $1,500,000 to the endowment of the College for Women, evidence of his interest in the education of women as well as men, a far cry from his statement of twenty-six years before that he was not interested in education. Rhees wrote to a trustee,

> I think you can imagine that I have found it difficult to keep my feet on the ground and my breath at a normal rate of respiration since this thing happened. I remarked to Mr. Eastman when he first outlined the plan to me that I assumed he must realize what it meant to an institution to have such confidence reposed in it. He smiled and replied, "I have the confidence." It is our obligation henceforth to prove that the confidence was justified.

Eastman himself, in explaining why he was making large gifts to Rochester, MIT, Hampton, and Tuskegee said:

> A friend of mine who had advance knowledge of this transaction asked me why I selected these four institutions as beneficiaries of this distribution. The answer is easy. In the first place, the progress of the world depends almost entirely upon education. Fortunately, the most permanent institutions of man are educational. They usually endure even when governments fall; hence the selection of educational institutions. The reason that I selected a limited number of institutions was because I wanted to cover certain kinds of education and felt that I could get results with the institutions named quicker and more directly than if the money was spread. Under the best conditions it takes considerable time, sometimes years, to develop the wise expenditure of money in any line, no matter how well prepared one may be. I am now upwards of seventy years old and feel that I would like to see results from this money within the natural term of my remaining years.[153]

Eastman had no known religious affiliation and he never gave to strictly religious work, hence, perhaps his designation of education rather than religion as the phoenix surviving all manner of holocausts. Continuing his comments on giving to the University of Rochester, Eastman said,

> As to Rochester, the town in which I am interested in above all others, we are all set now to develop our university on the broadest lines and make it one of the outstanding universities of the country. By that I do not mean one of the largest, but one of the highest rank in all of the fields which it has entered. The citizens of Ro-

153. Slater, John R.: *Rhees of Rochester*, p. 171.

chester have never shown any inclination to "lie down" on any great civic enterprise or to "let others do it." This I suppose is one of the reasons that has actuated the General Education Board and other friends of the University outside of Rochester to aid in large undertakings for the University here. But for the fine response of our citizens in the recent University campaign, I should certainly not have allotted to the University of Rochester so large a proportion of the properties which I am now distributing.[154]

Clearly, Rhees' low-key campaign of slowly persuading his friend, George Eastman, to support education, was paying enormous dividends. Had he lost his temper in the encounter of twenty-six years before, when Eastman told him he had no interest in education, there is no saying what might have transpired. Rochester was blessed in having Rush Rhees at the right time in its history. He was its man of the hour.

Just as Rhees was the man of destiny for the University, so was George Hoyt Whipple for the medical school. He approached his new assignment with quiet enthusiasm and with very clear and unequivocal commitment to the highest standards. In his selection of faculty, he felt that American medicine had come of age, and he sought for the chairs young men with bright futures whose training had largely been obtained in American schools. The galaxy of stars he assembled is a tribute to his keen sense of horseflesh. He seldom picked a loser. The original faculty consisting of Nathaniel W. Faxon to head the new Strong Memorial Hospital, George W. Corner in anatomy, Walter R. Bloor in biochemistry, Stanhope Bayne-Jones in what was then called bacteriology, William S. McCann in medicine, Karl M. Wilson in obstetrics and gynecology, John J. Morton in surgery, Samuel W. Clausen in pediatrics, and Wallace O. Fenn in physiology reads now like a Who's Who in World Medicine but, at the time, most of these appointees were unknown outside of their own institutions; Fenn was only 31 years of age with Bloor 46,the eldest, the average age at appointment being 37.5 years and a little less than 40 when teaching began in 1925. No wonder that a well-known Austrian zoologist visiting the medical center in the spring of 1925 and chancing to meet three or four of the most youthful-looking professors remarked, "Vat kind of a place iss it? The buildings iss a barn, the professors are all boys!"[155] The "boys"

154. *Ibid.*, p. 172.

155. Corner, *Whipple and His Friends*, p. 154.

grew up and the buildings also grew, as did the institution that had won Eastman's vote of confidence.

Faxon subsequently became the director of the Massachusetts General Hospital and an outstanding leader in hospital administration. Corner achieved fame as an outstanding anatomist and embryologist, heading the Carnegie Institute of Embryology and in addition becoming an important writer and a leading historian of medicine. Stanhope Bayne-Jones left Rochester in 1932 to become professor at Yale Medical School, then its dean, and subsequently head of the Cornell-New York Hospital complex, plus military service as a Brigadier General in World War II. McCann, except for distinguished Navy service in World War II, spent his entire remaining career at Rochester where he built a strong department of medicine and developed many talented young men and women. He was an outstanding clinician and superb teacher capable of making complex matters seem simple, ideally suited for correlating basic science with clinical medicine. He stood for general internal medicine and looked with some skepticism on the trend toward subspecialization with consequent fragmentation of medical care. Bloor was a leading lipid chemist, pioneering in a field destined to attract some of the finest minds in medicine. Wilson established a strong department, and Rochester graduates have been better trained in obstetrics and gynecology than many of the graduates from other schools. Morton, quiet, modest, and extremely competent, developed a well-balanced division of surgery and earned high respect for his wisdom and judgement. Clausen, a humble, diffident man, extremely well trained in chemistry, was the head of pediatrics and had the respect of all who knew him. Fenn, the youngest of the group, has been characterized as the one with the finest mind. Under him, the department of physiology flourished and won world renown in the area of respiratory physiology, muscle and nerve function, and water balance. Whipple had reason to be very proud of his young staff. They more than lived up to their promise.

Whipple's first years at Rochester were devoted largely to building the new complex. Flexner had picked Rochester because it was possible to build a school from scratch without any prior or conflicting commitments. The concept of having the undergraduate school contiguous with the medical school, or nearly so, was revolutionary and had never been attempted before, not even at Flexner's revered Johns Hopkins. With Rhees working steadily at this approach, plans for the River Campus moved ahead. In the meantime, Whipple planned for the construction of Strong Memorial Hospital as an integral part of his medical school. The floor plans called for ease of movement between the hospital and the preclinical departments and their close functional integration. Whipple's New England capacity for thrift and lack of ostentation came to the fore and was greatly appreciated by George Eastman who wanted to see the most efficient use of his gifts. The six-story red brick buildings were very plain and lacked the ornate architectural trimmings then in vogue, leading Eastman to reply to a query on the style of architecture that it was "early penitentiary." The interior of the buildings was sound, the utilities and plumbing first-rate without glamour. So thrifty was the construction that most of the Rockefeller and Eastman gifts were untouched and left for endowment. Strong Memorial Hospital built by the two million dollar gift of Colonel Strong's daughters was paid off in its entirety by a brilliant stroke of financial wizardry or good luck, whichever story one may prefer, when LaRoy B. Thompson, then a young member of the University of Rochester financial team, decided to sell all of their common stocks just before the great stock market crash in 1929.

As opposed to other medical institutions that had overspent their dollars on architectural piles of masonry and then found themselves without the money to run them, Rochester was in the catbird seat of 1929. It hardly felt the crash or the ensuing depression. Its sound financial management made it possible for the medical school and the university to hold its staff and to move forward with their plans when others were folding up or faltering. This outstanding performance of the manager of the University of Rochester finances was not just a flash in the pan. Consistently, the University of Rochester has had superb financial management that has made it the envy of other institutions. Some years ago, one rumor had it that if Yale had Rochester's financial wizardry plus Yale's numerous and affluent alumni, there would be no limit to the growth of its endowment.

When Whipple came to Rochester, it was agreed that he would be spared from the demands of community service and outside medical affairs. Years later he recalled that "I told him (Rhees) that meeting important people at dinners, club meetings and the like took much time and energy and interfered definitely with my work the following day." He was to modify this position of his own volition when he became acquainted with George Eastman. There developed between these two giants a friendly relationship that cemented the bond between Eastman and the medical school. This was a process of education for both men, the Dean learning much from his brilliant business friend and Eastman, in turn, learning to admire Whipple as a human being and a leader in science. It was no wonder that Eastman's bounty, which might well have gone to MIT alone, was largely diverted to Rochester. The cultivation of George Eastman as a personal friend was an enormous service to medicine as well as a constructive contribution to his life. Eastman was a bachelor, living in splendor in his East Avenue mansion, but he was with all of his wealth a lonely man. He enjoyed good company and was especially fond of being surrounded in social gatherings by a bevy of bright, vivacious, and attractive young women of good character and breeding. The wives of the Rochester faculty played a leading role in this drama and faithfully attended Mr. Eastman's luncheons and social affairs. Prominent among the women involved in these activities was Katherine Waring Whipple, wife of the dean, a beautiful and charming participant, as was Nannie Bayne-Jones, wife of the professor of bacteriology. The dean often attended small intimate dinners in Eastman's mansion where he met important men of affairs. He was also a frequent guest at Eastman's Sunday late afternoon or evening musicales. In addition, the Whipples made trips with Eastman to Canada and to his hunting lodge in North Carolina. All in all, a warm friendship developed between the faculty of the medical school, especially George Whipple and Eastman. It was, as all true friendships must be, a mutually satisfactory and rewarding expression of regard and affection among compatible human beings.

I have told the Eastman-Whipple story in some detail because I believe that in it lies a lesson. Private philanthropy differs markedly from government disbursement. The personal contact between donor and recipient may be extremely important for the first and out of place for the latter. Cultivating and communicating with philanthropic individuals is essential if we are to sustain the existence of our private or independent institutions. The story of most of our great voluntary institutions is oftentimes that of a personal relationship between the donor and recipient. This fact has been lost sight of in recent years when it has seemed as if all good things in medicine simply have to come from Washington. Political clout has been substituted for idealism and charismatic leadership in some of our institutions, and they have suffered as a result. I am certain that George Whipple did not seek to curry favor from George Eastman. The events were fortuitous and dramatic in their consequences. The right people met at the right moment and together joined to promote an idea whose time had come.

Although some may disagree with me, I do not feel that the halcyon days of the 1930s are gone forever. Wherever human beings work in a free enterprise system, there will always be those who will amass wealth and wish to distribute it for the betterment of mankind. In an affluent society such as ours, there are many persons capable of contributing to philanthropic ventures that attract their interest. Given a broad enough base of donors, every fundraiser knows that even small gifts count up. Medicine must supply idealistic and charismatic leaders who will earn the confidence of these individuals and attract their philanthropy.

Whipple, allowed five years to complete the construction of his medical center, succeeded in doing this within four years, a truly major accomplishment! By September 1925, the first class of medical students was admitted to the University of Rochester School of Medicine and Dentistry, and the great experiment was truly on its way.

Chapter 16
FLEXNER QUARRELS WITH ROCHESTER

I do profoundly disagree with and regret what you have done, for I think that you are headed towards the second grade instead of making good on the first.

—Abraham Flexner to Rush Rhees
June 6, 1931[156]

Of all the medical schools aided by the General Education Board, the University of Rochester was regarded as almost personal property by Abraham Flexner who, if he did not exactly father the school, almost certainly delivered it into the world. His interest in the school was of a high order and he enjoyed advising the Rochester group on many details of the new venture. Correspondence indicates that Flexner's counsel was frequently sought by Rush Rhees, Whipple and other members of the University of Rochester medical school staff. Few major steps were taken without consulting Flexner. This he enjoyed while denying that he was really trying to influence policy. A favorite phrase of Flexner's when he was skating on thin ice, attempting to dictate policy, was "Please pardon my venturing to comment on this point. You know I do it in the spirit of helpfulness and with no desire to interfere with your final decisions."[157]

Problems with the full-time system for the clinical staff at Rochester began to surface soon after Strong Memorial Hospital was opened on January 4, 1926 and led to an exchange of letters with Flexner.

On April 6, 1927, Flexner wrote to Dean Whipple requesting a statement for confidential use, showing the salaries paid in the

156. Letter from Abraham Flexner to Rush Rhees, June 6, 1931. University of Rochester Archives 1921-1931, Vol. 82.

157. Letter from A. Flexner to Dr. N. W. Faxon, University of Rochester Medical School, April 20, 1925. General Education Board correspondence.

full-time clinical departments. Whipple sent the information and said that he thought the salaries were inadequate and would need to be increased if the clinical staff were to be kept in Rochester. Again, on May 31, 1927, Whipple expressed concern to Flexner over hospital deficits that were eating into endowment and once more expressed anxiety for the clinical full-time staff members who needed salary increases. Further correspondence between Flexner and Whipple stressed financial problems of the school and sought assistance to no avail. On December 12, 1927, Rhees entered the fray indicating his discontent with the financial treatment of the talented clinical staff at Rochester, stressing the need for higher salaries and requesting financial aid from the General Education Board.

In 1928, Flexner retired from the General Education Board and turned his talents to other endeavors, the first being the Rhodes Memorial Lectures at Oxford University. Since he retired at sixty-two, three years before the mandatory limit of sixty-five, newspaper reporters sought in vain to ferret out a rift with the Rockefeller Board. Headlines read, "Dr. Flexner to quit Rockefeller Board: Action Unexplained." "Board denies rift with Flexner." All individuals queried publicly denied there had been any problems leading to the resignation, but the gossip would not be stilled. Finally on May 31, 1928, Flexner sent a letter to his friends confirming the explanation offered by the General Education Board that his resignation was wholly voluntary, that the Board had spent nearly all of the $50,000,000 given by John D. Rockefeller for medical education and was embarking on a change in its work, that he had been offered a post of equal dignity and importance by Mr. John D. Rockefeller, Jr. and had declined. This denial quieted down the press but for those behind the scenes it was not the whole story. Flexner, as we have seen, was in hot water with some of his best friends and had made important enemies. Despite his retirement, we shall see that he continued to pursue his interest in full-time medicine, choosing to treat as heretics any who dared to stray ever so little from the strictest interpretation of this concept, which by now had become Flexner's obsession. With Flexner gone from the General Education Board, Rhees and Whipple would now be dealing with Mr. Trevor Arnett and Dr. Richard M. Pearce of the

Rockefeller Foundation, who fortunately were open-minded about the full-time concept.

On January 3, 1929, Whipple saw Dr. Richard M. Pearce in New York and discussed full time for clinicians, indicating that he was having great difficulty in filling lower ranking positions. Pearce notes,

> Peculiar difficulty exists in the case of Medicine; men from other institutions decline as in the case of several Harvard men because there is no opportunity for occasional consultation and practice even though salary offered at Rochester is greater than that offered at Harvard. Wonders [Whipple] about success of full time in Rochester under the circumstances.[158]

The following day Pearce discussed this matter with Trevor Arnett who:

> stated that some time ago [in 1925], all restrictions and conditions in the gifts of the General Education Board for medical education were removed, and that the questions of conditions of employment of men in the Medical School at Rochester must be settled by the authorities at Rochester according to their best judgement. It was understood, however, that the full-time principle was the objective and that every effort should be made consistent with the welfare of the institution to seek it.[159]

Arnett authorized Pearce to write to Whipple "giving him the information regarding the release of restrictions." My question is why the great secrecy? Why didn't Whipple, a trustee of the Rockefeller Foundation since 1927, know of the 1925 decision to rescind any restrictions on grants? Pearce's reply did not satisfy Whipple, who answered,

> In reply to your letter of January 7th about the original letter covering the Deed of Gift I may say that that letter is so vague as to give no assistance whatever. It states that the money is to be used for establishing a "school of medicine, surgery and dentistry of the highest order." There is no question but what we are interested in attaining this end but details about clinical teachers obviously are not covered.[160]

Rhees and E. D. Ball, treasurer of the University of Rochester, met with Arnett and Pearce on January 28, 1929 "for the purpose of inquiring regarding the application of the principle of full-time in the Medical School." Once again, Rhees was advised that

158. R. M. Pearce notes, January 31, 1929.

159. Pearce to Arnett, GEB, January 4, 1929.

160. Letter, January 10, 1929, G. H. Whipple to R. M. Pearce. Rockefeller Archives.

he was free to make his own decision.

Rhees had the ball in his hands, but he exhibited the same hesitancy that Welch had when Flexner was hounding him for a decision on full time at Hopkins. This time, the problem lay in an opposite direction. Strict full time was not working, and the clinical staff was agitating for liberalization of the terms. Rhees' problem was that he felt he had a moral obligation to comply with the unwritten conditions imposed by Flexner even though Flexner was no longer with the General Education Board. Rhees' nature was such that he could not bring himself to renege without thorough consultation and, hopefully, agreement on all sides. The problem of full time in the clinical chairs would not fade away; it had to be faced. On March 10, 1930, Whipple sent Flexner a list of rather sticky questions whose format suggests the sort of interrogation medical students would undergo at Whipple's teaching conferences as he looked over his half-glasses. This could be a terrifying ordeal, and I think Flexner must also have been shaken up. The letter starts innocently enough.

March 10, 1930

1. A University professor of economics is asked to give an authoritative review of his field before a city club—a fee is charged.
2. A University professor of chemistry is asked to make a difficult and accurate analysis of material for a city corporation—a fee is charged.
3. A University professor of engineering is asked to give expert consultation relating to bridge construction—a fee is charged.
4. A University professor of music takes part in a musical production, chamber music—a fee is charged.
5. A medical school professor of bacteriology is asked, as a duty, to give expert testimony relating to blood typing in a murder case—a fee is charged.
6. A medical school professor of pathology is asked to give a consultation on surgical material, coming from the family of a trustee—a fee is charged.
7. A professor of pharmacology is asked to give expert opinion in a poisoning case—a fee is charged.
8. A hospital director in a medical school is asked to give consultation relating to hospital construction—a fee is charged.
9. A professor of medicine or surgery in a medical school is asked to see a prominent citizen in consultation—he states that he is occupied all that day with teaching—he is asked as a favor to see the patient that evening at patient's home; a fee is charged.

All these people are full time University appointments. What dis-

> posal should be made of these fees?[161]

Flexner's reply was evasive with no attempt to answer Whipple's specific questions.

The culmination of these discussions was in a long meeting of the Advisory Board of the University of Rochester School of Medicine and Dentistry held on May 26, 1930, chaired by President Rush Rhees and, fortunately for us, meticulously transcribed and recorded. This document runs to twenty-six typed pages and is a storehouse of valued judgements and opinions on full time expressed with eloquence and clarity by this group of talented physicians. Those who participated in the meeting were, in addition to Rhees; Dean Whipple; Karl Wilson, Chairman of Obstetrics and Gynecology; John Murlin, Chairman of Vital Economics; Stanhope Bayne-Jones, Chairman of Bacteriology; Samuel Clausen, Chairman of Pediatrics; John Morton, Chairman of Surgery; Walter Bloor, Chairman of Biochemistry; William S. McCann, Chairman of Medicine; Wallace O. Fenn, Chairman of Physiology; George W. Corner, Chairman of Anatomy; and Nathaniel Faxon, Director of Strong Memorial Hospital. They represented an unusual team of dedicated, outstanding medical educators, scientists, administrators, and clinicians, known far and wide for their integrity, fairness, and idealism. We may never again be privileged to join so distinguished a gathering, privy to their frank and open discussion of the full-time controversy, as current as the morning's newspaper despite the passage of fifty years.

President Rhees opened the discussion with a brief review of the circumstances surrounding the establishment of the medical school at Rochester and paid tribute to Abraham Flexner for his key role.

> It was taken for granted all through negotiations that the policy to be adopted in this school would be that of so-called strict full time. There never was a written condition attached to the appropriation of the General Education Board nor, as far as I can recall—I haven't gone through the correspondence—was anything in the nature of an implied condition incorporated in the correspondence. On the other hand, there was no question in our minds here that it was expected that the policy adopted by this school would be the policy favored by the General Education Board, Johns Hopkins,

161. Rockefeller Archives: Whipple to Flexner, March 10, 1930.

> Washington University and Yale. Therefore, we organized this school on the basis of strict full time clinical men.

Rhees continued, saying he felt there was a moral obligation to comply with full time under the conditions of the Rockefeller gift but, since problems had arisen, he welcomed open and frank expression of opinion on this matter, "without the slightest hesitancy as to the desirable course to be pursued in the interest of the furtherance of scientific medicine."[162]

The discussion was initiated by Doctor McCann, the brilliant young internist heading the department of medicine, an effective faculty leader and spokesman who had been Harvey Cushing's intern at the Brigham and in charge of metabolic diseases at Johns Hopkins.

> I might introduce what I have to say with the remark that I came here with the full understanding of the desire of the institution to adhere to the full time plan as it was then in operation at Hopkins—with which I was familiar because I had been there.
>
> I am willing to continue in the future to give that plan a trial. I don't think we have ever had it since we began operation. We have had it in name but not in fact because those of us in the clinic have gradually been swept into a considerable amount of private practice which I didn't contemplate in the beginning, and which I never saw done by the full time men at Hopkins. During the year prior to my appointment, Dr. Longcope was there as Professor, in his first year, and he had a minimal amount of private work. Dr. Robinson had had none at all. Those men as full time professors had no concern except the administration of their department, conduct of teaching and rounds on their own wards.
>
> At the time I came up here, I had visualized full time professorship as one which might call for a certain amount of demand on a man's time but certainly not as much of it as it has come to be in the last year or two. I think we can't say that we have ever lived up to what I conceive the idea of the Flexner plan to be.[163]

The discussion continued:

> Dr. McCann: It seems to me that the question is pretty clear cut; I think here there are two main possible solutions: First, that we might decide that it was in the best interests of the institution to start out afresh, to try to live up to the Flexner agreement. Personally I don't think it is practical to do so; I don't think it can be carried out without a great deal of grief to all parties concerned.

---

162. Minutes of the Advisory Board of the University of Rochester School of Medicine, May 26, 1930. University of Rochester Archives, pp. 1-3.
163. *Ibid.*, p. 3.

> Dr. Rhees: You mean if the full time men were simply to decline to take any private cases?
>
> Dr. McCann: I think that would undoubtedly be an embarrassment to them and a source of great annoyance to the institution.
>
> Dr. Rhees: Reviewing it objectively as far as you can, do you think that policy if practical would be advantageous to the institution?
>
> Dr. McCann: I think it would be very distinctly disadvantageous. I think that undoubtedly the whole time professor would have more time to devote to scientific study and his teaching than now. I think practically all of us have continued to function as nearly as possible as we would, by the sacrifice of the normal amount of leisure time. I don't know whether you men have any idea how many times for instance my Sundays, holidays, evenings are taken up by telephone consultations, requests to come out, received during the daytime when I have replied that it was impossible to go because of University duties and countered by the request to come at night or on Sunday or on a holiday.
>
> The other alternative I think is the adoption of the Harvard plan, which means I think that there they maintain the spirit of whole time in the sense that they want their professors to be in the school at all times, to engage in no outside practice, carry on about as we do with regard to private patients. I think except for the method of compensation for work, we are practically on the Harvard plan now; the only difference is what becomes of the fee.[164]

There followed questions by Rhees and answers from McCann on medical staff performance at Harvard, Hopkins, and the Hospital of The Rockefeller Institute under their systems of employment. McCann felt that the staff of the Rockefeller Hospital was cloistered and limited in its experience by the restriction of admissions to only a few patients representing examples of diseases selected for study, a system not contributing to broad clinical knowledge or experience.

Wilson, the professor and chairman of obstetrics and gynecology, a man of great wisdom and wide experience, who had been on the Hopkins staff and in private practice in Baltimore for ten years, said:

> There are a good many angles to this question. If it were possible to have absolutely no private patients at all, I suppose from the academic standpoint it would be ideal, that is from the standpoint of time. On the other hand I don't think it is possible for this reason: We are dependent to a very considerable extent on the good will of a certain group of doctors whose practice represents a cross

164. *Ibid.*, pp. 6-7.

section of the communities in which they live. Probably the bulk will be frank clinic patients. On the other hand, there will be some private patients. If a man is pleased with the clinic, he will want to send those patients too. I see no way of declining unless we drop all the interest of the doctors all around. We admit we have got to have a certain number of private patients. It seems to me that after all the spirit of this thing is the important thing. We are not rigid full time, we are the Harvard plan—as to time but not compensation. If we do have to see a certain number of private patients now, as long as that can be done without interfering with the University duties and investigation one is trying to carry on, I don't see that the detail of where the money goes is vital one way or the other, and it might well go to the doctor who sees the patient rather than interfere with his work in any way.165

Morton, the quiet man of the staff, noted for his courage and integrity, then spoke up. He was a Hopkins graduate, had interned under Cushing, and was associate professor of surgery at Yale before being called to Rochester.

Full time as applied to clinical medicine is just a good name; that is, it is supposed to free the clinical chief and the men concerned from the duties of private practice outside, to make available to them leisure for contemplation, for research, for reading. It doesn't do it. There is no such thing as full time except in the amount of time you put in, because we all have to see private patients. This is not true of this institution alone; it is true of Yale, because I was there and worked under the full time system. At Yale I saw a great many patients, so many that I was unable to do anything in an investigative way. In fact from the point of view of a younger man down at Yale, the full time system was a failure, because just as soon as you developed your clinical ability to any extent, it was called on for use in treating private patients, and the better you became, the more you had to handle. There was no way out of it, so that any investigation or reading that you might wish to do would have to be done in supposed off hours; your leisure time was cut into; you had no home life, you had to write papers or study, and the time which was nominally yours in the terms of the contract was taken up with seeing private patients. The same thing is true here. I am getting more and more, and the other men in my department as they become known in the city are getting more and more demands on their time for handling private patients. I think from the point of view of younger men on the staff, they don't have the full time positions—they have the pay of it, that is all.

There is another point of view. Not every man in the department can be on the same standing. There is not sufficient money in the

165. *Ibid.*, pp. 9-10.

> world to budget a clinical department on a full time system. These men who head the specialties will be on this rating. Some will be allowed to see pay patients, others not, and that very fact creates a good deal of hard feeling one way or another in the department. A younger man will say "Why is it that I am not allowed to see private patients when so and so is, who apparently does the same amount of work as I do?" There isn't any answer; they are not on the same rating. They have that situation at Yale

Later Morton said:

> There are a good many other points I haven't touched on at all, but just from my own point of view, there is no such thing as full time; I don't think there is any such thing.166
>
> Dr. Rhees: In other words, you and McCann and Wilson agree on that.

Dr. Nathaniel W. Faxon, the Director of Strong Memorial Hospital, then spoke up for the first time. He was a native of Massachusetts and a graduate of Harvard Medical School, who had been a family doctor in Stoughton, Massachusetts, from 1906 to 1917, before he became assistant director of the Massachusetts General Hospital to which he would return in 1935 as its director. A highly respected and seasoned administrator, he brought to the conference knowledge of the importance of having the new institution relate effectively and well with the community and its laymen as well as its physicians.

> Dr. Faxon: It was my understanding when the hospital opened that we were committed to a fair trial of the so-called full time system, in which the men engaged in teaching and occupying higher positions were to be protected from private practice as much as possible. Immediately after the hospital opened, we began to get demands from people who wanted to be seen by those men. We recognized that there would be a certain amount of that demand when we put in twenty-six private rooms. The demand has increased . . . . What I wanted to point out is that if we expect to receive the good will of this community, we must accede to some of their requests—usually that they should be able to see the very best clinical men we have here. If we refuse, we are going to get into difficulties with the community; we will not have their good will; I think that is something we want to build up very carefully. Although we have started out with a very liberal endowment, nevertheless for increase of that endowment we must depend on that community good will.

Faxon then emphasized a very important condition.

---

166. *Ibid.*, 11-13.

> Another point I feel very strongly upon is the effect upon the clinician of seeing private patients. That has been brought out by men who have stated it much more forcibly than I; all I can say is that I agree heartily with their feeling that it does have an effect upon the man's attitude towards his patients, and on his teaching. I think the discipline impressed by private patients upon clinicians is advantageous and I believe it is a wise thing to foster to a certain extent.... In regard to fee, I think that it is important it should go to the man who does the work. I think it makes better feeling all around. A man dislikes to work for nothing. A doctor is altruistic to a certain extent, but nevertheless I think it would make for much better and much more contented feeling if in seeing a private patient, they would receive the fee. Not only that but the patients themselves object. One man who came out here complained bitterly to me because he was unable to pay any fee to the doctors who took care of him. I explained it, but he felt just the same, and others have expressed the same feeling. So I believe from the standpoint of the relation of hospital to community, and of the doctors here, it would be a great advantage to give up our rigid full time system and take on the Harvard plan.[167]

Whipple then said:

> I have tried very hard to find out exactly how Mr. Flexner would solve some of our problems, because after all theories are easy but when you come to applying a theory to the solution of a definitely distinct problem, your difficulties begin. Having thought about this a good deal, I proposed a number of questions to Mr. Flexner which I believe apply not only to this institution.

Whipple then presented the list of questions to Flexner previously mentioned and indicated his unhappiness because Mr. Flexner failed to answer them and merely stated that he thought all departments of the University should be on a strict full-time basis. Whipple continued:

> He didn't answer the question as to where the money was coming from to finance departments in the University. As I see it today, various and sundry departments in universities are choosing not of necessity but because they wish their teachers to do part time. Mr. Filene in Boston, who has written a very illuminating discussion of this whole thing, says it is highly desirable for professors in all departments of all universities to be encouraged to do part time work. So why should the other departments of the university be encouraged to do this and the professors of clinical practice not? That is the question I have not yet been able to solve.[168]

---

167. *Ibid.*, pp. 15-18.
168. *Ibid.*, pp. 19-20.

At the conclusion of the conference, President Rhees expressed satisfaction with the discussion saying,

> I think I have got to conclude as Dr. McCann indicates, that having started out on the hypothesis of clinical full time, we never have lived up to it, and therefore either should become practically similar to the Rockefeller Hospital or face the facts. There remains to us the necessity for considering how certain things would be ordered.

Rhees then stated that at Hopkins where two of the clinical professors, Barker and Kelly, had been judged to be exploiters of their positions, a drastic cure had been imposed, i.e. the full-time system. Whipple had said earlier in the conference that if Barker and Kelly "had played the game like Professor Osler there would never have been any full-time problem." Rhees continued saying, "I talked with Mr. Eastman just before he went away because I wanted to learn whether in his mind his contribution toward this school was definitely tied to the maintenance of a specific policy of theoretic full time. What he said to me was, 'Why, I understood that that was what was in mind when the thing was undertaken but it never stood in my mind as a condition of the gifts that I made nor does it stand in my mind in that light today.' "

Rhees continued, "I have tried by all the wiles and devices of which I am capable to learn from the Rockefeller people whether or not they are seriously concerned with the maintenance of a specific type of full time. I know because of something that Mr. John D. Rockefeller once said to me that they are extremely sensitive with reference to any justification of a charge against them that they will dictate to the institutions they help; they only implicate 'We put that money into your hands, it is your responsibility, go ahead and do what you think right!' If that means that they do not feel keenly about any particular form of academic medicine as Abraham Flexner does for instance, that is one thing; if it means that they are not going to put their fingers in and get scorched with it, that it is up to us to take this money and work out the problem that is another thing."[169] Whipple added that he had the impression "that Mr. Gates and Mr. Flexner were the ones who cling to the old-fashioned methods and the other members of the Board were more inclined to believe that the local representatives whose judgement they trusted were

169. *Ibid.*, p. 21.

perhaps better able to work out the details than by definite pronouncements from a central office."[170]

This historic meeting must have been a gruelling experience for each of the participants with a good deal of soul searching and plain speaking. From the transcript and conversations with some of the participants, certain broad concepts emerge. It is amazing how poorly informed these men were about the rebellion and resistance to full time in the very centers held by Flexner as prize examples of how well the system was working. It had failed and still this information was not common knowledge. Each institution, including Rochester, had to go through its own period of trial and error before the truth would emerge. Was Flexner's obsession with full time at the bottom of it all? Given his capacity to do anything to achieve his goals, was he misinforming his Board and the heads of the various medical schools to gain his point? Something of this sort was undoubtedly responsible for the lack of information in the medical school faculties, but I believe there was something more.

Physicians of that era were trained and bred to feel that financial matters were below the dignity of a true physician. This was the era when almost no one spoke of fees and bills were seldom sent to patients. Most medical expenses were paid out of pocket, and there were virtually no third party payments. Collection agencies were anathema, and advertising of fees was only for quacks. I think physicians of the calibre of the staff at Rochester found it extremely awkward to discuss money among themselves and among their colleagues in other institutions. There was a conspiracy of silence on these matters that made it possible for the right hand not to know what the left was doing. Change would come slowly as modern concepts and views of the financial aspects of medicine would be more openly discussed and debated.

The result of the Rochester faculty meeting was slow in making itself manifest. Rhees, by nature an extremely cautious man, asked the faculty to present their report in writing and to take their time in doing it. The first draft, sent to Rhees on July 9, 1930, was characterized by him in a letter to Whipple on August 10, 1930, as—

> a very clear and rather bald abandonment of our policy hitherto,

170. *Ibid.*, p. 22.

> insufficiently qualified by care to preserve some form of strictly academic medicine. I know that such is not the intention; but we shall have to find some clearer formula before we can submit this as our proposal to the General Education Board.

Whipple's reply was almost instantaneous in a letter to Rhees dated August 13, 1930, in which he expressed complete agreement with Rhees' criticism and would return the memorandum to the faculty for revision.[171]

The final version of the memorandum, revised to meet with the approval of Whipple and Rhees, was dated September 4, 1930, and entitled: "To the President of the University of Rochester. Recommendations for modification of the 'Whole-Time Plan' in the School of Medicine and Dentistry." It began—

> Since the opening of the School of Medicine and Dentistry, an attempt has been made to "adhere to the provisions of the Flexner 'Whole-Time Plan.' " While the members of the staff have been guided in their personal activities by the regulations of this system, the requirements of the institution have prevented a complete application of the plan. Experience during the past five and a half years has indicated that a strict adherence to the plan would be disadvantageous to the Medical School and Hospital and that the existing partial application of the plan places unjustifiable hardships upon the members of the staff. The situation has been the subject of numerous discussions. A summary of these discussions and recommendations for changes in the plan, to improve the arrangements here, will be presented in this memorandum.[172]

The memorandum was a sensible and fair statement of the problems of full time in the clinical chairs presenting the views of a group of dedicated scholarly teachers of medicine no one of whom could by any stretch of the imagination, even Flexner's, be accused of greed, avarice or venality. As a student of these men, I am proud of the stand they took and regret that their memorandum was held secret for many years and not made available to other institutions until the battles were pretty well over. My professor of medicine, Doctor McCann, often discussed this problem with me and pointed out that liberal endowments had come to his department largely because of the fact that he took care of sick people, liked them, and they in turn wanted to help him to turn out more doctors like him.

171. Rhees to Whipple to Rhees, August 1930, University of Rochester Archives.

172. Memo, September 4, 1930, on "Whole-Time Plan," University of Rochester Archives.

McCann and the Rochester group had to expose themselves to criticism and cruel attacks in the cause of what they knew was the truth, but they were more than equal to the task. Flexner, as anyone might have expected, took after the faculty, at first in a short note to Rhees, on January 2, 1931.

> I hear rumors which, I hope, are unfounded towards some inclination to weaken your full-time clinical organization. Columbia took the same backward step for twelve months, after which it changed back. If your clinicians are not busy enough on full time, it must be for the lack of ideas. I feel sure that, as long as you are at the helm, there will be no backsliding. While legally possible, such action would be questionable from a moral and absolutely unwise from an educational standpoint. Surely nothing that has happened in the brief period since the School started would justify such a disappointment to those who played a part in securing its establishment.[173]

This outburst led to a letter from Rhees to Arnett, January 16, 1931, requesting his advice as to how to deal with Flexner. Arnett in his reply of January 20, 1931, said,

> I wish I could be of help to you in answering the questions you ask. But it is one which must, in my opinion, be settled by the University of Rochester authorities as they alone are familiar with all the circumstances. The course they decide upon will no doubt be that which in their judgement will best promote the objectives and welfare of the Medical School on sound lines.[174]

Why didn't the Board officials simply and in plain language advise the aging Rush Rhees to ignore Flexner, long since retired and in hot water in a number of other institutions over the same problems? On February 24, 1931, Rhees sent to Arnett a copy of a resolution adopted by the trustees of the University of Rochester on January 31, 1931, accepting the recommendation of the medical school faculty to go off strict full time and to permit limited private practice by its key staff. In an accompanying letter, Rhees stressed that academic full time was not being abandoned; it was being modified "in the interest of what we believe in Rochester will enable us more satisfactorily to pursue that ideal." On the same date, Rhees wrote to Flexner saying,

> It is a source of distress to me that we cannot see this question

173. Flexner to Rhees, January 2, 1931, University of Rochester Archives.
174. Arnett to Rhees, January 16, 1931, Rockefeller Archives.
175. University of Rochester Archives. Rhees to Arnett, January 31, 1931 and February 24, 1931.

> in exactly the same light that you do, but I assure you, with all seriousness, that in the action which we have taken in response to the unanimous recommendation of our clinical chiefs, and after long and most thoughtful study, we have surrendered nothing of our determination to maintain "a medical school of the highest order" and to protect our clinical men from the inroads of private practice upon the full discharge of their obligation for teaching and investigation . . . .
>
> I am imposing upon your time with all this written material simply because we here all recognize, with grateful appreciation, the very great service which you rendered in making possible the institution of our school for medicine and dentistry, and because of our determination, to the best of our ability, in the light of conditions actually existing in our environment and to the limit of our resources available for medical education, to continue to maintain a school of medicine of the highest order.[176]

This letter arrived while Flexner was off on a long absence in Europe and was not answered until June 6, 1931, when this explosive missile was sent to Rhees in Rochester.

> Dear Dr. Rhees:
>
> Returning to this country, I find your letter of February 24 and your note of March 30, in which you ask Mrs. Bailey to hold it for me. I have read with great care your letter to me and your letter to Mr. Arnett. We–you and I–have been so candid with one another that there is nothing that I can do except to make a perfectly frank comment on the change which you have made.
>
> There is, in my opinion, no doubt whatsoever–and in the single week in which I have been in this country I have heard the same opinion expressed by others, whose judgment you greatly value–that your Medical School has admitted the "thin edge of the wedge," as Dr. Buttrick used to say, and that the School cannot any longer continue to be classed with the full-time institutions. It is, I believe, no exaggeration to say that, if anyone could have foreseen such a change of policy in five years, there would have been no medical school at Rochester today.
>
> My own diagnosis of your situation is a very different one. If your medical and surgical staffs were made up of men bristling with ideas, some other solution for your problem would have been found and, in my judgment, could have been found. Full time itself is inadequate for a professor of medicine who wishes to keep up with the literature of his subject, to teach students, to manage a department, and to carry on research. If he has no considerable number of ideas, the first thing that goes is research, the second thing read-

176. University of Rochester Archives. Flexner to Rhees, June 6, 1931. Rhees to Flexner, February 24, 1931.

ing, and, as these go, the full-time clinical organization is weakened or dropped.

Five years are far too short a period within which to try an educational experiment. If the men in charge found themselves unable to make a success of it upon the basis upon which they entered, they ought to have stepped aside and allowed the University to put in their places stronger men. It was, I believe, a serious error to change the organization rather than the men. Financial difficulties inevitably arose in your school, as they have arisen elsewhere. They should, I think, have been faced in a far more determined and stoical manner. The University is undoubtedly acting within its legal rights, but that is the most that can be said for the change that has been made.

Please do not feel that either as respects you or Dr. Whipple or the clinical men I have any personal feeling whatsoever. I do profoundly disagree with and regret what you have done, for I think that you are headed towards the second grade instead of making good on the first.

With all good wishes and very high regard,

Sincerely yours,
Abraham Flexner

Dr. Rush Rhees
The University of Rochester
Rochester, New York[177]

Fortunately, Flexner's prediction was Cassandrian and those who knew about it smiled and knew it would be false. The University of Rochester's School of Medicine quickly rose to fame, Whipple winning the Nobel prize in 1934, others of the faculty rising to international fame, its graduates among the best in the nation. Flexner was not only mistaken, he was deluded in pursuing an obsession which was totally impractical. Flexner's downfall was that he was inflexible. Until the end of his long life, he continued to defend and espouse the cause of strict full time with undiminished vigor. Alan Gregg of the Rockefeller Foundation recorded in a personal diary kept secret for some years the following incident involving Flexner and the full-time concept.

October 10, 1950, I have just had a talk with Abraham Flexner, who asked me to come to see him in his office at 522 Fifth Avenue. He began by asking me whether I had heard that President Conant had told the medical faculty [at Harvard] that they could carry on with their own funds from now on. I said I had not. He said he was greatly troubled at the present stage (or condition) of medicine,

177. University of Rochester Archives. Flexner to Rhees, June 6, 1931.

> and asked how I felt about it. I said I was greatly troubled. He asked, "What does it need—what is the greatest need of medical education in the world or at least in the U.S. today?" I replied, "Adequate support for full-time clinical instruction in a few of the best medical schools."[178]

This answer was almost identical with that given nearly forty years before by Franklin Paine Mall to the same question posed by the same questioner! Flexner continued:

> He said, "I am going to do something about it. I am going to try and raise thirty to forty million dollars for it. These trifling grants-in-aid that you have been doing in the Rockefeller Foundation aren't big enough. Will you leave the Foundation and come in with me if I can get the money?"
>
> I said I would.
>
> He said he would let me know and that I was to tell no one but my wife.
>
> I find my handwriting jiggly right now—perhaps it is from excitement.[179]

Gregg continues, recording a number of reasons for his decision to join Flexner in this effort: "I can do more of permanent value for medicine [by this plan] than any other."[180]

Again, we see Flexner the supersalesman, still pursuing the will-o'-the-wisp of strict full time rejected as it was wherever it had been tried, declared a failure by some of the best minds in American medicine, and responsible for untold anguish and conflict in our leading medical schools. How could Alan Gregg, privy to all of this information through his activities on the Rockefeller Boards, still buy the concept? Or was he thinking, as he had inferred in other writings, of a modification of full time on the lines of the Harvard plan? Did he think he could persuade Flexner, supersalesman, to accept a compromise on full time? Would Flexner, now eighty-four years old, be willing to accept a compromise that he had fought, tooth and nail, when he was much younger? We shall never know the answer, because nothing came of the plan, presumably because of Flexner's inability to raise the enormous sums of money he had mentioned to Gregg.

---

178. Penfield, W.: *The Difficult Art of Giving: The Epic of Alan Gregg.* Boston, Little, Brown & Co., 1967. p. 297.
179. *Ibid.*, p. 297.
180. *Ibid.*, p. 298.

Chapter 17
NEW YORK CITY MEDICAL SCHOOLS

If we could plant a first-rate medical school in Rochester, perhaps New York City would wake up.

—Abraham Flexner, 1920[181]

In 1904, a new dean of The Columbia University College of Physicians and Surgeons was appointed who had many innovative concepts and the energy and drive to put them into effect. He inherited a faculty of distinguished practicing clinicians, an exceptional physical plant for those days and too many medical students, there now being 800 students or more enrolled in the school. The dean was Samuel Waldron Lambert, an 1885 graduate of P & S, described by Dr. Albert R. Lamb with reverence and affection as a character out of Dickens.

> Dickens could well have used such a character, and Sam Lambert would have read the description of himself with his contagious chuckle. He staunchly commended the moderate use of alcohol in old age and did not hesitate to speak out strongly and publicly against prohibition. He was a lover of books and a devoted fisherman. His collection of Izaak Walton's writings revealed his enthusiasm for fine writing and for a fine sport. He also made a unique contribution to medical literature with his translations of the Latin writings of Andreas Vesalius, the sixteenth century Flemish anatomist. Many of us also remember another facet of his talent with language. "He barked, but never bit. He knew with Robert Louis Stevenson that it is the natural act of a sturdy man to inveigh. This he could do in full-bodied words"[182]

Another colleague, Dr. Edward L. Keyes, had this to say:

> The most characteristic yarn about him tells how a patient of another doctor in the Presbyterian Hospital begged that Doctor Lambert come to her room and, when he came, said: "Doctor, I had to see you. For days I have listened to you swear so beautifully

181. Flexner, Abraham: *Autobiography*. New York, Simon and Schuster, 1960, p. 181.
182. Lamb, A. R.: *Presbyterian Hospital and Columbia-Presbyterian Medical Center: 1868-1943*. New York, Columbia Univ. Press, 1955, p. 151.

at the patient in the next room that I just had to have you in to swear at me a little. I do so need to be cheered up."[183]

With appointment in 1904 as Dean, Lambert moved quickly to improve the teaching program. The number of students was gradually reduced to a manageable level. He instituted recitation classes in every subject, seeking to avoid total dependence on didactic lectures that lacked the give-and-take so essential to medical education. He introduced the system of clinical clerks and surgical dressers and brought his students to the wards of some New York hospitals at a time when most hospital authorities opposed the practice.

> His other accomplishments were many. In 1904, in his Department of Applied Therapeutics, at his own expense he started the first real system of medical histories in Vanderbilt Clinic. Also at the Clinic, he installed one of the first visiting nurses for tuberculosis and one of the first social workers in New York. For some time, he himself paid their salaries. He established in Vanderbilt Clinic the first clinical pathological laboratory which his colleagues at the time thought an interesting but impractical innovation. He found funds for this too.

In Doctor Lamb's opinion,

> Sam Lambert had become dean in 1904, and his accomplishments at P & S did nothing less than revolutionize medical education . . .[184]

In 1976, Dr. Samuel W. Lambert, Jr., in reviewing his father's fine record concluded by saying, "And all this was achieved by one Dean, who also maintained a very extensive medical practice, and by one secretary, Miss Wheeler, a most remarkable woman."[185]

Dean Lambert, eager to bring medical students to the wards and to the bedside of patients and realizing that a strong affiliation with a great hospital was essential to the future development of P & S, looked about for a solution. The obvious one lay across the street from P & S, the Roosevelt Hospital, and with President Nicholas Murray Butler of Columbia University, Dean Lambert initiated negotiations to achieve this end.

> The Dean first presented to the trustees on January 25, 1908, a resolution that the question of amalgamation of the medical school and the hospital be given favorable consideration, and on February

183. Keyes, Edward L. : *For Sam Lambert.* Proceedings of the Charaka Club, 15 April 1942, p. 135.

184. Lamb, *Presbyterian Hospital,* pp. 150-51.

185. Lambert, S. W., Jr.: *P & S Quarterly,* Winter, 1976, p. 11.

> 23, 1909, a joint resolution favoring cooperation between the two bodies was passed. On February 8, 1910, Mr. Edward S. Harkness, who had inherited a large fortune from his father, Stephen Harkness, offered to further the project by proposing to build on the site of old Ward V. a modern surgical pavilion with surgical and research laboratories complete, and to endow it. The conditions were amalgamation of the Roosevelt Hospital with P & S, the admitting of two to four clinical clerks to each ward for instruction and integration of the attending staff with the University faculty. These conditions were found unacceptable and the offer was rejected by six votes to four. A committee was appointed, however, to confer with Mr. Harkness to discuss it further. It was understood that many of the medical staff approved the project, particularly Dr. Joseph A. Blake, then consulting surgeon (and a close friend of Harkness), and Dr. George E. Brewer, while its chief opponent was President McLane. He took the stand that to use "the sick poor" for teaching purposes would be in contravention of the terms and spirit of James Roosevelt's will.[186]

Dr. Samuel Lambert, Jr. has another explanation for McLane's intransigence.

> The reason for Doctor McLane's antagonism to anything that Doctor Lambert wished to accomplish is based on the following incident. Dr. Edward Lambert and Doctor McLane lived in adjoining houses on 37th Street and were good friends. In Doctor McLane's backyard was a large tree with a branch which hung over the separating fence and which in a strong wind thumped against Doctor Lambert's library window. Doctor McLane's yard man suggested that he cut the offending branch off to which Doctor Lambert readily agreed. When Doctor McLane discovered this he was furious, the friendship ended and thereafter Doctor McLane was "agin" anything his successor as Dean wished to do.

> The committee appointed to negotiate with Harkness did not report and on November 29, 1910, Dean Lambert presented a lengthy resolution proposing amalgamation on much the same conditions as previously suggested by Harkness and requesting definitive action by the trustees. The resolution was defeated by a vote of six to five. Harkness resigned from the Roosevelt Board at the next meeting, December 27, 1910. In 1912, Doctor McLane died. In 1914, P & S students were admitted to the Roosevelt wards for bedside teaching as clinical clerks.[187]

By this time it was too late. Roosevelt Hospital had lost its

186. Cutler, C. W., Jr., et al.: *Roosevelt Hospital: 1871-1957.* New York, Roosevelt Hospital, 1957, pp. 52-54.
187. Lambert, *P & S Quarterly*.

prospective benefactor to another institution. Again we see great decisions and judgements leaning very heavily on personal reaction, oftentimes emotional. Had McLane agreed to accept the generous Harkness offer and risen above his emotions, there would have been a Columbia-Roosevelt Medical Center.[188]

On December 13, 1910, Edward S. Harkness became a trustee of the Presbyterian Hospital and within a week he submitted to the Presbyterian Board precisely the same offer he had made to Roosevelt Hospital. His generous offer was gratefully accepted by the Presbyterian Board of Managers and on April 25, 1911, the actual terms of affiliation with P & S was spelled out in a memorandum that was quickly approved by the governing boards of both institutions.[189] The highlights of this agreement were that the Hospital and the University maintain their independent corporate existence and control. The income of the Harkness Endowment Fund was to be paid monthly to the University to be applied by it exclusively to carrying on the scientific and educational work connected with the Hospital. The Hospital was to erect upon the East River site a new general hospital, including a surgical pavilion and having a total capacity of not less than 300 beds and all the usual accessories of a well-equipped general hospital, including a suitable outpatient department. The Hospital was to admit to its wards students of the College of Physicians and Surgeons to the extent and in the manner permitted by the most approved practice. The University was to make nominations to all positions on the Hospital staff. To make this privilege effective, the Hospital would make its appointments to such positions from persons nominated to it by the University except as otherwise provided. Persons occupying for the time being the ranking or foremost professorships in medicine and surgery in the College of P & S would always be nominated to appropriate positions on the staff of the Hospital and that so long as they held such offices in the Hospital they would have no official connection with any other hospital. The physicians and surgeons of various ranks and their assistants would have as full privileges as reasonably possible, consistent always with the welfare of patients, of instructing their students in the

188. Roosevelt Hospital, *History of Roosevelt Hospital*, p. 54.
189. Lamb, *Presbyterian Hospital*, pp. 75-78.

public wards and the various laboratories of the Hospital. The Departments of Pathology, Bacteriology, Biological Chemistry, and such other educational and scientific departments as might be hereafter created by mutual agreement would also have the like privilege of teaching students in the Hospital.[190]

Many years later Lamb was to say,

> The origin of the Columbia-Presbyterian Medical Center critically depended on as simple a thing as teaching medical students in the wards. Had Roosevelt accepted this principle, which proved to be so sound, there would have been a Columbia-Roosevelt Medical Center. Perhaps there should have been a statue of a clinical clerk on the grounds of our center. I once suggested it to Edward Harkness, and he laughingly agreed.[191]

Dean Lambert had finally succeeded in achieving his major goal, an affiliation with a first rate general hospital and an agreement bringing medical students to the bedside, not as passive observers, but as clinical clerks engaging in active clinical work under the close supervision of their teachers. The implementation of this contract was not a simple matter, and there were to be some awkward moments involving leading physicians and surgeons of the city. The clause requiring the key figures on the staff to confine their work to only one hospital may seem perfectly fair and reasonable today, but in 1911 it was a radical innovation that met with resistance.

It was Dr. Albert Lamb's opinion that—

> The manifold changes required by the agreement had to be effected at the very time when medical practice and medical education as a whole were undergoing transformation from the old order to the new. In the old order, most professors of medicine and surgery and consultants and attending physicians had been selected because of their reputations as famous consultants and successful practitioners. In the limited time left from their private practice, they often served several institutions simultaneously. They came to the hospitals for rounds, operations and usually one didactic lecture a week. In the new order, professors of various grades spent most of their working hours at the hospital—only one hospital—and shared attending duties with other members of the staff. Didactic lectures were being replaced by seminars and bedside instruction in the wards. Consultations, which had formed so large a part of many doctors' practices were losing importance. More often, perplexing and critical cases

190. *Ibid.*, pp. 415-21, abstracted from Appendix I.
191. *Ibid.*, pp. 79-80.

> were being sent directly to hospitals where the patients might have simultaneous advantages of careful examination by an eminent attending physician and of observation with the new methods available only in modern hospitals.[192]

This was one way of looking at the proposed changes, but there was room for differences of opinion and these soon became evident. Private consultations were still the key entry point of private patients to the health care system of that day, and most individuals who could afford the fees sought out private physicians and surgeons for advice. Hospitals in 1910 were not as popular as they are today, nor were they as comfortable or as well equipped. Privacy was hard to come by. For the indigent and the poor, a stay on a ward without privacy may have been better than in their humble homes, but for the rising middle class and the well-to-do there was no place like home with its comforts and family help and servants in ample supply.[193] The term "hospitalism," coined and popularized in 1869 by James Y. Simpson, defined as "the morbid conditions due to the assembly of diseased persons in a hospital" was used by surgeons of that day as a rubric for their discussions on erysipelas, septicemia, pyemia, and hospital gangrene, discussion hardly conducive to reassuring the public about its hospitals.[194]

It would be some years before the fear of the hospital would be replaced in the minds of lay people by the modern image of the hospital as a place of refuge and of first, rather than last, resort in illness. At the turn of the century, most illnesses, serious as well as trivial, were treated at home. Doctors made house calls. Nursing care of some sort was easily available. Operations were often performed in the homes of the well-to-do. Therapy of the day was empiric, with almost no specific drugs; diagnostic techniques were extremely primitive even in the best of hospitals. The fear of contagion was such that in New York City people with communicable diseases were treated at home under quarantine or sent to Willard Parker Hospital for Communicable Diseases. Some hospitals left much to be desired in their lack of

192. *Ibid.*, pp. 80-81.

193. Brieger, G. H. (Ed.): *Medical America in the 19th Century*. Johns Hopkins Press, Baltimore, 1972.

194. Simpson, J. Y.: *Hospitalism, its effects on the results of surgical operations*. Edinburgh, Oliver & Boyd, 1869.

cleanliness and the calibre of their personnel. The poor people of New York would not soon forget the sensational newspaper report in the spring of 1860 of a young Irish woman who gave birth on a Sunday night in Bellevue Hospital and the following morning the infant was found dead next to the mother, who had been too weak to prevent rats from devouring the baby's nose, upper lip, toes, and half of the foot.[195]

Clearly, the era of outside consultations, house calls, office practice, and home care was not yet at an end, although change was in the wind. The insistence that the key teachers confine their efforts to only one major hospital in a day when multiple hospital appointments were customary would prove to be the first of a series of constraints placed upon the practicing medical profession in their relationship to the teaching hospitals, all in the cause of improving education, training, research, and patient care. Criticism was raised by some who felt so long as they rendered good service, there was no harm and really some advantage in serving on the staff of several hospitals. Some questioned the isolation from other institutions that such a policy might entail. How could city hospitals be staffed by outstanding clinicians serving without pay if these men were denied appointments to the staff of the premier voluntary hospitals where they made their living? Others felt that compliance would interfere with their private practices and the freedom of choice their patients might have in going to the hospital they personally preferred. Some of the old guard, who had earned their spurs by the process of demonstrated ability, hard work, experience, and long years of practice, were reluctant to step aside and approve a change whereby the hospital might select junior physicians and surgeons and promote them to high positions, assuming that they would emerge eventually as great clinicians and teachers without having had to face the emery wheel of competition. Some farsighted individuals would predict that the denigration of the role of the private consultant in teaching might ultimately lead to isolation of the hospital and the medical school from the very community they were to depend upon for survival as independent or voluntary institutions.

Whatever the considerations may have been, Presbyterian

195. *The New York Tribune,* April 25, 1860.

Hospital, as the result of the affiliation agreement with P & S, lost by resignation some of its most distinguished professional staff, including Dr. W. Gilman Thompson, who preferred his position as professor of medicine at Cornell; Dr. Joseph Blake, President of the Medical Board; Walter James; John S. Thatcher; John A. Hartwell; George Woolsey; and Frederick Solley. Replacing these men, while not an impossible task, would nevertheless be difficult.

It should be stressed at this time that enormous pressures were being exerted upon the medical schools to improve their standards, chiefly as a result of the Flexner report, which was published in April 1910. When Flexner visited P & S in October 1909, he reported some good things, especially in the preclinical facilities, but he had many unkind words for the clinical facilities that he found to be seriously lacking despite the ample clinical material in New York City. Why, he asked have the great New York schools been in the main clinically unproductive? "The reason is a matter of history. The schools that are now called university departments grew up as proprietary institutions. They have never been adequately financed. They obtained, and still obtain, their clinical facilities at each other's expense: that is to say, what one gets, the other loses."[196]

Defeated in his attempts to affiliate with Roosevelt Hospital, Lambert now had a hospital for his medical students, but instead of being across the street from his medical school, it was across town at 70th Street on Park Avenue. For the present, he would make do with this arrangement, but exciting new plans were in the offing. By rejecting the medical students and virtually forcing P & S to go across town for its hospital, the Roosevelt Board had set in motion an extremely interesting train of events. The Presbyterian Board had decided to build a new hospital to cope with its increasing responsibilities and on February 8, 1909 purchased a site on the East River, the block between 67th and 68th Streets bounded on the east by the East River and on the west by Avenue A.

In the meantime, President Nicholas Murray Butler had plans of his own for the medical school and had persuaded several friends to furnish the money to purchase the block between

196. Flexner, *Bull. No. 4*, pp. 275-76.

116th and 117th Streets, Amsterdam Avenue and Morningside Drive. In 1910, Dean Lambert pointed out that this site was not large enough for a hospital plus a medical school and suggested that P & S might better merge with St. Luke's Hospital which already occupied a nearby site. In the meantime, the Harkness offer to build a new hospital and to endow it was causing Presbyterian to reconsider its plans and to think in terms of a great educational institution rather than a small general hospital. For this purpose, the East River site was obviously inadequate in size as well as poorly situated because of the presence of a large brewery and large numbers of flies, stench, noise, and an undesirable environment. Edward Harkness, now an important member of the Presbyterian Board, had caught the vision of a great medical center, the first of its kind in the world, and he was not to be dissuaded by financial problems or personality clashes. He was to need all his persistence, patience, and altruism to achieve this goal, for he had to deal with many powerful and highly opinionated individuals. First of all, Nicholas Murray Butler, President of Columbia University and nicknamed "Nicholas Miraculous," had his own notions about the medical school, and he would not take a back seat during any of the negotiations. In fact, Samuel W. Lambert, Jr. blamed him for obstructing and delaying the amalgamation of Presbyterian with P & S from 1910 until 1916, when the plan fell through, and not until 1919 and 1921 was a final agreement worked out.[197]

An idea whose time had come, the concept of a major medical center in New York, fired the imagination of lay people as well as professionals. Its scope was almost too much for mere doctors and needed the vision and resources of intelligent, informed and, incidentally, well-heeled laymen. The initial thought was to bring together the P & S medical school, Presbyterian Hospital, Vanderbilt Clinic, and Sloane Maternity Hospital. Soon these were to be joined by the Neurological Institute, Babies' Hospital, Squier Urological Clinic, New York State Psychiatric Institute, and later (1931) by the Institute of Ophthalmology, followed by the Board of Health Building on 168th Street and, in 1950, the New York Orthopedic Hospital.

The road to this achievement was by no means smooth; true

197. Lambert, *P & S Quarterly*, pp. 9-11.

to form in New York City, many pot holes would be encountered and serious clashes were to occur before the center could be constructed and occupied. The actions of President Nicholas Murray Butler were to cause much dismay and, in fact, seriously jeopardize the concept almost from its inception. Edward Harkness was to find dealing with Columbia University and its president a very difficult assignment, and there were times when he was tempted to drop the proposal of a medical center in anger and frustration. From the beginning, there was much jockeying for the site selection, starting with the East River plot that was ultimately dropped from consideration. Then Columbia, under President Butler, pressed for the Amsterdam Avenue and Morningside Heights site, which also was found to be wanting. Negotiations between Presbyterian and Columbia University for a combined site were characterized by inordinate delay, bickering, and a failure by the university to keep its pledges. Among other sites considered was the one in the Bronx on Gun Hill Road now occupied by Monetefiore Hospital. This would have been a disastrous move for the medical school in the opinion of many. Mr. Harkness had made up his own mind that the best site for the future medical center was in Washington Heights, at 168th Street, which had once been the home of the Highlanders, the professional baseball team that later became the New York Yankees. The stadium burned down, and the Yankees were sharing the Polo Grounds with the New York Giants until the House that Babe Ruth built could materialize across the Harlem River in the Bronx. The site of the burned-out stadium lay vacant for years and was used during World War I by the Armory of the 102nd Engineers, which was across the street. This area of New York City was almost rural then, and there was open land to the west and south of the center that would allow room for expansion, factors that Harkness and his advisors had taken into consideration when they selected this site. Below 165th Street, a large tract of land was owned by the Deaf and Dumb Institute.

Some years later when this institute moved to Westchester, the land was quickly and quietly purchased by Harkness for his pet project. Getting back to the initial negotiations for the Washington Heights tract, Presbyterian Hospital obtained an option to purchase it contingent upon the pledging of matching funds by Columbia University. For whatever the reason, President Butler stalled on meeting this commitment and was so high handed in his attitude that he seriously antagonized the Presbyterian Board and angered his most important philanthropist, Mr. Harkness, now strongly committed to the medical center. Fortunately whatever Butler lacked in his relationship with Harkness, was more than made up for by the understanding that Harkness had with his personal physicians and surgeons who were on the Presbyterian staff. Again, Harkness, the philanthropist, was finding that money alone did not solve problems. People had to be motivated to do good things. Personality clashes and the struggle for power were not peculiar to politics or the world of business. They existed, and still do, to a high degree in the field of medicine and health care. Harkness was of an even temperament, steady and tenacious, and willing to be patient in the face of difficulty and obstruction. He not only had the checkbook he also had the sense of commitment and the courage to pursue his goals and would brook no interference once he had seen the facts and made up his mind to proceed in a specific direction. Without Harkness, there would have been no medical center, at least one of the scope that developed under his aegis. The point is that it was not money alone, although this was essential. More than this, the concept of a great medical center needed a great leader of vision. Quite fortuitously, fate had provided this in the person of Edward S. Harkness, and mankind was to be the richer for it.

Harkness had an exchange of letters with Butler that was frank and to the point. Butler's answers were so unsatisfactory that the Presbyterian Board moved to dissolve the 1911 plan of merger of P & S and Presbyterian. The project stood in real jeopardy. Other alternatives were considered, among them a little publicized effort in 1917 of creating a Columbia-Cornell Medical Center on the East River. This was seriously considered and approved by the Board of Managers of Presbyterian Hospital and New York Hospital and conditioned upon bringing together the medical schools of Columbia and Cornell. At first, the four institutions agreed to the proposal but, in June 1917, Columbia reneged because of so-called "insuperable legal obstacles," and the project was dropped and the two medical schools and hospitals decided to go their separate ways.[198]

Why was Butler, an imperious but withall a very astute and practical university president, jeopardizing the relationship of the university with its greatest potential benefactor of all time? Was it merely his personality, his ego, and his demand that he dominate all decisions, or was something else troubling him? The something else may very well have been Abraham Flexner of the General Education Board. Flexner, in his 1910 Bulletin, had stated quite clearly his criticism of P & S as a medical school. He came out very strongly for a hospital controlled by the medical school under the aegis of the university, and he also spoke strongly for making drastic changes in the teaching staff. By 1917, now well ensconced in his position with the General Education Board, he was reaching for bigger game, namely the promotion of the concept of a full-time teaching staff in the clinical departments, seeking to introduce into New York City the concepts he had fought for and achieved at Johns Hopkins. His approach in New York was to attempt to work through the university. As we have seen, Flexner had a concept of the role of the university in medical education that looked to it as the panacea and the answer to all problems. Flexner himself, never the possessor of a graduate degree, was really quite limited in his experience with universities and saw in the European models a utopia that was never really there except on superficial examination. He was to learn very soon that Columbia University and its leaders were to prove as tough as he in moving toward changes in medical education. The bruising experience that Flexner was to have in the Columbia affair seems to have been of such severity that, in his autobiography, he appears to virtually ignore the subject except for a short reference.

On November 17, 1917, after meetings with President Butler, Dean Lambert, Trustee Newcomb Carlton, and Columbia University treasurer Frederick A. Goetze, Abraham Flexner prepared a memorandum on medical education in New York with special emphasis on P & S and its relation with the Presbyterian Hospital in which he made the following recommendations:

> The Presbyterian Hospital and the Medical School of Columbia should be rebuilt on a single site, and in medical teaching and re-

198. Lamb, *Presbyterian Hospital*, p. 125.

search Presbyterian should function as a university hospital.

The University should discontinue its practice of teaching its undergraduates in a number of hospitals and concentrate its teaching in the reconstructed Presbyterian Hospital. The enrollment of P. and S. should be limited to 400.

The clinical staff should be reconstructed on the full-time principle which was being followed or instituted at Johns Hopkins, Washington University, and the University of Chicago.

The agreement of 1911 between Presbyterian and Columbia should be revised and simplified.

The Crocker Institute of Cancer Research should be rebuilt as a part of the new plant in close relationship to the new Medical School and Hospital.

The site of the new center should be the property situated on Broadway between 165th and 168th streets.

A School of Graduate Instruction, separate from the undergraduate medical school, should be organized with Bellevue Hospital and perhaps certain other hospitals.[199]

On January 8, 1918, President Butler indicated in a letter to the General Education Board and the Carnegie Corporation that Columbia University would actively support the Flexner plan that was subsequently approved by the Board of Managers of the Presbyterian Hospital. By May 2, 1918, Butler had experienced a change of heart and had written to President William Sloane of the Presbyterian Hospital that four essential features of Flexner's scheme were completely unacceptable to Columbia. These were as follows:

1. The resignation of the Dean and all members of the present Faculty.
2. The institution of a system by which teachers of practical or clinical subjects would, if they accepted incidental service, pay any fee received therefor to the University.
3. The mechanical limitation of attendance of the Medical School to 400, and
4. The severance of all teaching and research relationships between the Medical School and other hospitals than the Presbyterian Hospital.

We deem all four of these proposals so reactionary and so antagonistic to the best interests of the public, of medical education, and of Columbia University, that they will not, under any circumstances, be approved by us. *Were the Trustees to assent to the suggestion that, as a condition precedent to receiving a large sum of money they would invite or require the resignation of the entire*

199. *Ibid.*, pp. 127-36.

> *medical faculty, they would thereby inflict a blow upon Columbia University from which it might not recover for a generation.* The Trustees have uniformly shown the utmost consideration for the teaching staff, and they have repeatedly asserted and upheld the independence and security of tenure of professors and instructors so long as they do their duty.[200] (Italics added by Doctor Lepore.)

The Columbia lion was roaring and asserting itself in no uncertain terms. Its principles and academic freedom were not for sale no matter how much was offered. Perhaps Butler may have been trying to support Dean Lambert who had a large private practice in addition to his position as Dean and had accomplished a great deal for the medical school during his tenure. There were equally powerful figures in the medical school faculty in private practice who would not easily be dislodged or replaced. There is enough evidence here to indicate that Butler was making every effort to preserve the status quo of the medical school, which, in spite of its failings, had become the outstanding medical school in New York and one of the country's leading institutions. It was the era of the great clinicians and P & S had a virtual monopoly on the outstanding New York physicians and surgeons of the day. Not only were they clinically competent, they also enjoyed great social prestige, included many of the Brahmins of American medicine, and exerted great influence in medical and community matters in New York. They were the physicians to the wealthy and powerful whose philanthropy and personal involvement in their hospitals and institutions would be strongly influenced by their personal relationships. Important matters having to do with hospital, medical school, and philanthropic commitments were being discussed at social gatherings and dinners. An impeccably arranged private dinner could do more to enlist philanthropy and cooperation than dozens of formal committee meetings. It was the era of personal exertion of power and influence in good causes by individuals with sufficient affluence and security to feel quite free to help the less fortunate. President Butler knew that Dean Lambert had advanced medical education significantly by his innovations and knew that P & S had become a great medical school largely because of his efforts. The fact that Lambert had accomplished so much as Dean on a

200. *Ibid.*, pp. 130-31.

part-time basis, while he was still engaged in a large private practice, may have led Butler to seriously question the validity of the full-time concept that could have removed Lambert from private practice. Was Lambert a great dean because he was also a busy practitioner, meeting the people of the city and the country and bringing to them the fruits of his wide experience and high clinical skills? Was he better able to administer the medical school and its curriculum because of this background? Was he a better role model for the medical students than a purely administrative type who would run the dean's office efficiently and without any daily contact with sickness and illness and patients?

These questions must have been raised for President Butler. The judgement of his response and his reversals of opinion on the medical school need to be made in the context of the times in which he lived and not in those of this day.

Also, let us not forget the story of Flexner and his personal animosity toward the Lamberts—one and all of them, stemming from his experience at the hands of Dr. Adrian Lambert in the incident of the fractured ankle. Butler must have been under heavy pressure and, at the same, time, he may also have felt that university privileges and obligations were being bartered for economic support. Whatever the reasons, his about-face caught the Presbyterian trustees off guard, and since this was not the first time, they reacted quite vigorously. Their exasperation was expressed in a firm letter to Columbia University, charging that since it had failed to cooperate with Presbyterian Hospital over a period of more than seven years, the Presbyterian Hospital wished to cancel and terminate the agreement of affiliation of April 28, 1911.

Fortunately, the cancellation of the affiliation agreement was not to occur largely because of a cooling-off period that ensued, part of it attributable to World War I and its inroads on staff and its heavy demands on all of our institutions. The influenza pandemic of 1918 added to the problems, and it was not until 1920 that attention would again be focussed on the affiliation of Presbyterian Hospital with Columbia University.

Flexner's proposals that had served to almost destroy the relationship between Columbia and Presbyterian were by no means a dead issue. They would surface again, and the first casualty would be a very important individual who would pay the price for being in private practice and at the same time head a major medical school.

Chapter 18
THE BATTLE OVER FULL TIME AT COLUMBIA-PRESBYTERIAN

The battle over full time at P & S began in earnest in 1919, and its first casualty was Dean Samuel W. Lambert, who resigned on March 3, 1919, when he was sixty years of age, well before mandatory retirement. A colleague said of his resignation, "He is probably the last dominating, predominating medical leader in practice, teaching and organizing ability we are likely to know."[201] He was, indeed, to be the last dean of a great medical school who actually had a substantial private practice and knew what it was in his day-to-day activities to actually take care of the sick. There was also the episode of Flexner's fractured ankle, his adverse experience with Adrian Lambert, brother of the dean, and Flexner's vow to never give money to any medical school with a Lambert on its faculty. Beyond this, Sam Lambert's robust and earthy personality may have rubbed Flexner the wrong way during the initial exploratory conferences held with President Butler. Curiously, while Flexner offered General Education Board support for full-time clinical department heads, he made no similar provision for the deanship, assuming that the job would simply be added on to the responsibilities of heading another department, preferably Pathology. It is a little odd that a man thought to be an authority on education would not have placed a higher priority on the deanship in a medical school and insisted upon adequate financial provision for it.

Dean Lambert was given the usual flowery written testimonials of gratitude by Columbia University and praised for his excellent performance during his fifteen years of tenure. I am not certain whether he was also given a gold watch or the equivalent. The choice of a new dean was accompanied by considerable bickering,

201. Coons, Horace: *Columbia: Colossus on the Hudson.* New York, E. P. Dutton & Co., 1947, p. 268.

jockeying for power, and bitter arguments. The war had disrupted the smooth running of the medical school, and a group of "Young Turks" had returned from military service with very definite notions about the role they should play in the hospital and school. With each war, there is always this phenomenon of the return to civilian life of a new breed of individual—often unwilling to accept the status quo and ready to fight for his rights and privileges. The deanship would no longer be a rather small part-time job dominated by a single individual who made most of the decisions, but it would have to represent the entire school and all of its many divisions and departments.

To step into this breach on July 1, 1919, Columbia designated Dr. William Darrach of its surgical staff, recently returned from military service in Europe, as the new Dean of P & S. Darrach lost no time in consulting with key representatives of Columbia and Presbyterian, as well as with the General Education Board, the Rockefeller Foundation, and the Carnegie Corporation, and on December 13, 1919, less than six months after assuming the Deanship, came out strongly and unequivocally for full time for the clinical departments in a carefully worded statement distributed to his staff. In this interesting document, he expresses the view, in essentially Flexnerian terms, that the men in the main clinical departments must be free to concentrate their energies on their university and hospital work, protected from the "distractions" of private practice, the purpose being to obtain a more truly university-type of clinical teacher. He considered five so-called full-time plans, listing them as follows:

- Plan 1. No private practice and no outside employment.
- Plan 2. Private practice at the discretion of the clinician but no fee is paid for such service.
- Plan 3. As in Plan 2, except that the fee is paid to the University.
- Plan 4. Private practice for fees allowed in such limited amounts that it does not interfere with the thorough, efficient and sincere fulfillment of his academic duties.
- Plan 5. Unlimited private practice within the hospital.[202]

202. Lamb, Albert R.: *Presbyterian Hospital and Columbia-Presbyterian Medical Center: 1868-1943.* New York, Columbia University Press, 1955, pp. 434-42.

After a brief discussion of the various alternatives, Darrach recommends the adoption of Plan 2 and in the summary of his memorandum says,

> The three-fold purposes of the School of Medicine are teaching, research and the care of the sick. To attain these there must be: a. An intimate geographical and functional union with a University Hospital. b. Such limitation of numbers of students as will permit the consistent pursuit of a definite policy. Increasing demands may be met by a complete duplication of the whole unit. c. Reorganization of the main clinical departments on a full-time basis.[203]

Flexner had won the battle, for these were the essential features of the plan he had submitted to the Presbyterian and Columbia trustees in 1917 that had met with violent opposition and caused great controversy. To sweeten the acceptance of his plan was a gift of two millions dollars proferred by the General Education Board and the Rockefeller Foundation for its adoption and contingent upon its full implementation. The latter phrase was to plague P & S in a few years and return to haunt it, placing in jeopardy the entire concept of a Columbia-Presbyterian Medical Center.

Following Dean Darrach's memorandum of December 13, 1919, a trial of Plan 2 of the full-time concept was initiated at P & S on July 1, 1921.[204] This was the scheme for full-time salaried clinical teachers who were to be allowed private practice at their own discretion with no fee to be paid for such service. Within a few months, it was evident that the plan was unworkable. Some patients hesitated to accept free service, while others took advantage of it and of the doctors. Physicians from outside of the Presbyterian Hospital resented the apparent monopoly of the full-time staff and complained of unfair competition. How could they charge their patients when the professors at a medical school could, because of the subsidy of their salaries, charge them nothing? Referrals from the outsiders to the insiders and vice versa were constrained by similar considerations, leading to a reduction in the exchanges known to be vital to the survival and growth of any medical center. In addition, full-time salaries were proving inadequate, and several of the participating key clinicians were

203. *Ibid.*, p. 442.
204. *Ibid.*, p. 189.

planning to resign to enter private practice for financial reasons. These and other considerations led to a special dinner meeting in Edward Harkness' home on January 17, 1922, attended by President William Sloane of Presbyterian, Dean William Darrach of P & S, and Doctors Hugh Auchincloss, C. Charles Burlingame, A. Raymond Dochez, Albert R. Lamb, Walter W. Palmer, Fordyce Barker St. John, Frederick T. Van Beuren, and Allen O. Whipple. Harkness, who strongly believed in the full-time concept, was surprised to find that it was not working out well. When the doctors expressed their criticism with frankness, sincerity, and facts, Harkness agreed with them that the concept of not charging fees to private patients was unsound and that the salaries for full-time positions were grossly inadequate. Following this meeting, the Medical Board submitted to the P & S Committee on Administration a special memorandum recommending that private patients be charged fees and that the Presbyterian Hospital should collect the fees and turn them over to the University's special fund for research and teaching. Salaries of several full-time men were to be raised to meet the cost of living in New York. It was proposed that a more elastic system than strict full time be installed including "(1) full-time men; (2) men with offices and sufficient private beds in the hospital, confining their work to the hospital, but receiving fees directly from patients; (3) part-time men, limited service to the hospital, with offices outside."[205]

On May 9, 1922, President Sloane reported to the Presbyterian Board of Managers that the Joint Administrative Board and Columbia University had agreed to the proposal. Beginning July 1, private patients would be charged fees that were to be assessed by the attending physician, approved by the Superintendent, and then billed and collected by the Hospital. The fees would go into a special fund for supplementing the salaries of full-time clinicians. The details for reimbursement were spelled out and the new experiment was on. The abandonment of free treatment for private patients was an important change, but the Hospital could now be accused of practicing medicine. Total control by the hospital of professional fees would set a dangerous precedent. But before these questions would arise, it became evident that

205. *Ibid.*, pp. 190-92.

this modification of full time was only a makeshift and would not serve the purpose for which it was intended. The clinicians involved were not able to generate the private fees that had at first been anticipated, and the hospital found itself burdened by its commitment to pay higher salaries. Dissatisfaction was so great that in the Spring of 1923, Dean Darrach appointed a Committee for the Organization of the Clinical Departments chaired by Dr. Walter W. Palmer, Bard Professor of Medicine, and consisting of Drs. Hugh Auchincloss, William Darrach, A. Raymond Dochez, James Jobling, Albert R. Lamb, Fordyce B. St. John, and Allen O. Whipple.[206] The concept of full time and its trial at P & S were subjected to close scrutiny by the committee, which considered various alternatives, and on October 29, 1923, presented a voluminous report before the P & S Committee on Administration, with President Sage of Presbyterian and Edward Harkness as invited observers. Almost every item of the committee report was reviewed and accepted, altered or discarded, and the first report was prepared by Doctor Palmer accompanied by a summary that was a masterful analysis of the full-time concept, its weaknesses, and its strengths. Entitled, "Summary of Report of Committee on Organization of the Clinical Departments," the memorandum is one of the most incisive and brilliant statements ever made on this topic.[207]

Doctor Palmer's report began with the statement that for two years the Departments of Medicine and Surgery had been reorganized upon a vocational basis that provided for a number of strictly full-time salaried clinicians who were denied the right to charge fees for private practice. This change was made because of dissatisfaction in many medical schools where the teaching and scientific productiveness in the clinical departments were considered inferior to those in the basic science divisions, the inferiority being attributed to the distractions and demands on the clinicians arising from their private practices. It was theorized that if the financial attraction of private practice were matched or bettered by a high salary and the individual's energies confined to university activities, "true excellence of teaching must result." But Palmer points out:

206. *Ibid.*, p. 193.
207. *Ibid.*, pp. 443-49.

> The theory took no cognizance of the fact that the nonclinical group were wholly devoted to the application of science while the clinical group must, in addition, practice an art or cease to be clinicians. Human nature was to be cut to fit an idea. Properly speaking this was not a real university basis for it was lacking in that essential academic freedom which is a primary requisite in university departments. But in acknowledgement of a financial honorarium at a higher rate than that given to nonclinical teachers, the clinicians agreed to the imposition of certain restrictions which have never been laid upon the officers of any other departments of the university. This double distinction immediately set them apart as objects of interest, admiration, envy or disdain according to the spirit and inclination of the commentator.208

This situation holds true even to the present day.

Palmer goes on to indicate how these "distinctions" came about, stating first that in the initial planning for faculty recruitment it was felt—

> that only by offering higher salaries could clinicians be secured of such character as to assure that their full-time devotion would place the Departments of Medicine and Surgery upon the high plane of teaching efficiency and scientific productiveness so ardently desired.

Secondly, by placing restrictions on the full-time salaried clinicians, denying them financial compensation other than their salaries for their practice within the hospital and prohibiting them from practicing at all outside the hospital, these individuals would be protected from the temptation and demands of private practice. Palmer's solid and scholarly criticism of these fallacies is phrased in these vibrant and telling remarks.

> There were two serious fallacies in this plan which had been lost sight of in that enthusiasm for better clinical teaching which caused its adoption. In the first place, as to compensation: the services of the most desirable clinicians cannot be secured by offering high salaries. Many universities can offer facilities and opportunities which will attract such men, but no university can buy their continued services under conditions which are burdensome and restrictive.
>
> In the second place, as to restrictions: if the university has secured the right type of man and if it has provided him with a fair salary and with facilities and opportunities commensurate with his needs and desires, he will neither want to do too much private practice nor will he have to. His tastes lie in other directions. There is no need for special prohibitions. One has only to recall the names

208. *Ibid.*, p. 443.

> of Delafield, of Osler, or Halsted and of others to confirm the statement . . . .
>
> In addition to these fallacies there was a certain disingenuousness connected with the imposition of the restrictions against private practice. This restriction was ostensibly to protect the clinicians from the demands of private practice, but there was inherent in the prohibitions an implication that the clinicians must be prevented from succumbing to their own weakness. Such an implication is not the best basis for continued cordial understanding and loyal service.[209]

That the full-time plan was not totally without advantageous features was clearly and fairly stated by Palmer who pointed out the advantages accruing to the department heads who could give adequate time to teaching and administrative activities when relieved of private practice responsibilities. By confining their activities to one hospital, the teaching staff could function more efficiently and more productively.

> In balancing the account between the advantages and disadvantages it would appear that most of the advantages must be credited to the clinicians who have done the work and that most of the disadvantages must be debited against the plan under which they did it.

The final pages of the Palmer Committee statement convey in unequivocal terms their position on the trial of the full-time concept at P & S.

> After a very careful and conscientious test of its merits by actual trial of more than two years, it is unanimously agreed that the drawbacks of the plan in operation outweigh its desirable features and that, in the best interests of medical education at this University, it should be discarded by these departments.[210]

Fully aware of the possible repercussions of this decision, especially when it would be viewed by Abraham Flexner and the General Education Board, Palmer sought to soften the blow by a conciliatory explanatory statement.

> Two years is not a long time in which to build up a tradition, but we cannot help feeling that a new tradition has arisen within those years: a tradition of Full-Service rather than of Full-Time; a tradition which has been founded by no one Department alone but which can be shared equally by all. We feel that the present Directors and their Associates in the Departments of our School are the type of men who will foster this tradition. And we confidently

209. *Ibid.*, p. 444.
210. *Ibid.*, p. 446.

> expect that, under their inspiring leadership, the troublesome distinctions between full-time and part-time will eventually disappear in the general desire to give full service: full-service which can be rendered by any man—whether he works one hour, or eight hours, or twenty—if he gives the best there is in him to the University.[211]

From my personal experience as a part-time member of Doctor Palmer's department starting in 1937, I can attest to the genuineness of his comments and the integrity of his message. He built his department on the concept of full-service rather than full-time, and each one of us knew what he meant and what he wanted and we were happy to play even minor roles in this great adventure. When Doctor Palmer retired in 1947, he had established one of the best-balanced and strongest departments of medicine in the country, and he could say with pride that he had struck the right chord when he brought together "a goodly company of full-time men combined with sympathetic and cooperative men in practice affording wide flexibility in organization."[212]

Palmer's capacities as a peacemaker and compromiser would be severely tested by Flexner who would soon attack P & S for what he interpreted as abandonment of the full-time concept.

The attack was precipitated on May 30, 1924 by a brief item that appeared in the *Columbia Alumni News* written by Dr. Walter B. James stating, "During the past year the faculty of the Medical School advised the abandonment of the 'full-time' teaching system in P & S, and a return to the part-time system now general throughout the University is being worked out."[213] The news came as a bombshell to the General Education Board and the Rockefeller Foundation and was regarded as a breach of faith, especially since they had not been consulted. So serious was this deemed, that they felt no longer under any obligation to keep their pledge of $2,000,000 to P & S, and in fact there was even some talk, but only talk, of a suit against Columbia for breach of contract. The Carnegie Corporation registered no complaint and made no effort to withdraw its contribution of $1,000,000. But the Carnegie, under its president, Henry Pritchett, never sought to influence university policy through its gifts. At any rate, the battle over the

211. *Ibid.*, p. 448.
212. *Ibid.*, p. 197.
213. *Ibid.*, p. 221.

full-time issue at P & S again became a very disruptive force. Harried meetings were held. Negotiations dragged along for more than a year, becoming increasingly bitter and dominated by personality clashes. By the fall of 1925, the Rockefeller Foundation and the General Education Board announced their intention to cancel their agreements with Columbia. Without the Rockefeller $2,000,000 gift, the financial viability of the Columbia-Presbyterian project was seriously threatened, and the Presbyterian trustees were gravely concerned. In the meantime, Doctor Palmer, who was respected by the Foundations as well as the University and who had been a member of the Rockefeller Hospital staff, had been working on a possible solution. With Presbyterian President Sage's approval, he embarked upon discussions with Abraham Flexner and correspondence with Stephen Baker, a Columbia trustee, and acted as a superb peacemaker.

> The solution which he proferred was not so important for any underlying principles. It was, rather, an excellent diplomatic compromise which placated the two Rockefeller institutions without really surrendering one jot of the important modification of full time for which Doctor Palmer himself had been largely responsible.214

In essence, the Palmer plan called for raising the salary of the full-time staff to more realistic levels and the addition of four new full-time men to the staff. If the salary increases were effected, all of the men would work on a form of full time though retaining the right to see private patients of interest to them, with the fees from such services going into a fund to be disposed of later as decided. The specific amount needed was a relatively small sum, $68,000, for the next two and one-half years, by which time the medical services would be fully established in the new hospital and the service would be able to pay the increases out of its regular budget.

> In mid-December, Doctor Palmer represented the Medical School and the Hospital at a decisive meeting which included Stephen Baker and John Millburn, Columbia trustees, Doctor (Sic) Flexner of the General Education Board, and Thomas Debevoise, legal representative of the Rockefeller Foundation. Mr. Debevoise had with him the papers necessary for canceling the agreement with Columbia. Backed by the memorandum, which had already been circulated, Doctor Palmer made the official presentation of his case. He declared emphatically that there had not been the slightest intention of

214. *Ibid.*, p. 222.

> abandoning the full-time principle, but on the contrary, a special effort to increase its usefulness. A number of men on the Medical Service were already working on full time, as the memorandum showed, and others wished to do so when the funds became available. His plan was accepted in short order. The papers to cancel the grants of $2,000,000 were not presented, and Doctor (Sic) Flexner agreed that the General Education Board would provide the $68,000.[215]

This was a great coup for Palmer and Columbia-Presbyterian, and it saved the day for the Medical Center. More importantly, Palmer was able to get Flexner to back down from his hard-nosed position on pure full time and to accept a compromise. That Flexner adjusted to this so graciously and, in fact, added more money to the till is an enormous tribute to Doctor Palmer's skill as a peacemaker and negotiator, owing to his integrity, calmness under fire, his fairness, and great sense of equity. His major contribution to the battle over full time was not only in developing a balanced modification of the plan but in his skill in selling his concept to the previously hostile and irate Abraham Flexner and the General Board of Education, using the language of a true university professor to win a landmark compromise that would serve to guide other medical schools faced with similar problems.

While the battle over full time was being fought to its conclusion, construction of the Columbia-Presbyterian Medical Center went steadily forward. One especially revealing error in the early planning was the failure to include any provision for private patients. Indeed, it was only as an afterthought that the omission was discovered, so carried away had the planners and professional staff been by the emphasis on full-time teaching, research, and a university clinic that they had been blinded to the need for facilities for the care of the sick who could afford to pay their bills. This failure in planning would have been a deadly blow to the medical center. Fortunately, Edward Harkness himself, one of the first to notice this deficiency, encouraged by several members of the professional staff whom he trusted, persuaded his mother to provide the funds for the construction of what was to become one of the most famous hospitals in the world, the Harkness Pavilion, in honor of her late husband, Stephen Harkness. Had this pavilion not been included in the plans, it would have been the death knell of Doctor Palmer's concept of a core

215. *Ibid.*, pp. 223-24.

medical staff of full-time salaried physicians with privileges to care for some private patients of interest to them, surrounded by a group of physicians interested and competent in teaching and research whose financial support would come from the fees they earned from the care of private patients. Some would be geographic full time, while others would have outside offices. Even worse was the failure to make any provision in the original plans for semiprivate rooms, all of the rooms in Harkness being designed for single occupancy. Remedial measures were not undertaken until the move into the medical center was imminent, and the solution was to prove unsatisfactory for the patients and their doctors for years to come. We used to joke that patients occupying a semiprivate room in Presbyterian were neither fish nor fowl, denied many of the nursing advantages of ward care and deriving very little from the privacy of a room without running water or a toilet.

On March 26, 1928, the new Columbia-Presbyterian Medical Center admitted its first patients, and on Columbus Day, October 12, 1928, this Center was formally dedicated in an impressive outdoor ceremony held in the garden south of the main buildings. It was a great occasion with kudos and credit being assigned to numerous deserving individuals. Honorary degrees were conferred by President Nicholas Murray Butler. Absent from the list of recipients was the name of an individual who, in his way, had done as much as anyone to bring about the birth of a great institution, Abraham Flexner. His reaction to the successful establishment of this medical center must have been to gloat over his statement of 1920: "If we could plant a first-rate medical school in Rochester, perhaps New York City would wake up." The New York City medical schools, meccas in medical education and proud of their prestige and heritage, were badly shaken by the diversion of Rockefeller philanthropy to Rochester and the establishment in that city of a Hopkins-type medical school. The handwriting was on the wall: New York City would have to get its plans under way or its dominant position in American medicine would be compromised. Seldom satisfied with being second best in any enterprise and eager to do things on a mammoth scale in keeping with its tradition as the nation's premier city, New York's physicians and laymen, stung to the quick and true to Flexner's hunch, set out to revolutionize medical education in New York to a degree never before imagined.

Chapter 19
MUTINY OF THE PALACE GUARD

ELIOT AND PRITCHETT QUESTION GENERAL EDUCATION BOARD POLICY ON FULL TIME

The philanthropic efforts of the General Education Board and the Rockefeller Foundation in medical education and research were attracting favorable comment in the press under the skilled guidance of an experienced publicist, Ivy Lee. The Rockefeller image, tarnished by the claims of "tainted money," the Ludlow Massacre, the Merrit controversy, and the dissolution of the Standard Oil Trust, was being steadily improved through imaginative and successful projects aimed at improving the welfare and health of people and by the accomplishments of the outstanding research scientists of the Rockefeller Institute for Medical Research and other Rockefeller-sponsored institutions. In the field of medical education, adverse comments were from practitioner-teachers who violently opposed full time, but whose opposition might easily be dismissed as self-serving. The public and the press, especially the cartoonists, seemed to enjoy then, as they do even now, flagellating the practitioners of medicine, their alleged venality, greed, avarice, and lack of dedication. Only a few voices were raised in the press in defense of the physicians of the day. But full time, an idea whose time had come, supported by a resourceful and determined band of laymen and medical educators with large sums of money at their disposal; swept away all objections, that is, for a time. Opposition by average practitioners could be easily dismissed with only the voices of great leaders like Osler and Cushing giving cause for concern. But criticism was developing among the central core of the lay proponents of full time, and soon it would surface to cause embarrassment and a reconsideration of goals by the General Education Board and the Rockefeller Foundation.

The first of the new dissidents was a layman, former President Charles W. Eliot of Harvard, who had himself been a great innovator in medical education in his university. On April 24, 1917, Eliot wrote to Doctor Buttrick of the General Education Board:

> There is one matter, however, which is relevant but which I did not wish to bring before the Committee, because my knowledge of it depends on my membership in the General Education Board. I refer to the policy of the Board which I heard stated with great distinctness by Mr. Gates when I first joined the Board and have often heard since, namely, the policy of the Board not to interfere with the domestic management of an institution aided, except as regards its prudent financial management. I observe in the memorandum you handed me on the 9th of February a desire or purpose to condition a gift from the General Education Board to the Harvard Medical School on the acceptance by the School of one method of introducing the full-time policy. This condition does not seem to me consistent with what I have always believed to have been the wise and generally acceptable policy of the Board. The Board seems to prefer to act in general through other institutions or public agencies. Ought not the Board then to adhere strictly to its original policy of not conditioning any gift on the acceptance by the institution or agency aided of directions from the General Education Board as to how the money given should be spent—except, indeed, such very comprehensive directions as for endowment or for buildings?

On May 16, 1917, Buttrick replied to Eliot's question on full time:

> To this I would say the Board has never departed from its announced policy of refusing to interfere with the internal affairs of colleges and universities to which it has made appropriations for general endowment.

Eliot, dissatisfied with Buttrick's answer, wrote on May 17, 1917:

> In your second letter dated May 16th, you state the distinction between the Board's action in making appropriations to colleges and universities for general endowment and their action in making appropriations for specific kinds of work. I recognize the force of this distinction.
>
> The committee which made an informal application to the General Education Board on behalf of the Harvard Medical School thought it was understood that it was making an application for aid in establishing full-time clinical departments in the Harvard Medical School. It asked that that School should be made one of the "selected institutions" in which such full-time clinical departments

> should be established. It described fully the manner in which the authorities of the School proposed to carry out an extensive programme for the introduction and maintenance of full-time clinical professorships.
>
> It infers from the negative conclusion stated in your letter that this programme is not acceptable to you and some of your colleagues in the Board; and it accepts this result as final.
>
> I cannot but think, however, that the result indicates that the General Education Board intends to enforce in all medical schools which they aid to establish full-time professorships one particular mode of instituting and conducting such professorships in connection with hospitals, and one authoritative status for full-time professors in the medical schools so aided.[216]

It is difficult to escape the logic of Eliot's reply but the General Education Board held to its position that it was doing its job at the request of the university making the application. It seems quite obvious that the General Education Board was going to great pains to persuade universities to modify their policies on medical education to fit the mold cast by the General Education Board. Apparently, Eliot chose not to pursue this issue any further at this time. The next critic was not so easily stilled as Eliot, and he too carried impeccable credentials. This was President Henry S. Pritchett of the Carnegie Foundation for the Advancement of Teaching, who startled Buttrick on November 11, 1919 with the following letter:

> I never looked carefully at the contracts between the General Education Board and the Johns Hopkins University and Chicago University until after I was talking with you and Flexner today. I must confess I was rather staggered by them. These contracts lay down a stated policy for conducting a medical school which the Board approves and then in a formal contract the universities bind themselves to carry out these policies, and agree not to change them except by permission of the General Education Board, and in case they do change without such permission the universities agree to return the money. Such a contract binding a university to a fixed policy laid down by the giver of money seems to me a dangerous thing. If these contracts were made public I am sure it would bring down on all educational foundations no less than on the universities themselves severe criticism. It seems to me a dangerous policy for those who administer trust funds to adopt.

Buttrick, in his reply dated November 21, 1919, tried to defuse

216. Harvard University and the General Education Board: 1915-1920, Rockefeller Foundation Archives (Eliot and Buttrick).

Pritchett in the same manner he used with Eliot saying:

> I fear that you failed to notice that the preamble to the contract with the Johns Hopkins University distinctly recites that the policy was proposed to us by the trustees and medical faculty of the University and that the terms of the contract were such as they themselves asked for. The General Education Board has no fixed policy regarding medical education, and certainly it did not presume to lay down a policy for the Medical School of the Johns Hopkins University. After this work was inaugurated three other universities sought our aid on similar terms and our pledges were made in accordance with their requests and suggestions. In fact, the contracts were drawn under the supervision of their own legal advisors.

Buttrick's explanation did not satisfy Pritchett, who wrote to him on November 25, 1919 as follows:

> I do not think the preamble to which you refer greatly alters the situation. Even though the trustees of a university came to one of the foundations and proposed a policy, it is, in my judgment, a very questionable proceeding to draw up a contract binding them to such policy which they may not change without the consent of the corporation giving the funds. Particularly does this seem a dangerous proceeding when coupled with the condition that the failure to accept this outside control involves the return of the funds. Looking at the contract even in the light of your statement it seems to me open to very serious objection, and I am inclined to think that it will sometime in the future bring upon all of us a kind of criticism difficult to answer.
>
> I am also inclined to believe that a university like the Johns Hopkins, for example, makes a serious mistake in accepting a contract defining in detail the policy of its Medical School which it cannot change without the consent of an outside corporation which obtains this power through a gift of money. Nobody believes the General Education Board will ever use this power in an arbitrary manner. But the contract is one that in critical or hostile hands could be made embarrassing both for the university and for the Board. Apart from all this, however, I think there is a sound reason why a foundation giving money to an educational or charitable agency should not bind it to a stated policy by a contractual agreement.[217]

By this time the fat was in the fire, and it would not be enough for Buttrick alone to deny that the General Education Board was interfering with University policy as a condition for making philanthropic gifts. The precedent was a poor one and soon other

217. University of Chicago and General Education Board Corrspondence 1919-1922. Rockefeller Foundation Archives (Buttrick and Pritchett).

voices on the General Education Board and Rockefeller Foundation would be heard. While Buttrick and Flexner were the most visible proponents of the full-time scheme, we know that Gates was completely sold on it and insisted on this condition for gifts to medical schools. John D. Rockefeller, Jr. backed the policy to the hilt and expressed himself in no uncertain terms in writing to Judson regarding prospective staff appointments at the new medical school in Chicago.

In 1924, Anson Phelps Stokes, of Yale, a trustee of the General Education Board, joined the dissidents, saying,

> It is not a question of whether we are right or wrong in our opinions regarding the university full-time basis of medical education. I think that where adequate funds are available, we are absolutely right in favoring this policy, and I am very proud of what has been accomplished by the Board under Mr. Flexner's leadership in the field of medical education. But it is a question of whether or not we can psychologically and morally afford–in view of public opinion, and our great wealth as a board–to be imposing, or at least requiring detailed conditions regarding educational policy in medicine in elaborate contracts which can only be amended with our consent . . . . Personally, I think this policy unwise and fraught with serious dangers.[218]

We have already described the situation at Columbia P & S in 1925, when the full-time issue became so explosive that it almost destroyed the plans for the great new medical center. The Columbia University conflict was one of several that led the Board to modify its general policy in 1925, "authorizing the revision of contracts with the medical schools to permit such modifications as educational and scientific experience might, in the judgement of each school, justify."

To top it off, Frederick T. Gates, next to Flexner the foremost protagonist of full time on the General Education Board, was to confess his unhappiness with the original GEB policy, which he himself had approved, to attach conditions on the Rockefeller grants. In a wideranging memorandum, included in his papers dated December 31, 1926, Gates revealed his change of heart in this passage:

> d. May I suggest in this connection that Mr. Rockefeller seriously review the practise of conditional giving by himself and his

218. Yale University and General Education Board correspondence 1924 (Anson Phelps Stokes).

> philanthropies. It has always been attended with distasteful and perhaps indefensible features. Dr. Eliot saw them and always argued against conditions. The contributing public does not like the conditional feature. That the conditional feature is often asked by the beneficiary is carefully concealed from the public. The public thinks it imposed by Mr. Rockefeller and some speak bitterly about it. They say they are not in his class. He can give without feeling it. Weighed down by a colossal fortune, giving some of it away must be to him a relief. They too are willing to give and their giving is more meritorious than his because they give out of their comparative poverty, he of his opulence. By reason of his unexampled wealth he is in the worst possible position to make his own giving dependent in the least on theirs. Is it for him to indicate when, where, how much, and for what they shall contribute, under penalty of his declining to give at all? Moreover the greater the Rockefeller conditional subscriptions, personal or chartered, the severer the pressure forced on the local constituency. After years of such complaints I can not doubt that it is for Mr. Rockefeller's personal interest that he and his philanthropies should give outright and cease to give conditionally.[219]

At this point, the full-time principle was being battered quite severely on several fronts; by many physicians, who did not believe in it, and by key members of the General Education Board, the Rockefeller Foundation, and other highly respected educators and foundation heads who opposed the imposition of requirements designed to modify university policy as a condition for approving any grant. Its prime proponent, Abraham Flexner, was on the ropes, reaching the end of his tenure as secretary of the General Education Board, now an enemy of Gates who characterized him as a bureaucratic officer, usurping the power of the Board, and at odds with his early mentor, Henry Pritchett.

---

219. Gates Private Papers, December 31, 1926. Rockefeller Archives.

Chapter 20
"MISTER, CAN YOU CURE FITS?":

Duke University Medical School

The story of the Duke University School of Medicine is the saga of a generous benefactor with great vision and the funds to implement his dream. My purpose in selecting it for presentation in this volume is that Duke is an example of a medical school that never embraced the Flexnerian full-time concept, choosing instead to develop geographic full time and group practice in the clinical departments and emerging as one of the nation's truly great medical schools. It is a prize example of what can be accomplished by teamwork and by the efforts of individual doctors working in a common cause under conditions controlled by themselves and not by government, bureaucrats, or the university.

James Buchanan "Buck" Duke is said to have become interested in medicine, especially rural medicine, through an encounter with a small boy at the construction site of a power plant at Lake James (Marion, North Carolina) where Mr. Duke, sitting in the shade of his private railroad car, was asking questions, giving orders, and making decisions. The boy was so impressed by this activity and thinking that a person so powerful and decisive must surely be able to solve any problem, asked, "Mister, can you cure fits?" Mr. Duke said, "Do you have fits?" and the boy replied, "Yes sir, and if something ain't done for me they'll kill me." While the engineers thought it was funny, Mr. Duke was so moved by the experience that he gave orders then and there that medical attention be provided for the little boy.[220] Surely, this was not the only reason for the brilliant, hard-driving, acquisitive tycoon to direct his philanthropy to medical education and medical care, but the fact that the story of this brief encoun-

220. Davison, Wilburt C.: *The Duke University Medical Center: 1892-1960.* Durham, Duke University Press, 1966, pp. 2-4.

ter lives on indicates that it was an event of some importance. Another incident narrated by Wilburt C. Davison, founding dean of Duke University Medical School, tells of Mr. Duke's treatment in 1904 for an infected toenail by Dr. W. Gill Wylie who took advantage of this opportunity to talk about a "hydroelectric plant that W. S. Lee, a South Carolina engineer, was then completing at Indian Head Shoals on the Catawba River near Rock Hill, South Carolina, with the financial backing of Doctor Wylie and others. Doctor Wylie told Mr. Duke that Mr. Lee had said that if anyone had the foresight to purchase the water rights on the long North Carolina and South Carolina rivers and build additional power plants, factories would spring up throughout the two states. Mr. Duke (whose initial fortune had been made in tobacco) had been interested in water power since 1897, so he sent for W. S. Lee, gave him a check for $100,000 and told him to start the project, which in 1905 became the Southern and later the Duke Power Company" which was to become a major resource of his great fortune.

On December 11, 1924, in his famous Indenture establishing the Duke Endowment, "Buck" Duke would spell out his philanthropic motives in these terms,

> For many years I have been engaged in the development of water power in North and South Carolina. In my study of this subject, I have observed how such utilization of a natural resource, which otherwise would run in waste to the sea and not remain and increase as a forest, both gives impetus to industrial life and provides a safe and enduring investment for capital. My ambition is that the revenues of such developments shall administer to the social welfare of the communities as the operation of such developments is administering to the economic welfare of the communities which they serve. I have selected Duke University as one of the principal objects of this trust because I recognize that education . . . is, next to religion, the greatest civilizing influence . . . . I have selected hospitals as another of the principal objects of this trust because I recognize that they have become indispensable institutions, not only by way of administering to the comfort of the sick, but in increasing the efficiency of mankind and prolonging human life —I hope that the people will see to it that adequate and convenient hospitals are assured in their respective communities. It is to these rural districts that we are to look in large measure for the bone and sinew of our country.[221]

221. *Ibid.*, pp. 2-4.

Before this written commitment would be obtained from Mr. Duke, much time would elapse and a number of disappointments experienced when a variety of plans for promoting medical education in North Carolina would be offered and would fail to attract financial support and the necessary joint approval of physicians, politicians, men of the cloth and administrators. The Duke family had early in its history been generous in its support of charitable activities. "Buck" Duke was proud of saying that if he amounted to anything in this world, he owed it to his "daddy and the Methodist Church." Washington Duke set the pattern by contributing substantially to hospitals, orphanages, colleges, and the Methodist Church, and he encouraged his sons to share in these projects. Even with this background of good will and ample financial resources, it would take great skill and imagination to direct good motives into specific channels for the public good.[222]

The road leading to the establishment of Duke University and its medical school was long and tortuous and beset with pitfalls. The major credit for engineering the success of this mission fell to a laconic and talented young man, William Preston Few, son of a physician and a graduate of Wofford College and Harvard University. Few had come to Trinity College in Durham, North Carolina, in 1896, to fill a temporary vacancy in the English department. This college, a Methodist institution, had been persuaded in 1890 to move from the small Randolph County community of Trinity, North Carolina, to Durham largely because of a substantial gift from Washington Duke, a staunch Methodist and loyal Durhamite. William Few did so well that, in 1897, B. N. Duke was persuaded by President John C. Kilgo of Trinity to endow a new chair in English to keep Few at the college. In 1902, Few became Trinity's first dean and in 1910, when Kilgo was consecrated a bishop of the Methodist Church, Few was elected President.[223] Kilgo, a fiery old-style preacher, had succeeded during his presidency (1894-1910) in raising Trinity's endowment from $22,500 to $441,339 and its assets from approximately $200,000 to $1,221,382, making it relatively free of financial problems and the best endowed college in the South.

222. Gifford, J. F., Jr.: *Evolution of a Medical Center: A History of Medicine at Duke University to 1941*. Durham, Duke University Press, 1972, p. 36.

223. *Ibid.*, Chapter 2.

The only reservation expressed over Few's election was that he was not a great orator, but he had other qualities that were destined to bring fame and fortune to Durham and its college, far beyond the imagination of those who had elected him to his post. Of more than passing interest is a statement by Few in 1903 supporting academic freedom when John Spencer Bassett, professor of history at Trinity, was attacked by Josephus Daniels, editor of the *Raleigh News and Observer,* for criticizing racism in Democratic party politics.[224] This memorandum brought Trinity College and Few to the attention of Dr. Wallace Buttrick, head of the General Education Board, and was to bear fruit in the near future. Most of Trinity's financial support had come from the Duke family and adverse newspaper publicity linking it to the "tobacco trust" hampered the approach to other sources of philanthropy. In 1911, Few succeeded in obtaining from the General Education Board through Doctor Buttrick a grant of $150,000 toward a drive for a million dollars in endowment, establishing an important precedent.

The Rockefeller Board and Foundation were now keenly aware of the existence of Trinity College of Durham, North Carolina, and the door would be open for further negotiations. More importantly, Few as president of Trinity was in a position to deal personally with the Duke family, and he exerted all of his skill in encouraging their interest in his plans, chiefly by establishing a warm and personal relationship with key members of the family. Trinity College was now the chief focus of the Duke benefactions, and by 1916 Few had become certain that James B. Duke's great fortune would be given away during his lifetime. Unquestionably, Duke himself was aware of the benefactions of Andrew Carnegie who had proclaimed that it was sinful to amass a great fortune and not to give it away before death. He was also well aware of the philanthropy of John D. Rockefeller, which was being directed largely to medical matters. How to channel Duke's generous motives from generalities to the specifics of supplying the needs of Trinity College, a university, a medical school, and hospital, was to be the major focus of Few's activities for years to come. If he failed to achieve his goals, his life as an educator

224. *Ibid.,* p. 24.

would have been a disappointment. If he succeeded, he would be making history. William Few was well aware of this, set about his task with tenacity and skill, and kept his cards well hidden from public view.

In 1916, Abraham Flexner's brother, Simon, Director of the Rockefeller Institute, showed him a letter from his old friend, William Preston Few.

> An increasing number of graduates of Trinity College are seeking a first-class medical education. For a large number of our graduates, the expense of four or five years at a good medical school is well nigh prohibitive. We are being urged over and over again to establish a two-year medical course that would be accepted at good medical schools . . . . I should be glad for an expression of your opinion as to the advisability of our undertaking this new line of work, and I should be glad for you to indicate in outline what you think we might undertake to do.[225]

An exhange of letters followed between Few and Abraham Flexner and, while no specific action was taken, the attitude of the General Education Board was one of considerable interest, but no money was offered. The advent of World War I caused all plans for Trinity College to remain in abeyance. Following the Armistice, there was an increased demand for expanded facilities for medical education, and Few resumed discussion with Abraham Flexner, members of the Duke family and the Watts family of Durham, and drew up a plan he felt might attract the widest possible support. The medical school Few proposed was to be a clinical one, offering only the last two years of study, and it was to be located in Durham as part of Trinity College. A United States Veterans Administration Hospital was to be built adjacent to the Watts Hospital in Durham where clinical facilities would be located. This plan met with Flexner's approval and in a letter to C. W. Toms, a close advisor to James B. Duke, Few said:

> Doctor Flexner and Doctor Buttrick said they ought to start with \$6,000,000 and that they would stand for \$3,000,000 of that amount and believed that their local board would, provided we can get another \$3,000,000. I told this to Mrs. Watts today and she said if we could get \$2,000,000 of this she thought \$1,000,000 could be got here. All of this looks pretty good. I think you ought to talk to J. B. D. If he will say he will give us \$1,000,000 with-

225. *Ibid.*, p. 26.

> in five years, I will undertake to raise the rest. If he will give us $2,000,000, success will be assured and I, of course, wish he would give three or more.[226]

Progress in the negotiations was slow and complicated by the effort of the University of North Carolina trustees to establish their own state-supported four-year medical school. This led again to intense wrangling among the cities of North Carolina for designation as the site of the medical school, with Charlotte putting on the major push. Governor Morrison feared that in the heat of the controversy appropriations for other university projects might suffer if the medical school failed to be assigned to Charlotte, and he was wary of taking a strong position. For similar reasons, President H. W. Chase of the University of North Carolina was wary, but he also knew that he had to press for a decision. Few, knowing that North Carolina needed only one good four-year medical school wanted it for Trinity and Durham under the combined auspices of the Dukes and the General Education Board. "Buck" Duke had intimated to him that he was going to make substantial gifts to Trinity, but had not as yet taken the necessary steps. The General Education Board would not act until the University of North Carolina's plan had been rejected or accepted. William Few came up with his second compromise, which was acceptable to both President Chase and Governor Morrison and was presented at a meeting of the University of North Carolina Board of Trustees on December 20, 1922. It called for a four-year medical school in Durham under the combined auspices of the University of North Carolina and Trinity College, with Wake Forest College and Davidson College also participating as two-year schools. A bond issue of $4,000,000 would be issued by the state and an equivalent amount would be raised by President Few from other sources. The teaching hospital would be Watts Hospital in Durham. When the plan was publicized in the press, it met with great opposition. The Baptists of North Carolina were adamantly opposed to any institutional union of church and state; the church they opposed being Methodist. The squabbles among the cities broke out anew. The University of North Carolina alumni felt they should control the school, while the Trinity alumni felt just as strongly that their

226. Woody, Robert H. (Ed.): *Papers and Addresses of William P. Few*. Durham, Duke University Press, 1951.

alma mater should be in charge. Whereas President Chase had at first agreed to dual control by the University of North Carolina and Trinity, he now reversed himself and insisted on sole control by the University of North Carolina. In this climate, the North Carolina Assembly, in January 1923, took the usual political step by approving the four-year school in principle, failing to designate any site and, finally, making no appropriation for it. The proposal was dead, the second cooperative plan sponsored by Few had gone down the drain. The time had clearly come for a unilateral plan, tossing caution to the winds and depending not upon the politics of the day but upon intelligent and generous laymen with philanthropic interests and no axe to grind. The politicians, medical and lay, had failed miserably, to the disadvantage of the sick and disabled of North Carolina. President Few's low-key reaction to the failure of his cooperative plan was that it "served two good purposes: it kept the road open for a first-rate School of Medicine later on, and it put Mr. James B. Duke on his mettle."[227]

By this time, 1923, William Few knew that he could not depend upon Abraham Flexner and the General Education Board for major capital. They had selected Vanderbilt University Medical School as their showplace for the South and were busy pouring money into it and did not feel that they could take on a major obligation in North Carolina. Faced with these facts and the double failure of the State of North Carolina to come forth with the necessary funds, Few knew that his main hope lay with "Buck" Duke, who had already indicated that he was well disposed toward Trinity, and since 1918 had joined his brother, B. N. Duke on its Board of Trustees. In fact, Few had gone so far as to draw up a proposal for Duke that needed only "Buck" Duke's signature and the ruling on such details as the number of millions to be given and when they were to be disbursed. The proposal read as follows:

> I, (James B. Duke) wish to see Trinity College, the law school and other schools expanded into a fully developed university organization. It has been suggested to me that this expanded institution be named Duke University as a memorial to my father (Washington Duke) whose gifts made possible the building of Trinity College in Durham, and I approve this suggestion. I desire this university

227. Gifford, *Evolution of a Medical Center*, 1972, p. 34.

> to include Trinity College, a coordinate College for Women, a Law School, a School of Religious Training, a School of Education, a School of Business Administration, a School of Engineering (emphasizing chemical and electrical engineering), a Graduate School of Arts and Sciences, and when adequate funds are available, a Medical School. I desire this enlarged institution to be operated under the present charter with only such changes, if any changes at all, as this enlargement may require. To this university that is to be thus organized I will give _____ millions of dolllars. I agree to pay with ___ years ___ millions either in cash or good securities.[228]

The report clearly states the provision that Trinity's name be changed to Duke, that the college be expanded to a university and, curiously, the last thing on the list is a Medical School "when adequate funds are available." The document establishes that President Few's primary interest was in getting Duke to fund a university with the medical school having a relatively low priority and without mention of a hospital or a nursing school. Were the heavy demands of a medical school and hospital so alarming to William Few that he hesitated to press this issue, especially in view of the rebuffs experienced by his cooperative plans for a medical school? Was President Few apprehensive lest he appear to be asking too much of his donor? Did he feel that once he had his university, other sources of funding a medical school would almost certainly materialize? As with all new plans, as several years went by William Few may well have altered his priorities, seeing in the medical school and hospital an opportunity for attracting the attention and support of his main benefactor who was becoming more interested in medical care than in general education. Duke's delay in expressing his formal commitment to Trinity was in part due to his prudent attitude toward his financial obligations. With the dissolution of his American Tobacco Company by the Supreme Court under antritrust laws in 1911, he expanded his investments in water power and related interests and awaited their development hoping that their success would ensure the generation of income from which obligations to charitable endeavors would be supported. The last of his major investments, a series of electric power plants in Canada, at first a little shaky, ultimately became extremely successful, leading to a merger with the Aluminum Corporation of America and

228. *Ibid.*, pp. 36-37.

assuring ample funds for what was to be Duke University, its medical school and hospital, as well as other charities.

That "Buck" Duke was not depending solely upon Few for information regarding medical care in North Carolina became especially evident in 1923, when he assigned his secretary, Alexander H. Sands, Jr. to survey the health care requirements of the Carolinas.

Duke issued specific instructions to Sands:

> to make a complete survey of the number and location of hospitals in the Carolinas, how they were controlled, the number of free and pay beds they operated, the percentage of the charges they collected from patients, and the net cost of the charity care they provided, as the basis for devising a philanthropic formula which would help to provide doctors and hospitals in the medically underdeveloped areas of these two states.[229]

It was by now obvious that Duke was interested not only in supporting education, especially medical education, but he was planning to attack the problem of health care delivery at the grass roots level. Sands asked Few to assist him with the study, and Few invited Watson S. Rankin, Secretary of the State Board of Health, to participate. Rankin was asked to recommend a plan for the development of small general hospitals in various areas of North Carolina, and he took as a model a project developed by Dr. M. M. Seymour, a health officer in Saskatchewan, Canada, for use in that province. The major theme was that modern medicine had grown to depend on advances in bacteriology, chemistry, physics, and instrumentation, and it was only in hospital settings that access to these advantages could be had. As a result, physicians crowded into cities where these facilities were available and refused to practice in rural areas. To reverse this trend, Rankin proposed that well-equipped small hospitals be built in communities willing to assume the building costs (estimated at $100,000 for fifty beds) and subsidized by having a portion of the maintenance cost (estimated at $3.00 per bed per day) provided for by the Duke interests. Rankin felt that health care was an important community responsibility not to be shifted to outside sources. With construction of local community hospitals, the drift of physicians toward the cities would be diminished, and the health needs of rural communities better provided. In addition, the

229. *Ibid.*, p. 37.

university hospital to be built in Durham would serve as a referral and consultation center as well as a center for continuing education and updating of skills.[230]

On December 1, 1924, James B. Duke, now sixty-eight years old, accompanied by personal counsel, William R. Perkins, arrived in Charlotte, North Carolina, for a meeting that was destined to revolutionize medical education and health care delivery in North Carolina. The culmination of many years of planning and discussion had been reached, and the time for vigorous action had arrived. On the following Monday, Duke spoke to the invited group of his key business associates and told them that he wished to create a charitable and educational foundation and that the group would remain in session in Charlotte until the plans had been drawn to his satisfaction. Perkins had come with a draft of a proposed charter of the new foundation that was thoroughly reviewed by all of the participants. In addition, while they worked on the charter, Duke drew up his last will and testament with his lawyer's guidance. Being a very private man, he did not permit his other advisors to see the will. In four days, the documents were completed and the charter ready for public inspection. On December 11, 1924, it was announced to the public that James B. Duke had, through an indenture of trust, created a perpetual foundation, The Duke Endowment.

> The beneficiaries, including orphanages, hospitals, educational institutions, and the Methodist Church, were those which the Duke family had supported for decades. He turned over to The Endowment securities valued at approximately $40,000,000 with the income to be distributed as stated in the indenture. Twenty percent was to be set aside until another $40,000,000 had accumulated. Of the remaining net income, Trinity College received 32 percent if and when it changed its name to Duke University. Few's plan for a university was included almost verbatim. Mr. Duke envisioned Trinity College as the undergraduate college for men in the new university. He suggested adding to it a coordinate college for women and graduate schools of religion, education, chemistry, law, medicine, business administration, arts and sciences and engineering. The Endowment trustees were instructed to provide $6,000,000 for building the university, once the name was changed, and Duke added a gift of $2,000,000 for this purpose. Davidson College and Furman University each received 5 percent and Johnson C. Smith

230. *Ibid.*, pp. 38-39.

> University, a school for Negroes in Charlotte, 4 percent.
>
> Thirty-two percent was set aside for the support of every hospital in the Carolinas not operated for private gain, according to a formula based upon Sand's research and Rankin's recommendations. Each hospital was allotted up to one dollar per day for every day of care given to charity patients.[231]

The publicity accorded this announcement was a mixed blessing for President Few who was subjected to a barrage of letters, unwanted advice, some criticism, and some question as to his fitness and Trinity's capacity to cope with the demands of this vast undertaking. William Few almost certainly knew about the contents of Duke's will, but since this had not been made public, he was unable to divulge what he knew. As a result, his answers to questions relating to the medical school and nursing school had, perforce, to be rather evasive. Mr. Duke, on the other hand, was making matters a little more difficult by openly confiding to his friends that he was going to establish the finest medical center between Baltimore and New Orleans.

The need for secrecy ceased on October 10, 1925, when James B. Duke died at the age of sixty-nine of what was reported as pernicious anemia, the successful treatment for which would be announced in 1926 and the Nobel Prize awarded for it in 1934. It seemed a pity that it was not available for Mr. Duke. The disappointment is somewhat lessened when we learn from Dean W. C. Davison that Doctor Frederic M. Hanes had a letter from Doctor George R. Minot, cowinner of the Nobel Prize for the treatment of pernicious anemia, in which he says that Mr. Duke had a rapidly progressive hemolytic anemia that was not pernicious anemia. Another authority diagnosed the illness as aplastic anemia.[232]

With the publication of the terms of the Duke will, certain key portions having to do with the medical school and the hospitals of North Carolina were now a matter of public record. In Item VIII of the will, Mr. Duke bequeathed ten million dollars to the Duke Endowment for Duke University, four million dollars of which was to be spent in erecting and equipping a medical school, hospital, and nurses' home at Duke University, the income

---

231. *Ibid.*, pp. 41-42.
232. Davison, W. C.: *Duke University Medical Center*, 1966, p. 6.

from the remainder to go to the University. Under Item XI, he bequeathed 90 percent of his residuary estate, which probably equalled the original $40,000,000, to the Hospital Section of the Duke Endowment.[233] He changed this item by a codicil dated October 1, 1925 shortly before he died, giving $7,000,000 for building at Duke University, 10 percent of the income from the remainder for support of Duke University, and 90 percent for expenditure under the hospital provision.[234]

President Few now had the financial resources to implement the grand Duke plan, and he set about it with vigor. From the very first, he realized that the sums of money allocated for construction of the medical school and hospital and the six million dollars in endowment, generous as they were, would be inadequate for the support of the major medical center envisioned by Duke. He again approached the General Education Board and Abraham Flexner who had at one time offered $3,000,000 for the first of Few's cooperative plans for a medical school in Durham. The answer was in the negative, the Rockefeller Board indicated that they were already deeply involved in supporting medical education in the South at Vanderbilt University. In any event, they wondered why Few needed any more money than the $6,000,000 endowment already committed by Mr. Duke. Despite the setback, Few proceeded with his plans, sought advice from Dr. William H. Welch of Hopkins who recommended that he appoint as dean of the new medical school a thirty-four-year-old pediatrician and assistant dean at Hopkins, Wilburt C. Davison. Other individuals of stature in medicine also spoke highly of Davison, and after deliberating for nearly a year, his mind made up, President Few arrived in Baltimore on January 19, 1927, in the office of Dr. Lewis H. Weed, Dean of the Johns Hopkins Medical School, where Wilburt C. Davison was summoned, and the following brief discussion ensued.

> Doctor Few greeted me with "I have come for you. Are you ready?" I replied, "Yes, sir." He then named the salary, the amount for building and for the endowment,and asked whether they were satisfactory. I replied, "Yes, sir." (They were in 1927.) Doctor Few asked if I could start in September and again I replied, "Yes, sir." He said he would ask the Executive Committee of the Duke

233. *Ibid.*, p. 4

234. Gifford, *Evolution of a Medical Center*, 1972, p. 43.

> University Trustees to confirm the appointment, and that was the end of the interview. Two days later (January 21, 1927), I received a laconic telegram: You have been elected. Delighted with prospect of working with you–W. P. Few. My reply was: Delighted with honor. Wish to express to you my great appreciation–W. C. Davison. To those who insist on contracts and written terms, this informality may seem amazing, but I found they were superfluous when dealing with the administration of Duke University[235]

Once the Dean was appointed, Few's policy was to let him run his division without interference. "Make you own policies, and when you get in trouble, let me know and I shall help you." With humility and candor, Davison, recalling the past said, "I was often in trouble and Doctor Few always helped."[236]

Having familiarized himself with James B. Duke's indenture and will, Davison realized that he was being called upon not only to head a new medical school. He would play a key role in shaping the destiny of hospital care and health care delivery for an entire region of the country, with special emphasis on rural areas. With the rejection by the General Education Board of the Duke appeal for additional funds for endowment of the medical school, the Duke Endowment trustees asked President Few to reconsider whether or not to start a four-year school or to be satisfied with a two-year school teaching the clinical years. Davison, of course, wanted the four-year school and felt that the breadth and scope of the Duke concept should prove extremely appealing to the General Education Board if it were reconsidered. Failure to obtain additional capital for endowment from the Rockefellers did not necessarily close off other avenues of appeal, among them annual grants and even support for individual departments of the medical school. Financial problems were mounting for Davison while the public was led to believe that there was simply no end to the millions provided by the Duke Endowment. What was not well understood was that "Buck" Duke had tied down his bounty in such a way as to provide generously for construction but relatively modestly for personnel. More significantly, so far as the medical school and hospital were concerned, he was committed to a policy of providing generous help (for those days) for Duke Hospital as well as other hospitals in the communities

235. Davison: *Duke University Medical Center,* 1966, p. 7.
236. *Ibid.,* p. 21.

of North and South Carolina. The state had one of the lowest per capita incomes of the entire nation and the economy, already depressed, would suffer even more as the Great Depression closed in. There was no health insurance of any consequence and medical expenses had to be either out of pocket or, as was usually the case for the poor, out of minimal public funds. Health care was regarded as a privilege or even a luxury. Many years would pass before it would be described as a right. Maneuvering in this climate proved difficlut for Davison, but he was more than equal to the task although there were many frustrations and delays before he was able to complete his assignment.

In preparing his case for review by the Rockefeller interests, Davison collected detailed estimates of the budget for the medical school and hospital during the first year. He estimated the total annual budget for the medical school at $331,500 with $30,000 in tuition fees from seventy-six students. He expected an average daily bed occupancy in the hospital by 100 patients who might pay one-sixth of the total cost of nine dollars per day. With Duke Endowment subsidy of one dollar per patient-day, the annual net cost of operating the hospital would be $244,000. The total net cost of operating the hospital and the medical school would be $545,000.[237] President Few was so horrified by the size of the deficit that he quickly persuaded the Duke Endowment Trustees to add a fourth story to the hospital to house more private patients which would increase the hospital income. He also wrote to Rankin that "we do not have either on hand or in sight sufficient resources to develop the other departments of the University as Mr. Duke expected us to develop them and also to support the sort of medical school and hospital that the public expects of us and that all of us want to see."[238]

For a time, Davison was concerned that because of inadequate funding, his only recourse was, for a period of at least five years, to cooperate with the ten regional preclinical schools and provide training only in the clinical departments, i. e. a two-year clinical school like those he had seen in London. When, in March 1929, the General Education Board turned down Davison's request for $250,00 annually for ten years, this seemed the only

237. Gifford, *Evolution of a Medical Center*, 1972, p. 55.

238. *Ibid.*, p. 55.

viable alternative. But Davison was not satisfied to settle for less than a four-year school and he felt that Duke and the people of North Carolina and its physicians were anticipating nothing less than a four-year school and would not settle for a two-year clinical school except as a last resort. He again appealed to the General Education Board, this time reducing the scale of his requests, hoping to get enough help so that he might carry the first two years until an increased enrollment and increased occupancy of the hospital might reduce the deficit. "Estimating the annual operating cost of preclinical instruction at $116,650, Davison requested five annual grants of $100,000, $80,000, $60,000 and $20,000, respectively, for the years 1930 through 1934, so that preclinical instruction could commence from the opening of the school in 1930." After a good deal of correspondence and persuasive discussion, the General Education Board, in November 1930, approved the Davison proposal and Duke was able to function from its beginning as a four-year medical school which was "Buck" Duke's expectation as well as of the people of North Carolina.[239]

Applications for admission to Duke Medical School were numerous, and for the first class all the decisions were made by Dean Davison. He stressed these qualities in applicants and sought to identify them: "honesty, intelligence, memory, accuracy, application, intellectual curiosity, charity, faith, humility, hope, compassion and patience."[240] He also sought rural students who might return to their home towns in the Carolinas to practice. His medical school was to stress service and work. It was not to be merely a high-powered research institute with a limited commitment to people. Davison himself was informal, people oriented, called others by their first names and expected to be so addressed himself, his nickname being "Dave." Davison expressed his creed in these terms, "The goal of the Duke University Medical Center from the beginning has been to emphasize the importance of sound teaching, good medical care, cordial and informal student-faculty relations, and mutually helpful public relations with the medical profession, and to orient the entire program toward the community needs of the Carolinas and Virginia." Later, Davison

239. *Ibid.*, p. 65.
240. Davison, *Duke University Medical Center*, 1966, p. 38.

was to say of his medical center, "The word *service* is to be carved into the corner stone."[241]

The selection of a faculty for the new medical school was to occupy a good deal of Davison's time for it would be critical to the success of both the medical school and the hospital. The first appointment was his professor of medicine, Harold L. Amoss, on February 10, 1929. Amoss had impeccable academic credentials and Davison, the son of a Methodist minister, was pleased when President Few told a Methodist clergyman Trustee, who had raised a question about Amoss' church affiliation, that his religion had nothing to do with his professional qualifications. Amoss was appointed and the freedom from religious control of Duke appointments had been clearly stated; a precedent had been set.

While Amoss' credentials were excellent from the point of view of research and academic standards, there were some deficiencies on the clinical side that became more evident after he arrived in Durham. Amoss had been Associate Professor of Medicine at Hopkins and was senior to Davison by six years. He had M.D. and Ph.D. degrees from Harvard, had been a chemist for several government agencies, and had been on the staff of the Rockefeller Institute for Medical Research where he had worked under Simon Flexner to establish the viral etiology of poliomyelitis. In 1922, he was appointed to the Hopkins staff where he continued with his research in infectious diseases, one of the projects being the development with Konrad Birkhaug of an antitoxin against erysipelas. He was not an outstanding clinician. Most of his effort and training, and his chief inclinations, lay with the laboratory investigation of disease rather than patient care. Be that as it may, this background was considered ideal for a chairman of a department of medicine in a new school, and the appointment was greeted with acclaim by the leading medical authorities of the day.

Amoss suggested that the City of Durham might be asked to build an infectious disease hospital adjacent to Duke Hospital where research in his specialty and treatment of patients with infectious disease would be conducted at a high level. Infectious diseases were not to prove to be major sources of admission to

241. Gifford, *Evolution of a Medical Center*, 1972, p. 54.

Duke Hospital in its early days. Many of these conditions were self-limited and had no specific therapy in the days before antibiotics and sulfa drugs and were treated at home. As a result, a small unit for infectious diseases built in Duke Hospital for Amoss' uses, remained under-utilized and eventually had to be turned over for other purposes. These factors and some administrative differences of opinion led to Amoss' resignation and his replacement in 1933 by Dr. Frederic M. Hanes, a practicing consultant in neurology, from Winston-Salem, North Carolina, a talented member of a distinguished and wealthy North Carolina family. The Hanes appointment will go down in the annals of Duke University Medical School as one of the wisest made by Dean Davison, although at first the comment of academicians was adverse—"Hanes, who is he?" Hanes was a graduate of Johns Hopkins, Class of 1908, and a student of Osler who had gone on to occupy positions as Assistant Professor of Pathology at Columbia University, P & S, briefly as a staff member of the Rockefeller Institute, and also the professional staff of Washington University Medical School. During World War I, he commanded the North Carolina Base Hospital No. 65, and on his return he entered practice in Winston-Salem, North Carolina, concentrating chiefly on neurology. While Hanes was not a research scientist, he was a superb clinical teacher, a perfectionist in the Osler mold. He had a commanding presence and knew how to handle the powerful and the rich as well as the poorest sharecropper. He could make decisions without vacillating, and he was one of the most frank and open men I have ever known in his discussions with patients. From him I learned a great deal about communicating with patients, responding to their needs and demands and, more than anything else, he insisted that there was only one class of patient, whether he was on the ward or in the most expensive private room. Davison, a staunch Oslerian, was now joined with an equally ardent disciple of Osler, and this was to influence a number of critical decisions that were soon to be made.

Davison was a Princeton graduate, Class of 1913, who was elected to Phi Beta Kappa, was on the varsity crew and water polo team, and in 1913 won a Rhodes Scholarship at Oxford, where he studied medicine. He planned his curriculum at Merton College, Oxford, to cover in one year at Oxford the first two years of the curriculum described in the Johns Hopkins catalogue. For this he received permission and encouragement from Sir William Osler, then Regius Professor of Medicine at Oxford. Out of this contact a relationship developed that was to influence young Davison for the rest of his life. He became a close friend of Osler and his wife and spent many happy hours in their home. In addition, starting in the very first year, Davison made weekly rounds with Osler at Radcliffe Infirmary, and he also attended informal seminars in the history of medicine held at the "Open Arms," Sir William Osler's home on the Oxford campus. He also studied anatomy at Edinburgh University, surgery at Sir Arbuthnot Lane's clinic at Guy's Hospital, London, and obstetrics at the Rotunda Hospital in Dublin, all outstanding units, the cream of British, Scotch, and Irish medicine. The advent of World War I disrupted Davison's education for a brief spell while he volunteered for service with an expedition to fight an epidemic of typhus in Serbia. On his return, he resumed his formal studies, also acting as Osler's intern; in 1915 he received a B.A. degree from Oxford and in 1916, a Bachelor of Science.

With Osler's strong recommendation, he was given credit for the first three years of medical school and returned in 1916 to enter the senior class at Johns Hopkins University School of Medicine. Here he came under the influence of John Howland, father of American pediatrics, a severe taskmaster, who rekindled in Davison an interest in pediatrics originating in his rounds with Osler at Radcliffe Infirmary. Following graduation from Hopkins, Davison served overseas in the U. S. Army Medical Corps and, in February 1919, returned to the United States to start a residency under Howland at the Harriet Lane Children's Clinic of Johns Hopkins Hospital where he remained until 1927 when he was called to Duke. An important career decision was influenced by Howland, who advised him in 1925 to become Assistant Dean at Hopkins under Dean Lewis H. Weed, "with the argument that it was better to have two strings to my medical school bow, and that some position might arise in which double training–administration and pediatric–might be needed."[242] This in a nutshell is the background of the man called to head the construction and development of the new medical school in North Carolina. The

242. Davison, *Duke University Medical Center,* 1966, p. 4.

Osler relationship and experience would be extremely critical to the decisions Davison would have to make almost at the start of his deanship.

Davison Opposes Strict Full Time and Endorses Geographic Full Time

The first confrontation was with the concept of full-time *versus* part-time, the *bête noir* of many a dean and as we have already seen, the cause in numerous other institutions of wrangling, arguments, and serious discord. When Deryl Hart of Hopkins was approached by an intermediary, Samuel Crowe, regarding the offer of the position of Professor and Chairman of the Department of Surgery at Duke, he refused the offer. His immediate reaction was that he did not want a full-time salaried position because he wanted to have the experience of developing and carrying on a private practice. One week later, Crowe told him that the Duke appointment would be on a part-time basis and Hart indicated that he was interested. Soon after this, Hart was offered the position of Professor of Surgery and Chairman of the Department at Duke by Dean Davison and was invited to visit Durham. The offer was accepted and on March 9, 1929, Hart became the third member of the Duke medical faculty. Hart says, in recording the history of these events, that the decision to insist on part-time rather than full-time was entirely of his own making and "I have no knowledge as to the part it played in the decision on one of the most important policies established in the development of the Duke Medical School—namely, placing most of the clinical faculty on so-called geographic full-time, rather than on a completely full-time status."[243] Davison's decision to place one of his chief departments under a geographic full-time head was a critical one and I am certain it was not undertaken lightly. Davison, a disciple of Osler, admired him as a person and a physician and looked to his way of life as an ideal. Osler's strong opposition to the full-time concept is imprinted indelibly on the minds of his followers and epitomized in his famous letter to Remsen.

In an essay, published in 1973, entitled *Osler's Opposition to*

---

243. Hart, D.: *The First Forty Years at Duke in Surgery and the PDC.* Durham, Duke University Press, 1971, p. 2.

Whole-Time Clinical Professors, Davison said:

> As a medical student, I saw Sir William Osler frequently during 1913 to 1915, and almost daily as his intern during 1915 to 1916. During that time I heard him say many times that "whole-time clinical professors" would be appointed on the basis of their laboratory and research reputations instead of on their humanistic interest in patients and students, and that research would supplant clinical training and experience. He chuckled in 1913 when he heard that Lewellys F. Barker, the anatomist who succeeded him in 1905 as professor of medicine at The Hopkins, and a one time advocate of "whole time," refused to go on whole-time when the Rockefeller Foundation financed the whole-time clinical program, which Franklin P. Mall, the Hopkins Professor of Anatomy, had been trying to install ever since his original appointment in 1893 . . . .
>
> . . . He also probably resented Barker's establishing three laboratories which were concerned primarily with investigation and not with the instruction of students nor with the supervision of patients.[244]

Later in this essay, Davison says: "Osler was not as opposed to 'whole time' as he was to the appointment of laboratory men without clinical experience to teach the practice of medicine." Of course, the real issue is that under the full-time system, as advocated by Flexner, there was little or no demand for the physician to acquire, develop, and utilize clinical skills. For young men in a hurry, the message was to virtually ignore clinical medicine, which was time consuming and slow in securing promotion. Anyone can be a good clinician, proponents said, while only the first class people can master the laboratory. What was being forgotten and neglected was the art of medicine, while a lemminglike migration of young physicians was under way toward the laboratory.

In still another essay, entitled *Memories of Sir William Osler,* Davison has this to say about full time from the perspective of the deanship of Duke Medical School in addition to his student exposure under Osler.

> The statement which I had heard Sir William Osler make many times while I was a medical student at Oxford, namely, that full-time appointments would lead to clinical training being supplanted by research has been thoroughly substantiated in almost every American medical school when the deluge of research grants by the

244. McGovern, J. P.: *Humanism in Medicine: Essay IV.* Springfield, Thomas, 1973, pp. 30-31.

National Institutes of Health started after the Second World War in 1946. This flood shifted the minds of many of the faculty from teaching students and creative thinking to grant-chasing, empire-building, supervising hordes of Ph.D. graduate students and other technicians, and persuaded many young physicians so greatly needed in community hospitals as well as in medical practice to remain in the ivory-towered medical schools. Osler believed that a man did not have to be a research person in order to teach; in fact, he put it more strongly: "a research man often was not fit to teach medical students."[245]

Faced with heavy obligations and limited funds, Davison made the decision to place his clinical staff on a part-time basis and to proceeded with the development of a geographic full-time clinical faculty, a concept that was anathema to Abraham Flexner and the General Education Board, and had already been responsible for major battles at Columbia, Harvard, and Rochester, as well as other medical institutions.

Davison knew that despite the magnificent Duke benefactions for buildings, there simply was not enough money to support a strict full-time salaried clinical staff. It was all he could do to provide full-time stipends for the basic science staff. In addition, he had grasped the significance of the enormous scope of the Duke proposal and its commitment, not only to education but to health care delivery in the Carolinas. For this he would need a very strong and ample staff of clinical teachers who would be the role models for his students, inspiring them to seek to emulate them. If the role models were disinterested in the actual practice of medicine, this would influence the medical students and would almost automatically be a deterrent to the Duke plan to provide practitioners for the rural and other communities of the Carolinas.

The movement of Duke to clinical part time and geographic full time may well have played a role in the failure of President Few and Davison to generate more financial assistance from the General Education Board. How else does one explain that at one point in 1921, Few was offered $3,000,000 by the Board for a medical school under the auspices of the University of North Carolina and Trinity College and then, in 1930, only after much argument and discussion, a mere $300,000 be given to help support the Duke Medical School over a period of five years?

245. Davison, Wilburt C.: Memories of Sir William Osler. *JAMA, 210:*2219-22, Dec. 22, 1969.

By 1930, the cat was out of the bag and Duke University was simply not about to embrace Flexnerian conditions on full time in the clinical departments.

Fortunately, Duke was to work out its own salvation, showing the way to a new approach for developing a great medical center by involving the active participation of its professional staff on a day-to-day basis in the generation of substantial funds from private practice to be used for the good of the entire institution and its concepts. On September 15, 1931, the Private Diagnostic Clinic was opened at Duke University Hospital for the use of the clinical teachers in the diagnosis and treatment of private patients. The space was limited, but it was at least a start. Arrangements were made for the faculty to function as a group with the pooling of fees and facilities under a mutually satisfactory formula. Financial matters were handled by a business manager. The name of the unit was the Private Diagnostic Clinic (PDC) without adding the Duke name, thereby avoiding the possible accusation that the University or the Hospital might be in the corporate practice of medicine.

> The administrators of the Medical Center (the President and Treasurer of the University, the Dean of the Medical School and the Hospital Superintendent) assured the staff that such a program, with increasing concentration of financial information, *would not be used to pry into their earnings or to limit in any way their income from private practice as long as they fulfilled their University responsibilities.*[246] (Italics added by Doctor Lepore.)

The PDC flourished and expanded to include not only diagnosis but the treatment of patients and their follow-up. In 1937, the need for additional space and the emergence of newer concepts of financial management led to the separation of the PDC into a Surgical and a Medical Division. The story of the PDC has been told in interesting detail by Deryl Hart, one of the pioneering faculty and the individual whose personal decision to insist on part time rather than full time as a condition of acceptance of the chair in surgery was almost certainly the critical first step in this direction at Duke. The voluntary diversion of millions of dollars in PDC income to new buildings, new facilities, equipment, research, and staff is now a matter of official record. The Duke faculty has shown that the altruism and idealism of a staff can be

246. Hart, *The First Forty Years*, 1971, p. 9.

sustained in a voluntary system and harnessed for the betterment of the institution and its lofty goals.

Let the record speak for itself. Duke has reached its eminence by working within the free enterprise system, developing a climate of mutual respect and faith among the University, the Hospital, and its Staff. It has given its Staff a sense of purpose and direction in selecting its own destiny. Private practice and private enterprise have supplied the capacity and resources for taking care of the poor and well-to-do alike, the same staff serving both groups. Contrary to Abraham Flexner's beliefs, part time can work better than full time when it is given an opportunity to compete. That is the Duke message, and it should ring loud and clear across our nation as other institutions and individuals seek to make changes in our system of medical education and health care delivery.

Chapter 21
THE MEDICAL SCHOOL OF THE UNIVERSITY OF CHICAGO:
Franklin C. McLean Sacrificed on the Altar of Full Time

I have no doubt that Mr. Rockefeller would favor an Institution which was neither allopathic nor homeopathic, but simply scientific in its investigations of medical science. That is the ideal.

–Frederick T. Gates
January 12, 1898[247]

The Medical School of the University of Chicago represents one of the greatest benefactions of John D. Rockefeller. Here again, as we have seen on repeated occasions in the past, the full-time principle was installed as a condition for the granting of vast sums of money that served as the leverage for controlling university policy.

Following a period of prolonged delay, procrastination, indecision, and problems with finances and, after much prodding by Abraham Flexner, the search was instituted for a dean to head the new medical school. Many outstanding individuals were considered, and Francis W. Peabody of Boston was the overwhelming favorite. Despite all manner of pressure, Peabody declined the offer and elected to remain in Boston where he was Director of the Thorndyke Memorial Laboratory and Professor of Medicine at Harvard.

The person finally chosen in 1923 to head the Chicago medical enterprise was a very unusual individual, Franklin C. McLean (1888-1968), who earned his baccalaureate degree at the University of Chicago in 1907 and went on to work in the Department of Physiology under the great Anton J. Carlson, earning his Ph.D. and M.D. degrees simultaneously at the University of Chicago and Rush Medical College in 1910. A native of Maroa,

247. Corner, George W.: *History of Rockefeller Institute, 1901-1953.* Rockefeller University Press, 1964, p. 582.

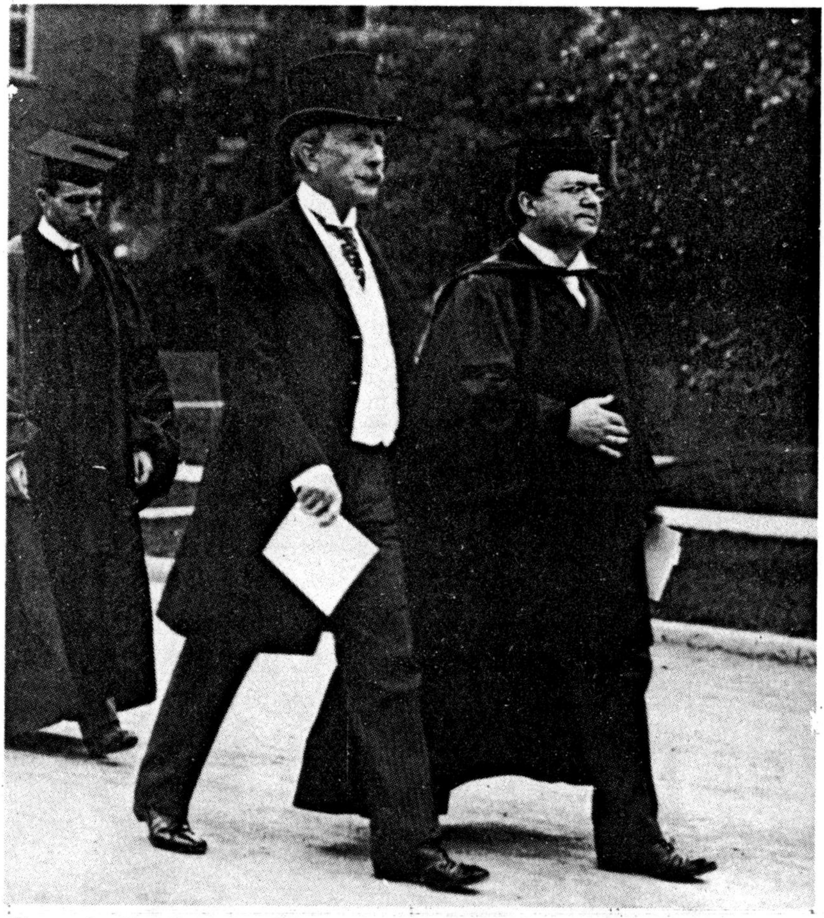

Figure 3. The Founder did not see the University until 1896, when he attended the celebration of its fifth birthday. This photograph was taken in 1901 during the decennial celebration when Rockefeller made his second visit to the University. Martin A. Ryerson, President of the Board of Trustees, follows Rockefeller and Harper. From: Storr, R. J., *A History of the Univ. of Chicago: Harper's University*, p. 328 in Chap. 36, Univ. Chi. Press, 1966.

a small town in Illinois, and the son and grandson of physicians, McLean, after internship at Cook County Hospital, settled in Portland, Oregon, where he was appointed professor of pharmacology in a wretched medical school characterized by Abraham Flexner as having neither resources nor ideals and having no justification for its existence. In this unlikely setting, McLean succeeded in accomplishing more than had others in more pretentious quarters. During 1913-1914, in a one-room laboratory classroom, he developed the first quantitative method for measuring blood sugar and, in addition, published one of the earliest papers on the mathematical calculation of urea clearance.

Marshall R. Urist, in a delightful essay on McLean, says of his mentor:

> As was the custom in the United States in the early part of this century, he traveled to Europe to study in medical centers in Austria and Germany. He found a place to his liking in Graz in the laboratory of Professor Otto Löewi where, in 1914, he worked for nine months. In Graz, in the tumultuous few months leading to World War I, he mastered the German language and witnessed the dawn of modern knowledge of the biochemistry of the transmission of nerve impulses.* . . . Filled with the excitement of laboratory science in medicine, he sailed back across the Atlantic and headed straight for the Rockefeller Institute for Medical Research in New York.[248]

The ensuing events could only have happened in America in 1914. An unheralded and virtually unknown physician—graduate of a midwestern medical school and teacher in a fifth-rate medical school in Oregon—walks unannounced into the front door of the Rockefeller Institute looking for work. Urist continues,

> Rufus Cole, director of the hospital and institute, interviewed young McLean and invited him to stay to luncheon to meet Donald Van Slyke. By coincidence, Van Slyke had just finished reading McLean's paper on quantitative measurements of blood sugar. As soon as luncheon was over, Van Slyke appealed to Cole to appoint McLean assistant resident to fill a vacancy in cardiology. Cole assigned him to Alfred Cohn to work on the biochemistry of edema, and to Van Slyke to devise quantitative methods of studying urinary chloride and nonprotein nitrogen. Cohn provided McLean with unlimited

* For his contributions to this field, Löewi, in 1936, was to share a Nobel Prize in Physiology with Henry H. Dale of Great Britain.

248. Urist, Marshall R.: Phoenix of physiology and medicine: Franklin C. McLean. *Perspectives in Biol and Med, 19/1:*23-58, Autumn 1975.

> funds for research and scientific equipment such as he had never seen before in a clinical laboratory. He went immediately to work and devised one of the first methods for determining renal function by an index of urea excretion. As he happily grappled with the mathematical formulae for kidney function, Cohn was busily experimenting with his future. Cohn indoctrinated him in the coming revolution in medical education in the United States. Cohn's experiment, as related below, was to take shape in the form of a Rockefeller Foundation project at the University of Chicago which would stir a major controversy in academic medicine in the United States. . . . Cohn lost no time in reporting to Rufus Cole about young McLean's perceptive mind and his extraordinary understanding not only of biochemistry but also of the sociologic aspects of medical science. Cole, in turn, sent news to Abraham Flexner and Simon Flexner of his young assistant resident from Illinois who by good fortune just walked into his office right off the boat from Graz. Abraham greeted the young man with his manuscripts on reform measures in medicine, probed his young mind for ideas, and proceeded to shape his career for the ensuing 16 years. Cole, who similarly began exchanging ideas with his assistant resident, continued to correspond with him for nearly fifty years about the philosophy of medical education[249]

This background and this indoctrination would, at the same time, be McLean's greatest assets and conversely would lead ultimately to his downfall as the head of the new medical school planned for Chicago. Before he would reach this milestone in his career, he would first be selected, in 1916, by the trustees of the Rockefeller Foundation, at the youthful age of twenty-eight, to build and develop a modern western-type medical school in China, the Peking Union Medical College and Hospital. Here, his preoccupation with laboratory investigation created some problems and, by April 1920, he gave up his duties as director of the hospital and dean of the medical school to become chairman and professor of medicine to devote more time to his research laboratory.

When McLean was recalled to the United States in June 1923 by the Rockefeller Foundation, he anticipated reassignment to laboratory research. Instead, he was asked to head the new medical school at the University of Chicago, and he accepted the challenge to return to his Alma Mater to establish a full-time program in a university medical school on the lines long envisioned by

249. *Ibid.* pp. 25-26.

Abraham Flexner and his colleagues at the Rockefeller Institute. This was no small project and it was beset with many traps and pitfalls, testing McLean and his mentors to the utmost. The enemy in China had been the practitioners of traditional Chinese medicine, whereas in Chicago the enemy would be entrenched and powerful men in private practice who would fight the full-time system tooth and nail.

Was McLean the best all around choice for this undertaking, or was he chosen because of his availability and his commitment to scientific medicine and to the precepts of his supporters at the Rockefeller Institute and the General Education Board? Alfred Cohn, Rufus Cole, and both Flexners had expended considerable effort in programming McLean for a chair in medicine in a university medical school and saw the new school of the University of Chicago as an ideal opportunity to put into effect their theories of medical education. Committed, as they were, to medicine as a science, they saw no flaws in McLean, paid little or no attention to his lack of clinical experience, and promoted his candidacy as a rather ideal prototype of the university dean and professor of medicine of the future.

The hand-picked choice of the Flexners, Alfred Cohn, and Rufus Cole, McLean arrived in Chicago toward the end of 1923 as Professor and Chairman of the Department of Medicine and Chairman of the Committee on Organization and Development of the Medical School. His mission was "to plan and organize the building, faculty, and curriculum of a full-time hospital and school of medicine." Much of his time was to be spent on administrative details, staffing, committee meetings, and planning for construction of the new school.[250] In spite of the generosity of the Rockefellers, Rosenwald, Billings, Lasker, and many others, financial insecurity was to plague the new institution from the very beginning, and there never seemed to be a time when the available funds were enough for its needs. Part of this could be attributed to rampant inflation, expanding new projects, and increasing costs of construction. In fact, the provisions for budget and carrying expenses of the institution were unrealistic and impractical from the very onset. New funds were sought but were difficult to obtain as the Great Depression developed.

250. *Ibid.*, p. 31.

President Judson of the University of Chicago seemed overwhelmed by financial problems and sought by retrenchment to keep the university viable. When he was replaced by Ernest D. Burton in 1923, there was considerable activity only to terminate with Burton's sudden and unexpected death in May 1925. Adjustments had to be made to a new administration and new presidency and these, of course, slowed down the momentum. Funds, originally donated by the Rockefeller boards for endowment had to be diverted to construction and bricks and mortar to solve immediate problems, the decision only postponing the inevitable day when these same funds would be needed for salaries of the full-time staff. Forward movement of construction was extremely slow. Not until October 2, 1925 was the cornerstone laid for the Billings Hospital, and it would be two years before the first patients were admitted.

By 1927, McLean who had been traveling abroad, working in Friedrich von Müller's clinic in Munich and then in Van Slyke's laboratory at the Rockefeller Institute, returned to Chicago to find many problems awaiting him. First in importance was a nasty argument over full time precipitated by the Rush faculty, which had been merged with the University of Chicago as a measure intended to safeguard access to the Presbyterian Hospital, the major source for teaching material for medical students pending the construction of a university hospital. A powerful nucleus of the Rush faculty pressed hard for abandonment of the full-time plan in favor of part time. The dispute was acrimonious and would not be resolved for many years. The most obvious reason for dissension was that at no time did the university have in hand the major sums of money needed to support a Flexnerian full-time clinical faculty. No matter what, in the struggle for mere survival, the university found that it had to rely upon the part-time practitioners for the clinical instruction and education of its medical students.

Those who were attracted to full-time clinical chairs were soon disaffected and unable to subsist on the modest salaries allocated to them. An example in point is Dallas Phemister, who left a lucrative and productive private practice for full-time service as chairman of surgery. This meant major sacrifices on his part as well as his family's. Living expenses had to be reduced, life-styles changed, and a smaller house accepted, etc. Despite all this, Phemister had to dip into his savings and was well on his way into insolvency when mild remedial action was taken by McLean by raising his university salary. The agony and distress of as idealistic and competent a man as Phemister, torn between the reasonable and not excessive demands of his family and his inability to provide adequately for them out of his salary, is a disturbing human aspect of the full-time concept that is bound to upset any fair-minded person sitting in judgement. Phemister knew that when he was in private practice he had earned enough to provide for his family, to support his research laboratory, and to not have to go begging for his subsistence. Trouble was bound to come, and it was not long before it really broke loose.

On July 29, 1930, McLean wrote to Alfred Cohn at the Rockefeller Institute, indicating his skepticism toward Flexner's claim that other institutions committed to full time were really following it rigidly to the letter, saying,

> I welcome comparison with an ideal and I also welcome comparison with other institutions. I do not regard it, however, as in keeping with realities to compare us with other institutions under an assumption that the other institutions are ideal unless it can be shown that they actually are so. Is this clear, and am I justified in my position?[251]

On February 3, 1930, Flexner, now retired from the General Education Board, sent a rather innocuous-appearing letter to McLean that was fraught with considerable evil.

> Dear McLean: I am assembling data for the purpose of finding out how much money has been turned into university clinics by the full-time men in the department of surgery in each of the medical schools on the full-time basis. I shall be very happy if you can send me a memorandum dealing with this item for the year 1929. I am making a similar inquiry of all other medical schools on the full-time basis.[252]

Rather than give Flexner a frank answer, McLean, smelling trouble, sought to parry. In his reply to Flexner, on February 5, 1930, he indicated that his institution had deliberately avoided accounting for income from professional fees by departments, in accordance with the principle that the income-producing power

251. Letter, July 29, 1930, F. C. McLean to A. Cohn, University of Chicago–General Education Board, Rockefeller Foundation Archives: 1930-35.

252. *Ibid.*, A. Flexner to F. C. McLean, February 3, 1930.

of an individual, or of a department, was not to be taken into consideration in fixing departmental budgets or individual salaries.

> At the cost of considerable work, we could undoubtedly answer the question raised in your letter of February 3, but so far as we are concerned, we would rather not know the answer. If, in spite of this you still wish to have the figure we would be most happy to get it for you.253

On February 7, 1930, Flexner bore down on McLean saying:

> I am sorry to give you so much trouble. The situation, however, is as follows: it has been frequently said that the full-time system results in the exploitation to greater or less extent of men on full time in behalf of the hospital or medical school. In my opinion, every medical school ought to be in position to meet this statement. As I wrote you, I sent similar letter to the Hopkins, Rochester, New Haven, etc., and I received answers practically by return mail.254

McLean's reply of February 11, 1930, continued to be rather guarded and defensive, and he took the precaution of sending copies to President Hutchins and Mr. Plimpton of the University of Chicago.

Flexner's next letter to McLean, February 21, 1930, was on the surface quite innocent and designed to keep the dialogue going, but he continued to press for data on full-time staff income. Finally, on February 24, 1930, Flexner received the specific information he had sought from the beginning. McLean reported that the total billed income for professional services rendered by the Department of Surgery during the calendar your 1929 was $83,726.50.

Flexner continued to play with his mouse, writing on March 1, 1930, requesting more specific information and was told by McLean that of the total of $83,726.50, "not less than $70,000 was turned in by the full-time members of the surgical staff, exclusive of Otolaryngology and Ophthalmology." On March 8, 1930, Flexner began to let the cat out of the bag, raising the question of why the Chicago "full-time" income was so much greater than Yale, Johns Hopkins, and Rochester where it amounted to $10,241.60, $4,770, and $6,650, respectively.

The information Flexner was really looking for is in McLean's reply of March 24, 1930.

---

253. *Ibid.*, McLean to Flexner, February 5, 1930.
254. *Ibid.*, Flexner to McLean, February 7, 1930.

> Mrs. McLean and I have just returned from two weeks in New Mexico and I find your letter of March 8 awaiting me.
>
> I suspected that you would find a very great difference between the figures from the University of Chicago and those of the other medical schools, and your letter confirms my suspicions.
>
> The reason for this is very simple since our figures reflect the clinical policy adopted at the time of the opening of the University of Chicago Clinics. You will recall that at that time we adopted a policy which would make it possible for us to collect a considerable proportion of hospital costs from patients. Our theory was that if we opened the hospital and out-patient department on a charity basis we would have little or no income from patients to offset the expense of operating the clinics, while if we opened the clinics on a pay basis somewhat similar to that of the Cornell Clinic we might expect at least a reasonable income from patients. In view of our urgent financial need the latter plan was adopted and is fully described in a folder reproducing our agreement with the Chicago Medical Society, of which I am enclosing several copies.
>
> Since we do not accept charity cases as a routine, most of our patients admitted either to the wards or private rooms pay some professional fee as adjusted by our Admitting Office, and since all of our general surgery is done by the full-time staff the income from surgical fees is correspondingly high. The majority of our patients are of the class received by the Cornell Clinic—that is, just above the charity class. Since we are the only institution in Chicago making provision for this class of patients the demand on us is very heavy and for nearly a year we have had to impose a system of selective admissions. In addition to this class of patients we accept charity patients when they are of particular interest to the staff and we have also a fair amount of work with so-called private patients the latter of course furnishing a considerable amount of income.[255]

Quite predictably, this letter of McLean's sent Flexner into a real frenzy causing him to mount a vicious attack upon his friend and protege. For some reason this exchange of letters is not mentioned in any of the historical documents available to me in 1978 covering the University of Chicago medical school, including the history written by Ilza Vieth and Franklin McLean. Perhaps the episode was too unpleasant to record, but accurate history demands that it be placed in the record.

In this rather startling and abrasive attack on McLean et al., Flexner said:

---

255. *Ibid.*, McLean to Flexner, March 24, 1930.

April 1, 1930

Dear McLean:

Thank you for your candid statement. I did not answer it promptly, because I was too disappointed and too profoundly shocked, but we must face the facts.

I persuaded Mr. Gates and others to participate in establishing the Medical Department on the Campus of the University of Chicago on the ground that we could establish there an institution following the model of the Johns Hopkins. On that basis, the General Education Board made its contribution, and on that basis I appealed to others. On no other basis would it have been possible to do anything at all. In the original contract this basis was explicitly set forth, but reflection having convinced us that, in the *long* course of time conditions might change, the contract was modified so as to leave the University free in its wisdom to do otherwise, if experience proved that doing otherwise was proper and sound. In the letter which I myself sent to every university in transmitting the changed contract, I made it quite clear that it was supposed that the spirit of the contract would be lived up to through a period of sufficient length to warrant modification, if modification there needed to be. Your letter quite frankly states that your motive was financial, though of course you naturally say in your own defense that the results have justified you. You will remember that I urged upon one president of the University of Chicago after another the importance of taking steps to finance the Hospital. No such steps were ever taken, nor have they been taken to this day. Instead, the purpose, for which the institution was founded, has been abandoned in order that the School and Hospital might become profit-making institutions. You have, in other words, instead of a full-time clinic on the Hopkins or another model, a Mayo Clinic on a small scale, simply limiting your earnings to what is needed to carry the Hospital and the Staff. I am not criticising the Mayo Clinic. I am simply pointing out that the Mayo Clinic and the clinics at Baltimore and St. Louis are different things. You were pledged to the latter, not to the former.

Now the whole full-time arrangement was meant to free the full-time staff from the necessity of doing uninteresting routine in order that they might devote themselves to teaching and research. Your arrangement, according to your own statement, puts your surgeons in a position where they have to operate, inasmuch as their services are at the command of anyone who enters the Hospital. It is an absolute surrender, and I shall so describe it in the volume on Universities which I have in preparation; for in this volume, as in previous things, I shall hew to the line no matter where the chips fall—a painful operation, you may well believe but I shall not sacrifice my intellectual integrity for any reason whatsoever.

I can now understand a number of things which have puzzled me in the past.

Please remember that I am writing you, not as an officer of the General Education Board, with which I have no connection and for which I have no responsibility, but as a student of university education in general and of medical education in particular.

Sincerely yours,
(Signed) Abraham Flexner

Dr. Franklin C. McLean
The University of Chicago
Department of Medicine
Chicago, Illinois[256]

Flexner followed this blistering epistle with a letter to the General Education Board requesting copies of the original memoranda of 1917 describing the terms of agreement between the University of Chicago and the Rockefeller Foundation and General Education Board. On receipt of these, Flexner commented in a letter of April 15, 1930, to Mr. W. W. Brierley of the G.E.B:

> Many thanks for your kindness in sending me the two memoranda. It is perfectly obvious from both of them that the Board subscribed its funds to the Medical Department of the University of Chicago for the purpose of creating there a school of the same type as the schools of Baltimore and St. Louis. Mr. Gates, to mention no others, would never have agreed to the appropriation of a dollar on any other terms.[257]

McLean's reply to Flexner, dated May 10, 1930, is a long point-by-point skillful rebuttal of the master by his pupil conveyed in ten and one-half pages of single-spaced type. It resembles a legal brief that systematically rejects most of Flexner's criticisms and claims. Of course, McLean was not adhering to strict full time as defined by Flexner, and in this sense he was breaking with his mentor no matter what the justification may have been.

The original sources attest that McLean was absolutely right when he said that Flexner had known about the private or group practice plan in Chicago from the very beginning and had raised no objection. Why then, the complete about-face in 1930 and the tirade against the University of Chicago and McLean? Was it perhaps that Flexner, immersed in his new book on medical education, realized in retrospect that he had condoned a breach

256. *Ibid.*, Flexner to McLean, April 1, 1930.
257. *Ibid.*, Flexner to Brierley, April 15, 1930.

in pure full time in Chicago and that he had to defend his rigid concept of full time to the death if necessary against the modifications and compromises that were springing up around the country? He would be reluctant to admit that his full-time policy in its purest form had never worked. He hated to compromise, and in the end this would be his undoing.

This was Flexner's reply to McLean on May 13, 1930.

> I am frightfully sorry that you felt called upon to prepare this elaborate memorandum. It reached me last night, and I am sailing for Europe tomorrow morning, so that I have to go through it more hastily than I like.
>
> I do not wish to argue the matter further, for there is really nothing that can be accomplished in this way. Let me only say that, whatever the merits or demerits of what the school is doing, you yourself clearly admit that you are not doing what the school and the University undertook to do. If you will look at the last page but two of this memorandum at the letter which I addressed to President Burton, you will see a reference to Dr. Welch's letter of October 21, 1915. You may not be aware of the fact that the *Rockefellers had determined absolutely to have nothing to do with medicine at Chicago after the University made its affiliations with Rush.* I overcame that opposition by persuading Mr. Gates and others that the University of Chicago would do what the Hopkins was doing. We were dealing with trust funds. The University was accepting trust funds, and people who give or accept trust funds have no right to depart from the terms upon which the transaction was based. I repeat what I said to you before that, if I had told Mr. Gates and the others the outlines of your present scheme, no medical school would have been established with General Education Board funds on the Campus of the University. All the argument on earth cannot get away from that central and absolutely irremovable fact. I would not have asked, and Mr. Gates and the others would have "turned me down," if I had asked it.[258]

By this time the correspondence had become too hot for McLean to handle alone, especially in the light of Flexner's accusations of betrayal of a trust. McLean placed the matter in the hands of his superior, President Robert M. Hutchins, who wrote to Arnett of the General Education Board on May 22, 1930[259]

> Dear Mr. Arnett:
>
> I enclose copies of correspondence between Mr. Abraham Flexner and Doctor F. C. McLean, Director of The University of Chi-

258. *Ibid.*, Flexner to McLean, May 13, 1930.

259. *Ibid.*, Hutchins to Arnett, May 22, 1930.

cago Clinics.

You will observe that in his letter of May 13, Mr. Flexner says that The University of Chicago accepted Trust Funds for the establishment of its Medical School and its Clinics and has departed from the terms upon which the transaction was based.

After you have examined this correspondence I should be glad to learn from you whether in the opinion of the present officers of the General Education Board the University of Chicago has diverted trust funds as charged by Mr. Flexner.

Very truly yours,
Robert M. Hutchins
President

Mr. Trevor Arnett, President
General Education Board
61 Broadway
New York City

On May 29, 1930, Arnett wrote in reply to Hutchins:

With regard to the question you raise whether the University has not used the funds given to it by the General Education Board for the purposes for which they were intended, I would state that it is the policy of the Board in connection with gifts made to educational institutions to rely fully upon the good faith of the trustees of the institutions to use the gifts for the purposes for which they were given.[260]

Arnett's answer was reassuring to Hutchins and McLean, indicating that the G.E.B. did not support Flexner's position and vindicating McLean. The price of victory was, however, high. McLean, already under attack by his enemies and those who favored part time over full time, was now abandoned by his mentor and vulnerable to attack. To compound the evil, both the nation and the university were faced with severe economic stresses.

The Great Depression that followed the stock market crash of 1929 created serious financial problems for the university medical clinics and led to further demands that full time be abandoned in favor of part time. Only the pledge of $500,000 for faculty salaries by McLean's good friend and patient, Julius Rosenwald, with Albert Lasker and Max Epstein saved the full-time plan for another year, but it was a losing battle that was becoming more acrimonious as the depression deepened. McLean as the leader of the full-timers and the representative of the

260. *Ibid.*, Arnett to Hutchins, May 29, 1930.

Rockefeller interests was more and more exposed to attack. Some of the attacks were fairly vicious. McLean had become tired of faculty feuds and wrangling and had taken steps to divest himself of some of his titles and authority. An idealist, not a Machiavellian, he forgot that the outside world was not yet ready to accept his concepts. In giving up his power, he committed a cardinal sin among rulers, for he placed himself at the mercy of his enemies before he had adequately protected his own position. McLean's main talents lay in the laboratory and not in clinical medicine or administration. His career was, in the words of a biographer, "to illustrate the wasteful practice of burdening a talented young physician with one administrative appointment after another during the most productive years of his life." The final episode of this scenario is told by Marshall Urist with the depth of feeling only a true friend and disciple could have.

> By 1933, the anti-full-timists were determined more than ever to eliminate the strange bird dominating the medical school policy. A. Baird Hastings, whom McLean had brought from the Rockefeller Institute and Peking to be the Lasker Professor of Biochemistry, was the decoy. Unwittingly, Hastings one day asked McLean to assist him and Dr. Lillian Eichelberger in setting up a heart perfusion apparatus on a dog. McLean had learned the method in Otto Lőewi's laboratory in Graz 20 years earlier. On that fateful day, McLean and Hastings found that minute variations from normal in calcium ion concentration instantly and measurably change the force of contraction of the heart muscle, whereas comparable small changes in other ions primarily modify the EKG . . . .
>
> Scammon stormed into Hasting's laboratory and accused McLean of being more concerned with investigations on mice, rats and monkeys than on sick people. Scammon called Hastings into the dean's office later in the day and declared that McLean had no business working on animals in a laboratory.[261]

Some years later, Hastings, still smarting under this rebuke, recalled the interview with Scammon.

> One day we were hard at work studying these ion effects in detail when I got a call from the Dean's office. It was certainly not the most propitious moment for me to call on the Dean. I was hot, sweaty, and dehydrated from several hours work in our 38° room which was, of course, saturated with water vapor. To my utter astonishment, I learned from the Dean that a condition of acceptance by the incoming Chairman of Medicine was that McLean was

261. Urist, *Perspectives in Biol and Med,* 1975, p. 44.

> not to work anywhere within the precincts of the Department of Medicine, which included my laboratory. Even today, I cannot recall this incident without my blood "boiling," as it did then.[262]

Following this episode in 1933, at a special faculty meeting, McLean's resignation was requested with only one dissenting vote. His resignation was greeted by some as a victory for the anti-full-time faction and by others as a tragic casualty of the depression that had made it impossible for him to fulfill his promises to the faculty. Urist characterizes him as "a sacrificial lamb for Flexner, Cole, Cohn and other evangelists of the full-time doctrine."[263]

In 1979, further light was shed on the McLean controversy by Walter L. Palmer in his essay, *Franklin Chambers McLean and the Founding of the University of Chicago School of Medicine.*[264] Here, Palmer, who was an active and distinguished member of the department of medicine, adds previously unpublished data and, for the first time, in a footnote, refers to the angry exchange of letters between Abraham Flexner and McLean on the full-time issue, crediting Cornelius W. Vermeulen, Emeritus Professor of Urology and Deputy Dean of Biological Division of the University of Chicago, with uncovering the correspondence which, independently, I had already discovered in the archives of the General Education Board, at Pocantico Hills, New York. Palmer states that in 1932, the department of medicine had great difficulty in selecting a new chairman to succeed Russell Wilder who had returned to the Mayo Clinic. Frank Lillie, Dean of the Division of the Biological Sciences, insisted that George Dick, his personal physician, be chosen despite the fact that the senior medical faculty did not want him and had voted on three consecutive occasions against his appointment. Lillie persisted and wore down the faculty and won out, but Palmer says, "Only later was it learned that the condition imposed by Dick for his acceptance of the appointment was that McLean should be 'off the premises.' " Documentation for this agreement was only recently uncovered by Vermeulen in a telegram dated, July 9, 1932, ad-

262. Nichols, G. and Wasserman, R. H. (Ed.): *Cellular Mechanisms for Calcium Transfer.* New York, Academic Press, 1971, pp. xxxiii-xl.
263. Urist, *Perspectives in Biol and Med,* 1975, p. 46.
264. Palmer, W. L.: Franklin Chambers McLean and the founding of the University of Chicago School of Medicine. *Perspectives, 22/2:*Part 2, S2-S32, Winter 1979.

dressed to Dean Lillie, reading,

> On the basis of the demand of Dr. Dick, I will withdraw unconditionally from my professorship in the Department of Medicine on or before the date on which his appointment begins and from all activities—professional, research or otherwise—directly or indirectly under the jurisdiction of that department. [Signed] Franklin McLean.[265]

Palmer, who was on the scene, professes not to know why Dick wanted to get rid of McLean and characterizes the action as "both ruthless and improper." Perhaps a partial answer is to be found in an anecdote related by Palmer.[266]

> McLean did make some unfortunate mistakes. One of these errors involved Joseph A. Capps, a protégé of Frank Billings and an elder statesman who had done a great deal for McLean. Capps, a member of the staff of St. Luke's Hospital, had been McLean's friend and senior advisor with an appointment as clinical professor in the Department of Medicine. His clientele included many distinguished Chicago citizens, of whom Julius Rosenwald was one. McLean had become a more recent friend of Rosenwald, one of the three philanthropists to whom McLean had turned when the full-time system was in financial jeopardy. One May day at the annual spring meeting of the Association of American Physicians in Atlantic City, McLean learned that Rosenwald was in Atlantic City and was ill. McLean took his friend Alfred Cohn, a cardiologist of the Rockefeller Institute, to Rosenwald's room for consultation without the prior consent of Capps, who was also in Atlantic City, perhaps unknown to McLean although both men habitually attended this annual meeting. Subsequently, Capps was superseded in his care of Rosenwald by the trio of Cohn in New York, McLean in Chicago, and one of the younger men in the Department of Medicine, Louis Leiter, who lived with the Rosenwalds for a few weeks or months. Capps, a genial, friendly, lovable man, was deeply hurt. The incident was doubtless exaggerated by McLean's enemies. Capps played bridge and golf with members of the ill-defined anti-McLean group, and was dearly beloved by his friends, so that any affront to him was magnified by them a hundredfold.[267]

That Capps was a good friend of George Dick did not make things easier for McLean. It is a strange thing that a leading proponent of the full-time system should meet his Waterloo by taking a private patient away from a part-time practitioner-teacher. In closing the McLean episode, I ask the question: Was it McLean

265. *Ibid.*, p. S20.
266. *Ibid.*, p. S21.
267. *Ibid.*, p. S23.

who failed, or was it the Flexnerian full-time system that failed to measure up to the needs of the era? Was Flexner's dream Utopian and completely out of touch with reality? Was it ever a workable plan?

Chapter 22
THE SECRET OF THE CARE OF THE PATIENT

One of the essential qualities of the clinician is interest in humanity, for the secret of the care of the patient is in caring for the patient.

—Francis Weld Peabody (1926)

We have already seen that staffing of the new school in Chicago was not easy. The first-line men had refused positions, and the bids had gone down the list. The offer to Francis W. Peabody has already been discussed. Peabody, whose credentials were of a high order, was so different from McLean in his philosophy and goals as to warrant further discussion at this point.

In 1923, McLean and his supporters stood for science in medicine with a capital S, while service to patients was low on their list of priorities. Peabody, with even more impeccable scientific credentials, including service at Johns Hopkins, the Rockefeller Institute and Hospital, Berlin, China, substantial research publications, Professor of Medicine at Harvard, and Director of the Thorndike Memorial Laboratory, had not neglected his clinical skills, and emerged from this background, or despite it, as a balanced physician, teacher, investigator, and clinician who believed that the prime obligation of a true physician was to the care of the sick. He felt that medicine was not a science but an art practiced along scientific lines.

Peabody, in the prime of his professional life, age forty-three, suffered a gastrointestinal hemorrhage in 1924. A victim of the lack of the technologic diagnostic advantages that we take almost for granted today, Peabody's bleeding was erroneously attributed to a benign gastric ulcer, the true cause being a carcinoma of the stomach. Diagnosed too late, in July 1926, it was declared inoperable at laparotomy. The anguish and grief of his many medical friends were almost beyond belief. Peabody knew his diagnosis and, despite his weakness and discomfort, continued to teach, make rounds, and to advise students, house staff, and other associates. Serious illness can seldom be kept secret, and before long it was common knowledge in the Boston community that their beloved and brilliant professor of medicine was stricken with a fatal illness. So it was that on a Sunday in November 1926, when he delivered a public lecture on "The Care of the Patient," at Harvard Medical School to his medical students and staff, they were joined by many of his lay friends and family who knew the facts. In the words of his father, The Reverend Francis Greenwood Peabody, Dean of Harvard University Divinity School:

> To those who listened to the address the scene was peculiarly touching, for they knew, as he did, that he spoke from out the shadow of disease, and that each allusion to the patient as a person, rather than as a "case" carried an unspoken and poignant reference.[268]

This essay expresses a philosophy of medicine and a Christian outlook that will live as long as we have a civilization and as long as medicine retains its hold on the art as well as its science. Every medical student should carry a copy of this essay in his pocket and refer to it whenever there is a need for renewal of faith, idealism, and concern for his fellowman. It should be read and reread by all physicians and, in fact, by all who dream of a career in medicine. Peabody began his talk by saying,

> It is probably fortunate that most systems of education are constantly under the fire of general criticism, for if education were left solely in the hands of teachers the chances are good that it would soon deteriorate. Medical education, however, is less likely to suffer from such stagnation, for whenever the lay public stops criticizing the type of modern doctor, the medical profession itself may be counted on to stir up the stagnant pool and cleanse it of its sedimentary deposit. The most common criticism made at present by older practitioners is that young graduates have been taught a great deal about the mechanism of disease, but very little about the practice of medicine—or, to put it more bluntly, they are too "scientific" and do not know how to take care of patients.
>
> . . . Medicine is not a trade to be learned but a profession to be entered. It is an ever-widening field that requires continued study and prolonged experience in close contact with the sick. All that the medical school can hope to do is to supply the foundations

268. Peabody, F. G.: *Francis Weld Peabody, 1881-1927: A Memoir.* Cambridge, Riverside Press, 1933.

> on which to build. When one considers the amazing progress of science in its relation to medicine during the last thirty years, and the enormous mass of scientific material which must be made available to the modern physician, it is not surprising that the schools have tended to concern themselves more and more with this phase of the educational problem. And while they have been absorbed in the difficult task of digesting and correlating new knowledge, it has been easy to overlook the fact that the application of the principles of science to the diagnosis and treatment of disease is only one limited aspect of medical practice. The practice of medicine in its broadest sense includes the whole relationship of the physician with his patient. It is an art, based to an increasing extent on the medical sciences, but comprising much that still remains outside the realm of any science. The art of medicine and the science of medicine are not antagonistic but supplementary to each other. There is no more contradiction between the science of medicine and the art of medicine than between the science of aeronautics and the art of flying. Good practice presupposes an understanding of the sciences which contribute to the structure of modern medicine, but it is obvious that sound professional training should include a much broader equipment.[269]

Finally, in the culmination of this magnificent essay, Peabody expresses in immortal phrases, his philosophy of patient care.

> There are moments, of course, in cases of serious illness when you will think solely of the disease and its treatment; but when the corner is turned and the immediate crisis is passed, you must give your attention to the patient. Disease in man is never exactly the same as disease in an experimental animal, for in man the disease at once affects and is affected by what we call the emotional life. Thus, the physician who attempts to take care of a patient while he neglects this factor is as unscientific as the investigator who neglects to control all the conditions that may affect his experiment. The good physician knows his patients through and through, and his knowledge is bought dearly. Time, sympathy, and understanding must be lavishly dispensed, but the reward is to be found in that personal bond which forms the greatest satisfaction of the practice of medicine. One of the essential qualities of the clinician is interest in humanity, for the secret of the care of the patient is in caring for the patient.

269. Peabody, Francis Weld: The care of the patient. *JAMA, 88:*877-82, Mar 19, 1927.

Chapter 23
THE SOUL OF THE CLINIC

Francis Weld Peabody vs. Alfred Einstein Cohn

The practice of medicine is an art, not a trade; a calling, not a business; a calling in which your heart will be exercised equally with your head.

—Sir William Osler
The Master Word in Medicine[272]

"The Care of the Patient," widely read and well received, appeared during a critical period when medical educators and practicing clinicians were engaged in a raging battle over full time in the clinical chairs. So persuasive was Peabody's essay that stalwart believers in full time, and in medicine as a science, came to have second thoughts. Among the first, and one of the most prominent, was Warfield T. Longcope, a warm friend and full-time professor of medicine at Hopkins, who wrote to Peabody:

> Dear Francis—I waked up rather early this morning, and had some thoughts on our medical clinics,* and particularly the full time clinics. As they were probably wakened by your paper, I must find out how much truth you think there is in them. I wonder whether almost an impossible thing is not demanded of the full time clinic, the general movement in this country; and I wonder also whether you have not come nearer to solving the problem than any one else! I do not mean from the purely material side, for I think that is secondary; but from another side which is of greater value. There must be something in all of us which makes us want to be physicians rather than pure scientists; and I am sure that the thing which you have highly developed, and have given not only to your clinic but to all of us, is far more important for the clinic than experimental research. Is it possible to develop that in the clinic; or is it possible for the head of the clinic to develop it to the highest extent, and at the same time make important contributions to science?

* Clinics = departments in present day terminology.

272. Osler, Sir William: *Aequanimitas with Other Adresses.* Philadephia, P. Blakiston's Sons and Co., Inc., 1932, p. 368.

> You have come nearer to it than any one else . . . . Nobody before has formulated it as you have. None of us has been quite so conscious of it before; and we must all strive to put this into the clinics so that we may develop better clinicians and better scientists, and not turn out machines that grind out cold, spiritless facts.237

Peabody's father continues the story.

> The answer to this generous letter became a document of not less than eighteen typewritten pages, dictated by Francis from his reclining chair, and surveying the whole field and future of the practice of medicine. It would seem as if he were consciously giving a last message to the profession which he loved, and reporting the lessons of his wide experiences; and when, some months after Francis's death, Dr. Longcope read the letter to an assemblage of physicians, the entire audience rose in silent and reverent approval of its teaching, and of appreciation of its writer.

The title of the letter was "The Soul of the Clinic."[274]

On April 23, 1928, Alfred Einstein Cohn, M.D., research cardiologist and eminent proponent of medicine as a science and now the unofficial philosopher in residence at the Rockefeller Institute, initiated correspondence with Simon Flexner concerning Francis Peabody and "The Soul of the Clinic," stirring up a controversy that persists to this day.

Cohn was a most unusual person. Dr. Thomas Rivers, of the Rockefeller Institute who knew him well, described him in these terms:

> He wrote beautifully, and he loved to argue from the privacy of his study or at the lunch table at the Institute. To sit with Cohn at lunch was always an experience because the youngsters at the Institute have no respect for age and when Cohn threw rocks he always got some thrown back at him. Which is just the way I would have it—you bang at ideas and people as long as you are able to. When folks get too old to stand or do this they should quit.275

Cohn wrote to Simon Flexner:

> Francis Peabody's paper called "The Soul of the Clinic," appeared in the April 14th number of *The Journal of the American Medical Association*, page 1193. Had I given it a title, it might perhaps have been called, "The Evil Genius of the Clinic."276

In the same letter, Cohn complained about the republication of Theodore Janeway's paper criticizing full time, which had ori-

273. Peabody, *Francis Weld Peabody*, pp. 75-76.

274. Peabody, Francis W.: The soul of the clinic. *JAMA, 90/15:*1193-97, Apr. 14, 1928.

275. Benison, *Tom Rivers*, p. 108.

276. Letters of Simon Flexner: 1922-1939. American Philosophical Society Archives.

ginally been published in an obscure journal[277] and not seen by many medical educators. Cohn continued to Flexner:

> No doubt you will have seen the republication of Dr. Janeway's paper with an introduction by Henry Christian also in the *JAMA*, April 21, 1928, on page 1344. Are the low brows going to be in full swing?[278]

Flexner's reply on May 7, 1928, took issue with Cohn's appraisal and it is of considerable interest that the arch prototype of the physician-scientist should disagree with his disciple, asking "just what it is in the letter that you find objectionable."[279]

Cohn was obviously nettled by this comment from his mentor, and he was extremely deliberate and slow in replying. In a handwritten letter to Flexner on August 6, 1928, he commented:

> I have noticed carefully what you have said on the subject of the Peabody letter. Even if it were, as you say, and I don't doubt the accuracy of your prophecy, that time and the plethora of literature will dilute it beyond recognition, the issue will still remain as to the place of the study of disease in the scheme of academic things. I'm afraid I'm enough a person of words to care what ones are used in this connection.[280]

The issue was not diluted by time and the plethora of literature. It is as alive today as it was fifty years ago and still unsettled in the minds of many.

Peabody's message had hit the target, and Simon Flexner, totally committed to full time and to medicine as a science, was a little shaken and as a sound investigator wondered whether there might be something to be said for the other side of the argument. He had read both of the Peabody essays and was deeply touched and impressed. He had a high personal regard for the author and was distressed that the career of one of his most eminent students was ending so tragically. Flexner saw in Peabody's message the wisdom, charity, idealism, and vision of a master clinician who, accepting his early death with courage and calm, sought to leave to posterity a distillate of his thinking and experience in the care of human beings. The essays have a lyrical

277. Education in Review: March 1918.
278. Janeway, T. C.: Outside professional engagements by members of professional faculties. *JAMA, 90/16:*1315-1318, Apr. 21, 1928.
279. Flexner, Simon: Letters 1922-1939. American Philosophical Society Archives. S. Flexner to A. E. Cohn, May 7, 1928.
280. *Ibid.*, A. E. Cohn to S. Flexner, August 6, 1928.

quality, expressing deep religious commitment to the personal care of the sick from the perspective of a physician who actually rendered it and did not merely talk about it. Presented with calm eloquence and deep conviction, they constitute the best argument I have ever read for a balance between the science of medicine and its art. Long after the medical world will have forgotten Peabody's not inconsiderable "scientific" publications, he will continue to be remembered and admired as the author of these essays, which I predict will continue to inspire oncoming generations of medical students and physicians to rededicate their lives to the personal service of their fellowman.

On August 1, 1928, some three months after receiving Simon Flexner's request to explain his position on the Peabody essay, Cohn replied in considerable detail. The letter is so important in the still-smouldering conflict between the scientist and the clinician in medicine that it deserves close analysis and almost a point-by-point rebuttal. To accomplish this, eight key points in Cohn's letter have been selected for review and rebuttals derived from Peabody's letter.

1. Cohn

> The difference between Peabody and me is that to him the center of interest in medicine is practice and the care of the sick; to me it is the enlargement of the confines of knowledge. His is not an unworthy object. But its center of gravity is not one which places the medical clinic in the heart of a University. His might be a preparatory or an apprentice school. It makes of the Professor the father of his children, and of knowledge a decoration. But in a University knowledge is not a decoration but a passion and indeed life itself. The University does not neglect the care of the sick nor ignore teaching how this end may be accomplished—it has a function here just as it has assumed one in respect to engineering. At the same time though it cares for mathematics and physics. But to care only for engineering is to erect a Stevens Institute; to be concerned only or principally with the care of the sick is to found a school like the College of Physicians and Surgeons of the year of grace 1900. Very good objects these, but not the one to which I thought I was devoting my life.[281]

Rebuttal: Peabody

What did Peabody actually write on this subject? Were Peabody and Cohn talking about the same thing? I think not. Pea-

281. Benison, *Tom Rivers*, p. 106.

body was expressing his views on the role of a chief of a medical department concerned mainly with the education of students for the practice of clinical medicine, and in fact he so stated.

> I believe that the primary function of a department of medicine is to teach students those things that will enable them to practice the best contemporary medicine and will give them a foundation on which to superimpose the advances that will come during their professional life. They must be taught medicine as a vitally expanding subject, and must be stimulated to keep abreast of its growth.[282]

Cohn was speaking for the role of the scientist and investigator advancing knowledge, not for the physician and healer. As Peabody said later in this lecture,

> The medical clinic should encourage its staff to use methods of any sort, no matter how difficult or specialized, that are needed for the solution of their immediate problems; but their first interest should center about the general subject of disease in man. The first interest of the "scientist," on the other hand, is in the development of his own particular field. Each has his proper role, but in the medical clinic it is better to have an inspired "internist" than a skilled chemist.[283]

There can be very little argument with these statements that are as valid today as they were fifty years ago. What a pity that this sane and balanced attitude toward the education of physicians was soon to be overwhelmed in our leading medical schools by an overemphasis on making of every physician a scientist to the neglect of clinical medicine.

When Cohn lamented that proficiency in the care of the sick was a very good objective, "but not the one to which I thought I was devoting my life," he really let the cat out of the bag, for this is where he and Peabody parted ways. And still, the voices of Cohn, Flexner, Cole, and their associates were going to dominate the education of medical students for the next fifty years, while Peabody's would be, at first, a voice in the wilderness. There is no need to impugn the motives of the Flexnerians and their opponents. Both groups were sincere and prepared to battle hard for their beliefs, but someone had to be wrong. It would be years before we would find out what really went wrong in medical education. The Flexnerians were well organized and well heeled, while their opponents, on the defensive, lacked unity and

282. Peabody, *JAMA*, p. 1194.
283. *Ibid.*, p. 1196.

a good battle plan and the funds to wage war. The outcome was clearly predictable, and for many years the Flexnerians would control the argument with little or no opposition.

2. *Cohn*

> Perhaps I have been in error in believing that the meaning of our activities was not even remotely directed to making the Professor feel more comfortable and intimate with his patient when he had established a relation with him on the basis of the coin of the realm. Or has the doctrine of materialism so taken possession of the puritan tradition that the meaning of *noblesse oblige* has completely departed from the belief of our society. But this is a trifling matter. It points, however, to an interest in action and in human relations rather than to one in knowing and in science. This is the interest which lies at the basis of Peabody's position.[284]

Rebuttal: Peabody

Let us examine Peabody's actual words and decide for ourselves whether Cohn's statements were in order.

> A complete "full-time" system is impossible from an economic point of view even if it were desirable medically, which I do not think it is. Experience has made it perfectly clear that the men who are in successful outside practice have something very definite and important to contribute to the teaching, and, as already indicated, they must be regarded as an integral part of the teaching service and receive proper recognition in the way of titles, salaries and clinical opportunities. . . .
>
> . . . There is no question in my own mind that I am a much better teacher for having had a limited number of such patients in recent years. These are the patients to whom I talk at length personally, and they are apt to be the cases that stick in my mind so that I refer to them continually in talking to students. One can always say that the same thing may be done as well if the patients belong to the clinic and if, for instance, their fees are paid to the clinic; but I fear I do not agree to this. If they had been the patients of the clinic I should have had most of the work done by my assistants and I should have missed exactly that personal relationship with patients which many people say cannot be obtained in a hospital. . . .
>
> . . . In all of this, moreover, I do not believe that I am very different or more sordid in attitude than most men. It is not wholly a question of to whom the fees are paid (often there are no fees), although this certainly is a factor in establishing and maintaining the personal bond. The main point is that the patient has sought you or me personally and not the hospital.[285]

284. Cohn, A. E. to Flexner, S.: American Philosophical Society correspondence.
285. Peabody, *JAMA*, p. 1197.

Once again, we have a statement by Peabody, in this instance, on full time and private practice which is as sound today as it was when it was first printed, fifty years ago. How could anyone take issue with this calm, objective and honest statement, and how could anyone impugn the motives of the writer?

Any seasoned clinician knows that the best way to test the performance of his hospital is by having under his personal care a limited number of private patients whose treatment and management are not by surrogates or committees but by the physician himself. In this setting, the physician finds out very quickly how well his orders are being followed, how the laboratory and radiology divisions are functioning, whether nursing care is good or bad, and if the performance of the aides is up to snuff or disaster prone. There is no better way to test the performance of the hospital than by monitoring it meticulously and personally on daily, or twice daily, rounds on one's own private patients. The point is that personal private practice has great advantages for the patient as well as the doctor.

3. Cohn

> You [Simon Flexner] suggest that if the system cannot stand the criticism to which it has been subjected it must be either too young or too weak to survive. It is not so much that the system can or cannot stand criticism as that the system which is under criticism is *not* the system we are proposing. If there is any slaying to be done it makes a difference whether the victim is a goat or a sheep. Their swan songs sound different and may make a different appeal.[286]

Rebuttal

In this paragraph, Cohn seems carried away with his emotions even to the point of mixing metaphors. The significant comment is his reference to "the system we are proposing." Here he shows his hand for he is not merely defending the Rockefeller Institute and his own way of life; he is speaking of the plan which the Flexnerians proposed to impose upon selected medical schools in their attempt to upgrade medical education. More specifically, he was talking about the plans for the University of Chicago and young McLean.

4. Cohn

> It seems unnecessary to analyze Peabody's letter in great detail.

286. Cohn to Flexner, S., American Philosophical Society correspondence.

> The error, foreseen by many of us at the beginning and still uncorrected, concerning the functions and choice of professors, is an error of judgment, only of historical interest; it does not cut to the root of the issue nor invalidate our proper aims. Time and a deeper insight may be counted on to correct it—provided loyalty to the initial aims remains.[287]

Rebuttal: Peabody

Let us reexamine Peabody's actual words on this subject.

> One of the first problems to be considered is the kind of man who ought to be selected as professor of medicine. I quite agree with you that the requirements which are now generally put forward are so impossible to fulfil that they become almost ludicrous. May we perhaps take pride in the fact that we have been called to fill the shoes of such supermen even if we do rattle around in them! When a professorship falls open, the committee in charge of filling the position usually says somewhat naively that it is looking for a man who has had an intensive scientific training, has done important research, is a good administrator, is a competent teacher, and finally has had clinical experience. We have heard this string of specifications so often that they are becoming rather hackneyed. Such a man is, of course, almost impossible to find, and I have been wondering where the ideal originated. I think it results from the fact that in recent years—since what we may call the Reformation—the selection of professors of clinical medicine has been more and more influenced by laymen and by professors of nonclinical subjects.* Both may be excellent pedagogues and experts on education and yet fail to grasp the difficulties and complexities which confront this particular type of position.
>
> "Clinical experience" is apt to be put last among the specifications. This is because some of our friends think that clinical medicine can be "picked up" very easily by the prospective professor. while others believe that if a man is well trained in such sciences as chemistry, physics and physiology he has only to learn the technical clinical methods of percussion and auscultation.[288]

Cohn is entitled to disagree with Peabody on this issue. His description of Peabody's position as "an error of judgment, only of historical interest" is pompous and unscientific. Again, Peabody was expressing wisdom and sound judgment from a background much superior to Cohn's for evaluating this issue. Any clinician who has served on a search committee for a chairman of medicine will back Peabody's statements to the hilt.

---

287. *Ibid.*

* An obvious reference to A. Flexner, Franklin P. Mall, et al. (author).

288. Peabody, *JAMA*, p. 1193.

5. Cohn

The wards are not "the backbone of the clinic"—at least of a university clinic. They represent merely one of the vertebrae. Whatever part of the argument depends on this assumption must go the way of all syllogisms based on incorrect premises.[289]

Rebuttal: Peabody

Here again, as Mark Twain has said, it is a difference of opinion that makes horseracing. Peabody actually wrote:

> If it be true that preparation of students for a career in clinical medicine, and more specifically for the practice of medicine, is the first duty of a department of medicine, then it seems clear to me that the backbone of the clinic is the general ward and the outpatient department, for it is here that one finds or can readily create conditions which most closely resemble those which are found in actual practice.[290]

I find this analogy most interesting and, once again, regret that this balanced approach to the medical clinic gave way to a system of excessive subspecialization leading to the fragmentation of medical care and medical education. The general medical ward should indeed be the backbone of the clinic. The trouble is that for many years this backbone has been afflicted with severe osteoporosis and not infrequently there has been collapse of its componenets with pain and disability and loss of function.

6. Cohn

The description of "the head of the clinic" is trivial. This conception of the professor is more like that of a Y.M.C.A. secretary than of a person with vital purposes in life. I can find little compensation for intellectual curiosity in the excellence of his proposed manners or in his sartorial perfection.[291]

Rebuttal: Peabody

Peabody's description of the head of the clinic does not merit Cohn's critique. Here are Peabody's own words.

> If the general ward is the backbone of the clinic, then the head of the clinic must be close to it; indeed, it ought to be directly under him. The importance of the general ward and what it stands for as representing the general practice of medicine can be impressed on the younger members of the staff and on the students only if the relation of the chief to the ward is real and not fictitious. The whole atmosphere of the general ward, and thus the attitude of

289. Cohn, A. E. to Flexner, S, American Philosophical Society correspondence.
290. Peabody, *JAMA*, p. 1194.
291. Cohn to Flexner, American Philosophical Society correspondence.

> the future practitioners to the profession of medicine, is here set by the chief of the clinic, for it must always be remembered that standards of thought, as well as of action, are set from above.[292]

Where did Cohn get his ammunition for his crack on "the excellence of proposed manners or in his sartorial perfection?" Not from Peabody, except by inference. Peabody's actual words ran this way when he was discussing his interns.

> This arrangement leads directly to a consideration of the status of the interns. On this point I feel very strongly. They should be regarded as advanced students, and as perhaps the most important group of advanced students that we have. They come with minds, characters and personalities in the most pliable and receptive states and can be affected in an extraordinary degree even by the atmosphere of the clinic. Their very manner of dress and parting their hair changes. Social ease, and manners that will play a large and legitimate part in medical practice, develop. At the same time intellectual changes of a far deeper character are going on, and the chief has an opportunity to set his seal on them. Provided the chief has anything in himself to offer, here is his chance to turn out every year a group of selected men who shall represent his ideas and his clinic all over the country, and it is to be hoped that they will gradually affect the type of medicine in many remote communities. Again, however, this cannot be done as successfully through subordinates as if the chief undertakes to keep himself close to the interns. It takes time, but it seems to me that the results are well worth striving for.[293]

For those of us who have witnessed the decline of good manners and the advent of uncouth, hairy, and often unkempt and sloppily attired young men and women into our wards as representatives of the profession of medicine, Peabody's words should be emblazoned in neon lights on all of our wards—for a while anyway—perhaps with a switch to turn them on and off.

7. *Cohn*

> On the subject of research it is impossible to say much but in order to do so, Peabody's conception of research itself requires analysis for he does not seem to regard it as an integral function of the good society nor to comprehend its essential nature.[294]

Rebuttal: Peabody

I find Cohn's evaluation of Peabody's concept of research com-

292. Peabody, *JAMA*, p. 1194.
293. *Ibid.*
294. Cohn to Flexner, American Philosophical Society correspondence.

pletely unacceptable. How he can say this of Peabody, of all persons, is beyond me and suggests that he may not have read the essay as carefully as he should. Peabody's discussion of research, its place in the clinic, its role in medical education, is eloquent and exhibits the wisdom derived from his own many years of intensive exposure and active participation in clinical investigation. His comments place research within its proper perspective within the total program of the medical clinic. The reader is referred to the original essay for the details.

8. Cohn

> But I must stop. If I escape boring you I may be impaling myself on the other horn of the dilemma by being annoying. I wish an enemy rather than a friend had written that letter.[295]

Rebuttal

This exchange of letters was characterized by Tom Rivers as—

> interesting because they are part and parcel of a debate that is still going on (1967) in American medicine relating to the role of research and clinical instruction. . . . If the patient was the center of Peabody's medical universe, research was the heart of Cohn's world! It's an argument that still goes on in medicine today, and perhaps with a little more intensity.[296]

The Peabody-Cohn letters are more than interesting, they reflect very different philosophies of two brilliant men. One was sought after to be dean of the new medical school in Chicago, a position he turned down, perhaps fortunately, for he was soon to die of carcinoma well before he could have lived to see the medical school come to life. The other, Cohn, with his friends the Flexners, was to play an important role in setting academic policy at the University of Chicago through his pupil and admirer, Franklin C. McLean. The scientists were set to control the medical school along the lines they felt should be followed. Or, at least, that is the way it was for a while.

Finally, I ask the reader, if you were sick and needed a doctor would you want a Peabody or a Cohn? If you were choosing a leader to set medicine's educational policy would it be Peabody of Cohn? And, finally, if you had a son or daughter studying

295. Cohn to S. Flexner: American Philosophical Society correspondence.
296. Benison, *Tom Rivers,* p. 101.

medicine, would you rather have the role-model be a Cohn or a Peabody? These are not idle questions for the answers are at the basis of what may be wrong with modern medicine. Have we not gone too far in the direction of the scientific to the neglect of the humanitarian aspects of medicine? Is it too late to advance to Peabody's high ground?

Chapter 24
WORLD WAR II AND FULL-TIME MEDICINE

World War II put more doctors on full time than ever before in the history of the country, dwarfing in magnitude the Flexnerian efforts of the preceding three decades. The majority of able-bodied physicians in the United States were in military service except for those too old to serve, those with physical disabilities, and others in so-called essential positions in civilian life. Of 85,000 doctors under the age of forty-five, over 60,000 served in the Armed Forces during World War II. By and large, the medical profession set a magnificent example for the rest of the population by volunteering to serve at considerable financial and personal sacrifice and personal risk in the greatest holocaust of modern times. Those who remained behind had to work long hours, struggle with civilian discomforts, gasoline rationing, meat rationing, and so forth and were denied the personal satisfactions of wearing the uniform and being considered something of a hero. In exchange, many in private practice were kept very busy going to the bank to make deposits, and some in academic positions enjoyed promotions with increases in prestige and power beyond their fondest dreams. At any rate, many thousands of the nation's doctors entered military service and found themselves practicing full-time medicine under government control, a new and unsettling experience for many.

The military services were ill-prepared for the enormous influx of highly individualistic, ambitious, and competitive professionals, all of whom wanted to be chiefs and few willing to be Indians. Assignment and rank were at first on the basis of seniority in the Reserve or National Guard, age, date of entry into service, and table of organization rather than competence or civilian experience. The Surgeon General of the Army set up a clearing house in Washington for all assignments, and valiant attempts were made to assign physicians to positions in keeping with their skills and competence. Those in charge of the distribution developed criteria for selection that would be acceptable to the profession as a whole. With the great volume of medical officers, it was impossible for each individual to be personally investigated and reviewed for clinical competence, and there were bound to be some bad assignments. The various specialty boards were now in existence, but they had not enjoyed the prestige in civilian life they were later to assume. In fact, I recall that many of our professors did not encourage us to take the board examinations, their feeling being that performance in one's institution and academic recognition were far more important than a board certificate. This would soon undergo a drastic change, one of the main reasons being the policy of the military services to use board certification as a more efficient and practical method for classifying medical officers. Each medical officer in the Army of the United States (AUS) had a Military Occupational Specialty (MOS) classification and was assigned a subclassification, A, B, or C, depending upon the level of competence achieved by the individual as judged by higher authority. Subspecialties were also classified, and all of this information was in the hands of local or higher authority for use in assignment and promotion and placed in each officer's "201" file. All of this was a far cry from the situation in World War I when the Surgeon General found so many of the self-designated civilian "specialists" to be overrated that specialist appointments were made conditional on examination.

> The results were appalling. Some of the "specialists" examined were found to be unfit to practice any branch of medicine in the service. A study of the examination results at Camp Greenleaf in 1918, revealed only one medical officer in three qualified to do independent surgery, and only about 6 per cent were rated as high-class surgeons; there was a similarly small proportion of really high grade men in internal medicine. Seventy per cent of the otolaryngologists, 51 per cent of the ophthalmologists and 38 per cent of those who said they were plastic and oral surgeons were rejected.[297]

In World War II, doctors who had paid relatively little attention to board certification soon found that it carried great weight in

297. Stevens, R.: *American Medicine and Public Interest.* New Haven, Yale University Press, 1971, pp. 127-28.

the military services. Those who were not certified lost no time in applying for examination. With rare exceptions, assignments in major Army Hospitals seldom went to nonboard-certified men. The message, delivered to the older and more seasoned physicians, that more attractive assignments, higher rank and pay would go to those with board certification was quickly relayed to younger physicians in residency and training programs to overlook no opportunity to qualify for American Boards. A pattern was established that would extend into civilian life when military physicians returned to private practice. They had learned that a government-controlled medical profession would lean very heavily on credentials, and certification and doctors were quick to read this as the wave of the future. At the end of military service, large numbers of physicians would seek residencies and fellowships to qualify as specialists in private practice. Few would choose to be family doctors or GPs. The lesson had been learned, and it would influence career decisions for years to come.

Military service showed the doctors what it meant to work an eight-hour day, have weekends off, and little night work except for occasional duty as OD (Officer of the Day). There was little or no contact with patient's families or relatives. The patients had little to say about their care, they had no freedom of choice, and neither did the doctors who had to accept each and every patient assigned to them. In the General Hospitals much time was occupied by paper work and administrative duties, including service on various boards that rendered decisions to separate men from military service, with or without a pension, limited service for others, or return to full duty after an illness or an injury. These functions were time-consuming and had to be reviewed by higher authority. The result was that the General Hospital had many patients merely awaiting administrative disposition mixed in with those with acute or chronic illnesses.

The plight of the doctor, assigned to a dispensary or outpatient work, was undesirable and almost always professionally unrewarding. Many soldiers sought to ride the system for all that it was worth, filling the queues on sick call. Faced with fifty or 100 "patients" to examine on morning sick call, many of them for minor or no real ailments, the doctor would feel frustrated and angry, and the few patients who were really sick might be glossed over with the two-aspirins-and-return-to-duty routine, sometimes inviting catastrophe. The system of providing everything for nothing was bound to be abused and overutilized; the desire to evade unpleasant military duty was too much for many soldiers to resist. There was little or no time for the physician to relate well to his patients, and "functional" disorders were poorly handled. Physicians of this period had been taught to emphasize organic or physical illness and sought to understand ailments in biochemical terms Their experience and training had geared them to diagnosing and treating organic illness while functional disorders were dismissed out of hand as being unimportant. The average practitioner's knowledge of psychiatry and treatment of nonorganic illness was primitive, and he usually associated psychiatrists with insane asylums. The confrontation in military service of many physicians by large numbers of patients with anxiety, depression, psychopathic behavior, hysteria, and psychoses was an uncomfortable one for the physician as well as the patient, the former feeling inadequate and insecure in the handling of these problems so far removed from civilian experience, undergraduate and postgraduate training.

The temptation was to refer these patients to the N-P (Neuropsychiatric) Section for appropriate care. These sections were soon overloaded and unable to cope with the demand, and other solutions were sought. General William Menninger, the well-known and respected psychiatrist and consultant to the Surgeon General, realized early that there would never be enough psychiatrists for the needs of the Army and decided that every medical officer should become psychiatrically oriented and competent in handling most neuroses and the milder anxieties. He made personal visits to the larger hospitals, made rounds with the staff, and did not limit his contacts to psychiatrists alone. His subordinates, many of them psychiatrists of considerable competence and reputation, served as regional consultants and helped to implement General Menninger's concepts.

Gradually, this led to a lessening of the load on the N-P Sections, and each of the specialty sections carried its share of psychoneurotics and persons with psychosomatic disorders. The stigma of being classified as an N-P patient was thereby avoided by some individuals who felt with good reason it would be harmful to either their military careers or to their future in civilian life. When a nonpsychiatrist took care of a patient with a functional disorder, he usually sought consultation with the available psychiatrist and there was an interchange of information and experience that was beneficial for the doctor as well as the patient. Soon, many of the general medical officers became quite proficient in dealing with patients with functional illness and, indeed, some were better at it than those with formal psychiatric training.

It must be remembered that the educational background of many psychiatrists was as inadequate for the demands of military service as that of the average physician. Many adjustments had to be made, and psychiatry had to exert itself to win its spurs in a new setting. Major advances were made but perhaps the most important of all was the psychiatric orientation of thousands of physicians, who were perforce, treating patients with functional, emotional and nonorganic illness, not because they wanted to do so but because they were ordered to do so. In the process, these physicians acquired an experience that would stand them well when they returned to civilian practice with attitudes and some skills improved over those with which they entered into military service. American psychiatry really came into its own during World War II, and the beneficial effects would be felt for years to come, especially in the postwar period. Returning veteran medical officers accustomed to working effectively with psychiatrists would be responsible for creating a demand for better teaching and training in psychiatry, more easily available treatment and consultation, and more personnel committed to this field. Psychiatry had come of age and was ready for a renaissance.

Another important aspect of the military experience of physicians in World War II was the emphasis on the specialties and subspecialties. It was more efficient to assign patients to beds in sections in cardiology, infectious diseases, gastroenterology, chest disease, etc. than to place all of them in general medical wards. Surgery was similarly divided. This division of labor was accepted by the medical staff as advantageous and efficient and permitted each physician to exercise his skills in areas of personal expertise and to continue with his own medical education. Teaching rounds and grand rounds were conducted in the large general hospitals at levels fully comparable to those in renowned voluntary teaching hospitals and attendance was compulsory. Overseas, similar policies were followed even in the midst of rather primitive surroundings. Where there were good teachers, educational efforts were sound and good for staff morale as well as patient care.

The overall impact of military service on the physician was to teach him to work as part of a team, under close supervision of his peers and superiors, obliged to keep good records, and to participate in administrative decisions and judgements, and to have little or no concern over the costs of medical care. The regular hours of duty, the freedom from the problems of dealing with anxious families, the absence of house calls, the security of being part of a group, would influence the careers of many physicians after they left military service. Many would opt for group practice and the specialties. Few would return to family or general practice. This experience would be felt for years to come in the practice and teaching of medicine in America. Full-time positions in hospitals and medical schools would be eagerly sought, but they were in short supply chiefly because of limited endowment funds. The institutional explosion of full time would come only when new sources for funding would appear, and they were in the offing.

Not all physicians in military service were enchanted with the system of practice. In fact, many abhorred it and couldn't wait for the day of their return to private practice. Very few chose to remain in military service despite the alleged attraction of job security, retirement in twenty years, and other inducements dreamed up by military recruiters. Perceptive and dedicated physicians bemoaned the depersonalization of patient care, the fragmentation of care, and the lack of recognition or adequate reward for work well done. With some exceptions, the doctor-patient relationship was brief, episodic, and oftentimes superficial, and there were seldom experienced the warm attachment, affection and respect of the patient for his doctor, and vice versa, which characterizes private medical practice at its best. Few of those who had been successful in private practice would choose the way of life of the military physician or surgeon. Doctors are individualists and are chosen for their capacity to stand on their own feet and to make independent decisions. They can adapt to all sorts of conditions, but deep down they resent regimentation, paper work, bureaucratic controls, and the intervention of third parties between themselves and their patients, be they government, insurance companies, politicians, or institutional administrators.

Most doctors think of themselves as the advocates of their patients, fighting their battle for them against sometimes overwhelming odds. This is the role that has attracted some of the finest minds to medicine. The military setting is hardly the place to attract and hold the majority of the best in American medicine. Many who emerged from military service having given loyal, dedicated, and magnificent service and care, swore they would never accept any form of socialized medicine or government-run medical system. Having seen it first-hand in military service, they would avoid it like the plague and fight it tooth and nail.

Chapter 25
PHYSICIAN-VETERANS ADJUST TO CIVILIAN PRACTICE

The return of the doctors after four years of military service called for major readjustments. For most it meant starting over again, rebuilding a practice, reestablishing hospital connections, and reembarking on the hard road to professional success. By and large, the veterans were welcomed by their colleagues, and their hospitals were solicitous and helpful in assisting them to resume their work. Professional office space in New York City was virtually unavailable. Housing was out of sight. Getting a new car, or even a good used car, was next to impossible, and there was no provision whatsoever for this to the shame of the car manufacturers of Detroit and their agents! Reestablishing credit was difficult. The butcher, the baker, the plumber, and the landlord had to be paid, and the M.D. degree was regarded as the key to affluence. In the large cities, the custom prevailed of soaking the doctor who would surely find the money somewhere.

For some physician-veterans, the experience was extremely frustrating and the adjustment rather difficult. Those in gynecology and pediatrics found that their skills had undergone deterioration through lack of practice and refresher courses were needed. The younger doctors, as a result of their hurry-up quasi-assembly-line education during the war years, felt very insecure and inadequately educated for civilian practice. They flocked to the residencies and specialty fellowships that were undergoing a massive expansion fostered by government funds for education.

Before World War II, hospitals were underutilized, and a great deal of medical care was rendered in the patients' homes. The house call was the way of life for many physicians. When these men returned to civilian practice, they found the hospital had become the base for delivery of medical care, there were fewer house calls, and it seemed more efficient to admit patients to the hospital for diagnostic studies and for special care, as well as for operations. In the prewar days, as prestigious a hospital as Harkness Pavilion, in New York City, was half empty and the staff was beseeched to admit its patients there rather than to other hospitals in the city. A good private room with bath in Harkness cost seven dollars a day, but very few people could afford even this. Blue Cross insurance was in its infancy and most people were not enrolled, only 9 percent of the civilian population being covered for any kind of in-hospital medical benefits.[298] By 1950, 51 percent had some coverage, and by 1960 the figure had risen to 81 percent. By 1976, over 93 percent of Americans had some form of health insurance. The success of big labor, especially steel and the auto industry, in securing health insurance through collective bargaining did much to propel the nation toward almost universal voluntary coverage.[299] Passage of the Hill-Burton Act, under President Harry Truman in 1946, authorized the construction and replacement of hospitals that had undergone serious deterioration during the Depression. The new hospitals looked more attractive, were better designed, more functional, and appealed to patients and their families.

Returning physician-veterans, accustomed to hospital-centered medical care in military service, found it easy to adapt to this new development and soon eschewed house calls, concentrating most of their efforts in offices or in hospitals. As utilization of the hospital for the practice of medicine increased, ground rules for Blue Cross disbursement had to be worked out and decisions made as to what costs were appropriate and allowable under the terms of the policies. A detailed study of this development has been made in "Blue Cross—What Went Wrong?" by Sylvia A. Law and several of the problems illuminated. The very controversial question of "the extent to which medical education and research are, and should be, allowed in third-party reimbursement" was avoided by Professor Law who felt that a separate and comprehensive study of this matter was needed and that it

298. Stevens, R.: *American Medicine and Public Interest.* New Haven, Yale University Press, 1971, p. 271.

299. Rogers, D. E.: *American Medicine: Challenges for the 1980s.* Cambridge, Ballinger Publ. Co., 1978, p. 19.

was beyond the scope of her monograph.[300]

In 1971, Herbert S. Denenberg, then Pennsylvania's Insurance Commissioner, challenged the Blue Cross reimbursement formula for hospitals on several fronts, among them the funding of internships and residencies, saying their costs should be borne by the attending physicians, a suggestion that fell like a lead balloon and evoked demands that Denenberg be removed from his position. In addition, he requested "disclosure of information and control of payments to hospital-based physicians" provided through Blue Cross. Neither of these matters has ever been fully aired, and sooner or later they will have to be brought into the open for free discussion. Whereas, in the 1930s, the best teaching hospitals boasted that they paid their interns not a red cent, giving merely room and board, the situation is now radically changed. All house staff now receive salaries, ranging for interns and residents between $15,000 and $20,000 or more per annum. Although the number of hospital beds has stabilized, the number of interns and residents needed to take care of the same number of patients has escalated. The salaries of house staff, an inconsequential item in the annual budget before World War II, is now a substantial item in large teaching hospitals, ranging into the millions each year. In the old days, few could afford to remain in residencies because the stipends were grossly inadequate. Young men were advised not to marry until they had completed their residencies and not even then if they were interested in academic medicine. Nowadays, the annual stipends for residents are in five digits, and there is less urgency to get out and make a living, encouraging many to continue in prolonged hospital training, usually focussing on a subspecialty. We have known for years that the longer one stays in the insulated and protected environment of the hospital, the more difficult it is to shake it off and to strike out for oneself. Is it any wonder that despite increasing medical school enrollments, fewer and fewer graduates are out in the community serving the people in primary care?

Many of the physicians who have undergone prolonged house staff training are inadequately prepared for the private practice of medicine with its emphasis on ambulatory care, primary care,

300. Law, Sylvia A.: *Blue Cross—What Went Wrong?* New Haven, Yale University Press, 1974, p. 66.

and the one-to-one relationship of a doctor to his patient. Many seek in institutional practice an escape from the demands of private practice. These individuals provide a large pool of candidates seeking full-time positions.

In addition to the support of interns and residents, the Blue Cross reimbursement formula provides for full-time salaries of some attending staff. The justification for this is that the presence of salaried hospital-based attending staff will enhance patient care by providing closer supervision of house staff and by more efficient administration and better teaching. Virtually every hospital administrator would like to have most of his doctors on salary and at his beck and call. The only thing that restrains him is the fact that there seems never to be enough money for this, and he accepts the part-time practitioner-teacher as a necessary evil. With the availability of funding from the reimbursement formula of Blue Cross, the temptation for the hospital administrator to hire salaried doctors is almost irresistible. If the trustees of every hospital had to actually dig the salary for full-time physicians out of their own pockets or out of endowment, there would be very few full-time appointments.

As it is, hospitals with little or nothing in the way of valid teaching or research programs, many of them unable to attract competent house staff from American schools, tend to solve this dilemma by appointing full-time salaried, hospital-based directors of departments and also chiefs of sections as well as other individuals for whom they feel the hospital has a need. There seems to be no real requirement for justifying these additions to the budget, no review by consumers and no real review by Blue Cross. In fact, the more expended on physician salaries, the more the administrator boasts of his full-time staff, and up goes the reimbursement with little or no incentive to control costs and expenditures. The Blue Cross reimbursement formula has opened up a source of funds for full time that would have made Flexner's mouth water. Whereas Flexner looked upon full time as an essential for a university medical school, he could hardly have envisioned that almost any community hospital of several hundred beds would because of Blue Cross have a substantial full-time staff with all of the money coming out of the pockets of patients.

Neither could Flexner have foreseen that salaries for full-time department heads in some nonuniversity community hospitals would dwarf those being paid to university professors of medicine or surgery. Even more startling are the salary levels of department heads in radiology and in clinical pathology in community hospitals, often based on a percentage of the take from a captive population of hospital patients.

The full-time salaried physician is a curious anomaly in a so-called community hospital for, by the nature of his appointment, his work is usually confined to activities within the hospital and seldom reaches out into the community that it serves. To be in touch with the community, the physician should be working in it, participating in many of its activities, and very much in touch with its problems and trends. In this respect, the community hospital differs sharply from the university hospital, which tends to avoid community service except as it relates to its educational and training programs. When and if the community hospital develops the ivory tower complex, it loses its effectiveness and fails to fulfill the role for which it really should exist. To staff community hospitals with full-time salaried doctors and to place in their hands the control of policy is asking for trouble. When the administrators of these hospitals complain that the only way they can attract house staff to man their emergency and other divisions is to have full-time salaried staff, their solution really does not aim at the problem. Their house staff programs need close inspection and review, and many of them should be cancelled out. Other solutions should be worked out, chief among them the feasibility of utilizing partially salaried attending staff who pledge themselves to give not full time but committed time to the educational, training, research, and patient care programs of the hospital. These are the men and women who will bring the community and the hospital together. They will set policy that will be relevant to the needs of the people in the community. They will help direct the education and training of house staff and other personnel in a constructive direction, stressing service to the sick as a primary goal. The present trend to isolate the doctor in the community hospital from contacts with the people and the community is not only inflicting undue expense on the hospital, it is supporting thousands of people who should be out in the market, competing with others and providing primary health care to those who need it. The situation has gotten out of hand. In seeking status by having full-time staff, the community hospital may well be losing sight of its real purpose.

When the community hospitals, with little or nothing going on in the way of solid educational programs, load their budgets with salaried full-time hospital-based clinicians, the public interest is not served and medical costs will escalate out of sight. Restraint and review are clearly needed.

Chapter 26
NIH FUNDS AND FULL TIME

At first the impact on full time of military experience, Blue Cross expansion, and specialization was to attract many individuals to institutional practice of medicine, with the main emphasis still upon patient care and teaching with research as a sort of by-product, done largely on the individual's available time and with limited funds and oftentimes primitive provision for space and technical assistance. The advent of NIH funds changed this picture dramatically through overemphasis on laboratory research on a massive scale and on the medicine of tomorrow to the neglect of clinical teaching and the provision of the health care of the day

During the early twentieth century, Federal involvement in health research was more talk than action. President Herbert C. Hoover recognized the need for a formal commitment when, in 1930, he was able to have the name of the Hygienic Laboratory, established in 1887, changed to the National Institute of Health and provided some funds for its operation. The appropriation for this purpose in 1931 was merely $43,000, and it increased very slowly over the ensuing decade. The real boom came with World War II and the establishment of the Office of Scientific Research and Development (OSRD) and the availability of substantial sums for medical research in problems related to the military effort. With the termination of World War II, wartime contracts were transferred to the NIH, with the Federal Government committed to their support as well as to extramural programs across the country. The subsequent dramatic growth of the NIH has been described by Dr. James A. Shannon who was its director from 1955 to 1969. Quoting from Doctor Shannon's article:

> In 1946 the national expenditure for medical research totalled

> 87 million, of which the federal share was 27 million, or 31 percent. The National Institutes of Health that year expended 8.3 million, or 10 percent of the national effort. For 1966, the national medical research expenditures are estimated at 2.05 billion, exclusive of construction and training.
>
> The federal component is $1.4 billion, or 68 percent; and the NIH portion amounts to $800 million, or 40 percent of the whole. A signal fact of this twenty-year comparison is that total dollars available for the nation's medical research have increased twenty-four times. If the Gross National Product deflation factor is applied to correct for price and wage changes over this period, the increase is still in the order of fifteen times.[301]

As Stevens commented in 1971:

> From these modest beginnings the National Institutes of Health developed into fourteen research institutes and major research divisions, together with the National Library of Medicine and five divisions designed to stimulate the research and training of health manpower. By 1968, the NIH employed over 13,000 full-time persons, and was responsible for a budget of $1.6 billion, of which $254 million was spent on its own direct operations.[302]

These numbers are simply staggering and beyond the comprehension of the average doctor. What was accomplished by these enormous expenditures? Was it all to the good or was it bad or was it a mixture of both?

Others have complained bitterly of the adverse effects of massive research expenditures on medicine in our leading medical schools. One of the most experienced and seasoned commentators was the late Dean Wilburt C. Davison of Duke University who delivered his message in an essay entitled, "Let's Give the Medical Schools Back to the Students." He criticized with telling effect the harmful results of excessive emphasis on research and the power falling into hands of those especially expert at grantsmanship.[303]

> Until sound knowledge and the skill and desire to impart it are given the same prestige and dignity as that of publication, research will be rampant, and will remind some of us of the old gag at the Rockefeller Institute under Simon Flexner, namely, "A paper a day

301. Shannon, J. A.: The advancement of medical research: A 20-year view of the role of the NIH. *J Med Educ, 42:*97-108, 1967.
302. Stevens, R.: *American Medicine and Public Interest.* New Haven, Yale University Press, 1971, p. 358.
303. Davison, W. C.: Let's give the medical schools back to the students. *The Pharos, 26/4:*98-104, Oct. 1963.

> keeps Simon away.". . .In fact, the younger members of the faculty are so busy with this pressure of research in order to justify a renewal of their grants that they have no time or inclination to accept invitations to assist with the school's problems of teaching, administration, and student contacts. They seem to expect all of the rights and privileges of a medical school without sharing its duties and obligations. In order to do more research, an occasional instructor will actually refuse to teach or to accept committee assignments, and the heads of their departments condone it. . . . Many American medical schools, including Duke, are being converted into research institutes similar to those of the pre-war Germans, but, even worse, the research programs with their herds of technicians and junior researchers, instead of being segregated into separate institutes like the Germans, are crowding out the medical students from the teaching space in the laboratories and hospital wards, and creating in the students the image that research is superior to medical teaching and patient care. The curriculum has been so distorted that almost every student is compelled to engage in the research program. Those who have no research skill are given special courses in gadgetry.[304]

Stevens described what happened in the medical schools in these terms:

> At the same time, the program of NIH subsidies to universities for medical research transformed the research functions—and altered the balance of faculty interests—in the nominally independent medical schools. By 1955, one-third of the income of medical schools was coming from outside research grants, chiefly from the federal government. Not only had the contributions by NIH become essential to the continued existence of the schools; the activities of the faculty had substantially changed. In 1949-50 the average medical school had a full-time faculty of approximately 70, a substantial increase from nine or ten years earlier. In 1959-60, the average full-time faculty was over 120 per school; of the total of 10,468 faculty thus represented, 1 in 7 received more than half of his salary from federal sources, with federal money concentrated in the lower academic ranks. By 1968-69, the total number of full-time faculty had reached 23,014, or over 250 per school. There was more than one full-time faculty member for every pair of medical students, *but many, if not most, of the faculty were not regularly involved in teaching medical students at all.* . . . [Italics added by Doctor Lepore.] While the AMA had been opposing federal aid for medical education, using as one argument distrust of increased governmental control over a traditionally professional responsibility, the medical schools had de facto become extensive-

304. *Ibid.*

> ly dependent on the government through the back door of research subsidy.[305]

The overall effect of large research grants to medical schools was to increase the number of so-called full-time teachers, while encouraging them to do little or no teaching and avoiding involvement in direct patient care! These were the role models for the students who could not fail to be impressed by the way of life and the attitudes of their teachers or nonteachers. The effect on susceptible medical students was as nothing compared to that on the clinicians responsible for ward and clinic patient care and teaching. The message quickly got around that being a superior teacher or a first-rate clinician was simply being a second-class citizen. Promotions, academic rank, and responsibility were begrudgingly given to the clinical teaching staff, especially those contaminated by their commitment to practice. There had always been a certain amount of this in the post-Flexner era, but the situation became worse with the NIH grants and their undue emphasis on the laboratory to the neglect of the clinic. The Flexnerian attitude was that practically anyone can teach clinical medicine or practice it and only quasi-geniuses can do laboratory research. One of the problems was that there were many mediocrities about and few geniuses. Someone in high authority had lost the sense of direction. The purpose of the medical school is to educate good physicians, most of whom will be taking care of sick people. Medical schools should not be primarily research institutes.

One specific example, worth a dozen generalizations, is now discussed in some detail. At Columbia-Presbyterian Medical Center in New York City, the delicately balanced and superb clinical faculty of the 1930s with its almost ideal makeup of full time, geographic full-time and part-time clinicians working harmoniously as a team had established its reputation as one of the finest if not the best center for clinical medicine in the world. The first of the large medical centers, it set the pace for all the others. On its staff were some of the foremost scientists in America as well as many of its best clinicians. The practicing clinicians were world-renowned and attracted patients from far and wide, not only the wealthy but also the poor. Vanderbilt Clinic was the

305. Stevens, *American Medicine*, p. 359.

best outpatient department I have ever seen or had the privilege of working in. Each patient was assigned to one physician whose name appeared on the yellow clinic card carried by the patient. Even in the subspecialty clinics, provision was made for the patient to be assigned to a specific doctor. Waiting time was not excessive, and each patient was seen in a private examining room. The personnel, from the nursing staff to the clerical staff, was superior in education and attitude. Compassion, dedication, and kindness were the order of the day. Social Service, under the direction of Miss Janet Thornton, was a joy to behold in action in the clinic. What was lacked in funds was more than made up for by the staff's dedication to service.

So attractive and prestigious was the institution that many of the best physicians in the city and the metropolitan area competed to work in the clinics and to participate in the Center's activities. On any given day, in the Medical Clinic alone, there would be a dozen or more attending, each qualified to be a professor of medicine in any medical school, contributing his services to the sick poor and teaching one medical student on a quasi-preceptorship basis. Side by side in the clinic were the professors of medicine, each taking his turn in helping with the care of the sick. The sight of Walter W. Palmer, the Bard Professor; Robert F. Loeb; Dana W. Atchley; Franklin Hanger; George Draper; Randolph West; Martin Dawson; and Dickinson Richards among others working in the clinic was enough to hammer home to any attending that ambulatory care was important and that the care of the sick poor was never below the dignity of any physician no matter how skilled or highly placed. Contrary to the situation in many other hospitals in the city, especially the so-called community hospitals, full attending physicians, as well as their juniors, were required to participate in the clinic as well as on the wards. The outpatient clinic was an important and key element in the teaching program of the medical center. To participate in it was not to be a second-class member of the staff, not when the key professors set the example by participating and being there in person. Occasionally, we would seek the counsel of our senior professors on a difficult case. They, in turn, would seek the advice of the younger staff, usually on a procedural matter or some little question to which we were more apt to know the answer.

One day, Doctor Loeb, who detested abbreviations, came out of his room holding a chart that contained a physician's note he was having some difficulty in deciphering. "What do you suppose he meant by the abbreviation describing the patient as S.O.B*? I hope it isn't the usual connotation." He knew and we knew what the doctor meant, but it was Doctor Loeb's way of letting us know how much he disapproved of abbreviations in the clinical record.

Robert F. Loeb, the son of the great Jacques Loeb, was without question the most brilliant all around clinician I have ever known. He was able to combine great clinical skills, productive and imaginative research, inspiring teaching, a superb basic science background, and the capacity to spur anyone within 100 yards of him to greater effort, qualities that set him apart from any of his colleagues I have ever seen in action. He was truly a charismatic figure. Once you met him, you never forgot his message. Even after relatively brief exposure, his students and staff would spend years of their lives trying to live up to his standards. If one came away from Doctor Loeb's ward rounds without wanting to go directly to the library to learn, the session had failed.

Having said this, and leaving much more unsaid, there was an aspect of Doctor Loeb's professional life that led to controversy, fear, and anxiety among his admiring colleagues. He was the most strongly committed man I have ever met to the concept of full time in the clinical departments. This should not have been unexpected in the son of Jacques Loeb, the contemporary of Franklin P. Mall at the University of Chicago, and unquestionably a participant in the early American discussion of full time in the clinical chairs. When Robert Loeb came to P & S, he was the only one of the initial cadre of full-time teachers of medicine who refused to go on part time when the short trial (described in an earlier chapter) was cancelled because of its failure to satisfy the doctors and their patients. Loeb stayed on full time and for his entire professional life was to remain one of its prime proponents. His advocacy led to some acrimony.

Fortunately, this hard-nosed position was not assumed by the Bard Professor and Chairman of the Department of Medicine, Dr. Walter W. Palmer, who took the middle road saying that it

* Short of breath.

did not really matter whether a man were part time or full time, what was really important was that he give committed time to his medical school duties. Doctor Palmer set the balanced pattern for the Department of Medicine with its central core of full-time salaried physicians, its geographic full-time members, and the largely voluntary part-time faculty. He was an extremely wise and fair New England Yankee whose skill in handling all sorts of prima donnas in his department was responsible for much of its great strength. Doctor Palmer knew that the men in private practice were essential to the teaching and service programs of the medical center, and he never lost sight of this. While he himself was on full time, he encouraged his staff to pursue their practices and rejoiced as his men and women achieved renown and recognition in the world outside the medical center. I am sure that Doctor Loeb understood these matters, but his Flexnerian scientific background was so strong as to make compromise on this subject very difficult. Still, I am certain that later in life, his experience with a few famous patients, among them Madame Chiang Kai-shek and Albert D. Lasker, must have had some influence on his thinking. The willingness to serve as Madame Chiang's physician may well have been influenced by international considerations. The Lasker case was different and is described in some detail by John Gunther in *Taken at the Flood.*[306] In 1939, Lasker arrived at Harkness Pavilion of the Columbia-Presbyterian Medical Center unannounced and without an appointment saying he wanted to see Dr. Robert Loeb. The secretary called Doctor Loeb who asked,

"Does he want to see me as a patient?" "Yes."

"Tell him that I don't take patients. It's the rule of the hospital."

"He says he knows that."

"Ask him the nature of his problem, and perhaps I can refer him to the proper doctor." Pause.

"No, he says he has to see you."

"I'm terribly sorry, but I can't see him."

"He says he has come all the way from Chicago to see you."

"Tell him that he should have written first, he should have made inquiries." Another pause.

"He says that if he had written to you, the reply would have been that you would not see him."

306. Gunther, John: *Taken at the Flood: The Story of Albert D. Lasker.* New York, Harper & Brothers, 1960, p. 257.

"I'm sorry, but you'll have to tell him again that I don't take private patients."

"He says that he's going to stay in New York and wait if it takes two weeks."

Loeb sighed. "I'll run downstairs and see him for a moment to get rid of him."

"Getting rid of him" led to a one and one-half hour luncheon and the beginning of a great friendship and one of the most important relationships of the century between a physician and his patient. The impact was to be not only of great benefit to the two immediate participants, but it was to spread almost beyond belief into areas of research and benefaction designed to help all mankind. Loeb made an exception to his rules and became Lasker's personal physician for the remainder of his life. The experience was rewarding in more ways than one. For Loeb, a "man of the most fastidious, intricate and sophisticated intelligence," Lasker was "altogether engrossing"—"he could not resist him and thought that he was probably the most intelligent man he had ever met. Not that he did not have defects. Loeb admired not merely his mind, but his sense of fun and *joie de vivre*. At sixty, he was still buoyant as a skiff, and he had the enlivening quality of always making everybody seem at his best. Loeb and his wife, who is also a doctor, were not social; they worked too hard; but they could never decline an invitation to dine with Albert Lasker." Said Loeb of Lasker:

> He had communicability, ... There was a bright cover on his book. He not only had faith in the capacity of man, but instinctive knowledge of man's limitations; he believed that people could surmount these, develop out of them, he had a marvelous instinct for concentrating on the valuable aspects of a human being and sloughing off the rest. *Voilà un "homme."*[307]

Lasker was never able to persuade Loeb to send him a bill, but he more than made up for it with substantial gifts, especially four commissioned paintings by Dali of Venice, Rome, Como, and Naples in Loeb's "favorite country." To top it off, Lasker had the satisfaction of leaving a substantial legacy to Loeb when he died on Sunday, May 30, 1952. The contributions of Albert and Mary Lasker to medicine are too many to list. I am certain that their admiration and respect for Robert F. Loeb played a

307. *Ibid.*, p. 261.

major role in their motivation to spend so much of their time, energy, and resources in medical research and improved medical care. What if Loeb had succeeded in rejecting Lasker as a patient at that fateful visit to Harkness Pavilion in 1939? Would the Laskers have neglected medicine and concentrated on their art collection? Or was it destined and foreordained that the greatest cigarette salesman of all time, the creator of the slogan, "Reach for a Lucky instead of a sweet" should repay mankind by subsidizing cancer research for his unwitting role in promoting the causation of carcinoma of the lung?

In retrospect, Loeb could not have failed to realize that the intimate relationship between a physician and his patient is at the basis of all medicine. The trials, tribulations, joys, and satisfactions must be experienced to be appreciated. To deny this role to any physician is to deprive him of much happiness and contentment. To deny it to teachers of medicine is to court disaster in setting the mold for the role model designed and needed to inspire the young medical student and the developing clinician. Any system of medicine that makes it impossible or impractical for a physician to establish a one-to-one relationship with patients is a second-class one that will fail because it satisfies neither the true physician nor his patient.

Any discussion of Doctor Loeb as a teacher and clinician would be incomplete without a comment on what we called Loeb's Five Laws of Treatment.* The first is the Golden Rule which needs no interpretation; the second stresses the importance of bedrest in illness, a concept now considered outmoded; the third is that when everything is going well, for heaven's sake let things be; the fourth, if things are not going all right, for heaven's sake do something different and in some cases stop all medication; and fifth, for heaven's sake, keep the patient out of the surgeon's hands. Loeb did not swear, his closest approach to it being, "for heaven's sake."

Doctor Loeb's antipathy for surgery was well known to all of our staff, and in a way it is unfortunate that some of his disciples in internal medicine were so carried away by the precept that it seemed to blind them to the importance of working as a team with their surgical colleagues. Indeed, all too often, in

* I am indebted to Dr. C. T. Vicale of the Neurological Institute for his lively version of these laws.

academic medical centers, the department of medicine acts as an armed camp toward the department of surgery, to the detriment of patient care. No physician who gives personal care to his patients can ever really bear the hostility toward surgery that prevails in some institutions. I have always sought in my teaching program and by my example to collaborate with my surgical colleagues and to work effectively with them as a team for the greater benefit of my patients. We must respect one another.

Despite the occasional acceptance of a patient on a one-to-one basis, Loeb continued to be the Medical Center's outstanding spokesman for the full-time concept, but implementation was sharply limited by lack of sufficient endowment and rising inflation. The advent of massive NIH grants for research served to open up the floodgates. Many new faces appeared in this center as well as others, their activities devoted almost entirely to special research projects having little to do with the overall direction of the institution. So it was that new additions to the full-time staff, funded by the NIH, felt their primary goals were those of research. It was not unusual for these individuals to refuse to work in clinics or with ambulatory patients. The decline of the outpatient department, already underway, was to become sharply accelerated. Even the ward services suffered. First, some individuals of competence were reluctant to give the ward service their energies, choosing to concentrate on their research projects. Secondly, and in a different vein, ward teaching assignments went to inexperienced junior staff or research staff because it was their only opportunity to gain experience in the practice or teaching of medicine. Seasoned attendings were bypassed and told they did not need the ward experience because their practices gave it to them. The fulltimers had to have it in order to maintain their medical skills. Heaven help the patients! How much of this did they really know?

The overall effect of massive NIH grants for research was not only to expand full time in numbers but to change its character. The new model was a research-oriented scientist with little or no interest in teaching or in clinical medicine. To the weaknesses of the Flexnerian full-time model, there was soon added a new aspect: neglect of patient care and clinical teaching. And yet, they were the faculty of the medical school. They ran it, and they set the policies. Even more ominously, they would be the department heads of the future, ill-fitted and poorly educated for the demands of their high ranking posts. The part-time teachers diminished steadily in influence and in numbers. Soon they would go on a slowdown, refusing to give as generously as in the past to the clinics and the wards, and to the students. They were accused of being too busy making money with their private practices, but the real truth was deeper than that. They were rebelling against a system that had reduced their prestige, identity, and power. The students were being abandoned to junior teaching staff, and the effects could be disastrous. Inexperienced and narrowly trained teachers taught by committee and tried to treat patients by consensus. Decision making, the way of life of every seasoned clinician, was seldom a personal act. Teams took over, and patient care and student teaching were to suffer.

As it is with many other endeavors, the massive NIH grants that sought to relieve human suffering and promote better understanding of disease would become so unbalanced over the long pull that they had the opposite effect. These results could have been anticipated. Why didn't the faculties of the medical schools, including their deans, realize this and take appropriate action? Where was our leadership? What went wrong? Why didn't more people speak out?

Chapter 27
FOREIGN MEDICAL GRADUATES (FMGs) FLOOD AMERICA

Catastrophe struck American medicine in the 1960s when enormous numbers of foreign medical graduates were imported to make up a doctor shortage at a time when thousands of our own highly qualified young men and women were being turned away from American medical schools, not because of incompetence but because there simply were not enough openings in the existing schools. How did this come about? Who set this policy? Who was to blame? What went wrong?

We have already described the burgeoning of residencies and house staff positions following WWII and the continuing increase in the years that followed. Good, as well as fifth-rate, hospitals now had approved internships and residencies, many of them poorly supervised, providing cheap labor and with little or no commitment to education or bona fide training. The medical schools, their energies absorbed by undergraduate commitments, failed to see the importance of getting into postgraduate medical education. They simply turned their backs on this problem except for their own closely affiliated university hospitals. Regulation and accreditation of house staff programs was left to the Joint Commission on Accreditation of Hospitals (JCAH) with its limited staff and feeble power to enforce rules and regulations. Hospital administrators, faced with the prospect and the reality of vacancies on their house staffs and seeking nothing more than cheap professional labor to supply service demands of their hospitals, looked about in desperation and at first could see no practical solution. In 1973-1974, there were 66,302 openings in residencies and internships in the American hospital system with only 41,765 graduates of American schools available.[308] Clearly, too many internships and residencies had been set up and the suppliers

308. American Medical Association 76th Annual Report: *Medical Education in the United States: 1975-1976. JAMA, 236/26:*2931-3146, December 27, 1976, p. 3051.

(the American medical schools) could never fill the gap. Never underestimate a desperate hospital administrator or ambitious doctors seeking to maintain a power base in their hospital services. They always find a way out—not necessarily the best but nevertheless a pragmatic solution. For some, the answer lay in foreign medical graduates (FMGs). The foreign medical graduates of U. S. origin (USFMGs) were numerically too few to supply the demand. The greatest relatively untapped source was the foreign-born graduate of foreign medical schools. It was to this group that the lesser hospitals and some of the greater ones looked for relief.

Before Flexner's day, the foreign medical graduate was not a problem in American medicine, he was a welcome asset. As the opportunities for obtaining a medical education in this country expanded, few Americans sought their undergraduate medical education abroad, but those who could afford it traveled to Europe for postgraduate experience. With improvement in the standards of American medical schools and hospitals and the development of residency and fellowship programs, it was not long before the position had become reversed, with foreign graduates seeking postgraduate education and training in this country with the intention of returning to their country of origin on completion of their assignments. This development received encouragement from educators and government officials who saw it as a wholesome and constructive effort by the strong to help the weak. With the post-Flexner elevation of standards of admission to American medical schools and the relative scarcity of available places, it was inevitable that some Americans would go to European countries for their medical education, only to return for postgraduate training or to enter practice.

The total of the two groups, USFMGs and FMGs, who applied for licenses to practice medicine in America was, at first, quite small: 437 in 1935, rising to 2,088 per annum in 1940, mainly from European medical schools. With Hitler's rise to power, large numbers of European Jewish physicians fled to America. They found hospitality and generous acceptance, expecially in New York City where thousands entered the practice of medicine, encouraged by liberal state licensing provisions that other states were unwilling to offer. Anti-Semitism was not confined to

Germany alone. These physicians were soon to provide a major portion of general practice care for the residents of the New York metropolitan area. Their smooth assimilation was a tribute to the tolerance and understanding of the physicians in practice, as well as to their patients who accepted them with relatively little bias. There were, of course, some problems, especially with those deemed unqualified for hospital appointments, but nevertheless the immigrants were soon incorporated into the health care delivery system of this country, their assimilation accelerated by the civilian physician shortage of World War II.[309]

By 1970, the number of FMGs entering the United States had risen dramatically to 6,236 per annum, equivalent to three-quarters of the total graduating from American medical schools that year. Not only had the numbers increased, there had also been a striking change in the ethnic and national origins of the immigrants. Whereas in 1966 three-quarters of our physician-immigrants came from Europe or the Americas, by 1971 over 70 percent came from Asia, with India ranking first in numbers, followed by the Philippines, then South Korea, and Iran.[310] Clearly, a great change had come about in the immigrant-physician profile. The United States was now being flooded with physicians from inferior medical schools, many of them poorly educated by our standards and often with a serious language barrier. The richest country in the world was depending upon the poorer nations for doctors needed to cope with health care demands of its own people. When we should have been educating ample numbers of physicians for our own needs and exporting to the poorer nations, we were taking advantage of them and draining them of a valuable resource.

All of this, while we were turning away thousands of well-qualified youngsters from our own medical schools because of a lack of space! How did such a policy develop? Who was responsible? The story is like many others, the tale of a program that was started on an idealistic plane that was subsequently subverted to perform a function it was never originally designed for—to provide a source of cheap medical labor for hospitals whose

309. Lippard, V. W.: *A Half-Century of American Medical Education: 1920-1970.* New York, Josiah Macy, Jr. Foundation, 1974, p. 85.

310. American Council on Medical Education*Physician Manpower and Medical Education II.* A Report to the AMA House of Delegates, June 1978, p. 37.

educational programs were, to put it mildly, rather primitive and virtually nonexistent. The letter of the act was used to destroy its spirit and true meaning. Let us trace the development of this disaster.

Following the end of World War II, seeking to implement the wishes of a nation to help those less fortunate, the U. S. Congress passed the Informational and Education Act of 1948, establishing an Educational and Exchange Program under the supervision and control of the State Department. The purpose was to assist the developing countries by allowing them to send "their experts and other professionals to the United States for specialized training." This made it possible for the graduates of foreign schools to obtain exchange visas for graduate training in the United States "including a one-year internship and additional years of residency training up to five years." At the end of the period of training, these aliens were expected to return to the country of origin where it was anticipated that their newly acquired skills and education would be put to immediate use as a seedbed for upgrading human resources.[311]

Of some interest in this connection is that, as of October 1948, The Council on Medical Education and Hospitals of the American Medical Association took the position that "there is no need of any great increase in the number of medical graduates from our own schools and the gradual expansion of facilities for medical education that is taking place will adequately meet the nation's needs."[312]

This was at a time (1950-1951) when the postwar boom in house staff openings was beginning to soar, with 28,734 internships and residencies approved and only 19,453 U. S. and Canadian graduates available to fill the positions. The situation was to become progressively worse and indeed, within five years, the figures had risen to 38,132 positions, with only 24,995 U. S. and Canadian graduates available. Obviously, the AMA had lost sight of the hospitals' dilemma and was basing its policy on medical graduates on a data base with faults that would soon become glaringly evident.

---

311. Mamot, P. R.: *Foreign Medical Graduates in America.* Springfield, Thomas, 1974, pp. 8-9.
312. *Ibid.*, p. 7.

The FMGs admitted to the United States under the Exchange Visitor Program were all too often so attracted by better conditions here that they resorted to all sorts of measures to remain as permanent residents, thereby defeating the purpose of the Act under which they had obtained visas. Marriage was for some the way in. Others, required by law to leave the United States for two years, would comply by going to Canada and then applying for readmission to the United States as new immigrants. In 1956, the first Fulbright Act was passed to further encourage international goodwill by exchanging students, some of ours going overseas while some of theirs came here. In 1961, the National Educational and Cultural Exchange Act (The Fulbright-Hayes Act) expanded the concept, its purpose being "The improvement and strengthening of the international relations of the United States by promoting better mutual understanding among the peoples of the world through educational and cultural exchanges."[313] It also included a very important clause giving "the Attorney General the power to waive the requirement of the two-year foreign residency abroad in the case of any alien whose admission to the United States is found by the Attorney General to be in the public interest." This really opened up the door, and many FMGs took advantage of the loophole.

Further liberalization of immigration policies soon followed, capped by the 1962 ruling that "foreigners with specialized skills and training who had applied for Permanent Resident Visas prior to April 1, 1962, were allowed to come to the United States without regard for national quotas." This was a very marked policy change for it emphasized quality and skill of the immigrants rather than their geographic origin. By the same token, it opened up the gates for immigrants from Asia for whom the old quotas had been a prohibitive barrier. The effects were soon in evidence, many FMGs taking quick advantage of the opportunity and forgetting whatever obligations they may have felt toward the people who had made possible their undergraduate education. They elected to remain in the United States. What had started as an idealistic scheme to enhance cultural exchange among countries had become a one-way ticket into the mainstream of American life. As if this were not enough, in 1965

313. AMA 76th Annual Report, p. 3052.

amendments to the Immigration and Naturalization Act (P. L. 89-236) really let the floodgates down for FMGs by granting preferential status to immigrants with close kin living in the United States or with professional technical skills in short supply in the United States. Among the preferences listed in this Act were:

> Third preference applying to "qualified immigrants who are members of the professions or who because of their exceptional ability in the sciences or the arts will substantially benefit prospectively the national economy, cultural interests or welfare of the United States." The Sixth Preference of the Act applies to "qualified immigrants who are capable of performing special skilled or unskilled labor, not of a temporary or seasonal nature, for which a shortage of employable and willing persons exists in the United States."[314]

These provisions are believed by competent authority to have been tailormade to accommodate FMG physicians. When this was followed by the Labor Department's 1965 declaration that a shortage of physicians existed in the United States, all hell broke loose.[315]

The quality of the immigrant doctor's education or his language impediment were not a concern of the policy makers. Any individual recognized as a doctor in his own country could qualify for admission to the United States—a prime example of what can happen when an inexpert bureaucracy deals with a complex issue as a routine matter. Who took this way out? Where were the pressures emanating from? Almost certainly from the hospital lobby, for the shortages were in the main of applicants for beginning internships and residencies, many of them unnecessary except to provide cheap hospital labor or service. Educational commitment of the hospitals to these house staff appointments was, for the most part, absent. Those FMGs who were coming to America for educational purposes were being shortchanged, but most of them were seeking desperately to get out of their native countries to become part of the affluent society of America. The idealists were, as they have always been, few and far between. For most, it was a matter of survival with strong economic pressures to move upward.[316]

314. AMA 76th Annual Report, *ibid.*, p. 3053.

315. Margulies, H. and Bloch, L. S.: *Foreign Medical Graduates in the United States.* Cambridge, Harvard University Press, 1969.

316. Mamot, *Foreign Medical Graduates*, p. 25.

There were, of course, voices raised against the indiscriminate flooding of the country by FMGs. It was pointed out that the education of these physicians was inferior, that language barriers formed a real obstacle to communication, that reliance on developing, chiefly Asian, countries to supply physicians for the world's richest country was a disgrace, and turning a significant part of our health care delivery to individuals from an entirely foreign culture was at best unwise and, at the worst, inviting catastrophe. To stem the tide and to monitor quality, various measures were undertaken to screen out the applicants for visas. In 1957, the Educational Council for Foreign Medical Graduates (ECFMG) was established, and examinations in English as well as in basic sciences and clinical medicine were made available to FMGs seeking visas through a worldwide network of 178 examination centers, with questions being selected largely from Part II of the National Board tests. One weakness in this screening procedure was that it was not mandatory that the test be passed before appointment to an internship. In addition, the test could be repeated until the candidate passed and, worst of all, the emphasis was on a written test to the exclusion of consideration of the quality of education acquired by the candidate. By 1970, 29,950 took the ECFMG examination and 39.8 percent passed. Of those who failed the examination, a substantial number hold positions in hospitals in the United States that are very unattractive to graduates of our own medical schools. These form what has been described as an underground group of FMGs who seem to be permanently unable to pass their examinations, the actual number being in the range of 10,000. They continue to be used by the system that led them into America. Too late, measures are being undertaken to prevent repetition of this tragic fiasco.

What are the people saying about this massive influx of foreign doctors? Do they care? How much do they know? An American seeking emergency medical attention in any one of our great cities is brought up to date in a hurry on this issue when he is confronted in the emergency room by FMGs chiefly of Asian origin, many with language handicaps and from a culture quite different from the patient's. The patient becomes apprehensive and fearful and wonders what has happened to the system of health care delivery that has brought this about. Why are these foreigners taking care of him when his own son, daughter, or sister are denied admission to American medical schools despite excellent grades, integrity, and high motivation? These questions are not easily answered, and sometimes the answers offered are grossly untrue and unacceptable. A common whipping boy is the AMA, blamed vigorously but certainly in recent years unfairly, for limiting the production of doctors in order to maintain a monopoly.

However, over the long pull, the AMA and our specialty societies must take a substantial share of the blame for permitting the country to be overrun by FMGs without raising an enormous outcry. Would the American Bar Association ever have permitted this to happen in the legal profession? Neither can the deans of the existing medical schools be absolved of blame in this development. Why did they not take vigorous steps to control and regulate postgraduate medical education? Why did hospital administrators and staff physicians allow house staff positions to proliferate without end, almost forcing their institutions to look to FMGs to fill the spots? What was the Federal Government doing to control the influx of FMGs? What sort of policy is it that defends the admission of thousands of FMGs with the claim that millions of American dollars were saved because we did not have to pay for the undergraduate medical education of the FMGs? Is this a policy or an invitation to disaster? When it became apparent that the idealistic original purpose of the Fulbright-Hayes Act was being subverted by those using it as an employment agency for American hospitals seeking cheap physician labor, why wasn't the loophole plugged before it was too late? Why was the matter left to the Labor Department? Who sets Federal Health policy? Is there a visible Federal Health policy?

The actual dimensions of the FMG problem are startling.

> Foreign medical graduates now compose almost 22 percent of all physicians in the United States. About one-third of all hospital interns and residents are FMGs. In the five-year period 1970-74, approximately two in five of the medical school graduates added to the licensure registers of physicians in the separate states were alumni of other than U. S. schools. In 1974, FMGs made up 50 percent or more of physicians licensed for the first time in 14 states or other jurisdictions and in 5, FMGs comprised 75 percent or

more of the new licentiates that year.[317]

Our people cannot understand why the richest country in the world has failed to give them enough doctors of their own culture and national origin. Where is all the money going that we are spending on our medical schools? Why does it cost so much to build a medical school and to run it? Do we really need to stay with the post-Flexner lockstep and the dinosaur model of medical schools? Why can't we try compact models? Like the American automobile industry, medical education may have to settle for smaller models without the chrome and with better fuel mileage. It is an idea whose time has come.

Would any other profession in the United States have permitted this to happen? Aren't the people of this country entitled to receive their care from their own, who speak their language, understand their goals and aspirations, and can relate to them with empathy and understanding? The close personal relationship of doctor to patient is difficult enough to achieve and maintain without the barrier of language and serious cultural differences. To what avail has been the Flexnerian elevation of standards of admission to our own medical schools if we create scarcity of output, turn our own young people away, and then seek to remedy the disaster produced by our own plans by robbing developing countries of their own brightest and best? Something really went wrong, and something must be done about it! Or is it already too late? Is there not already in our midst a potential Trojan horse of thousands of alien M.D.s, poorly educated by American standards and remote from our culture?

---

317. AMA 76th Annual Report, p. 3049.

Chapter 28
THE GREAT MEDICAL MALPRACTICE RIPOFF

And Jesus said, Woe unto you also, ye lawyers! for ye lade men with burdens grievous to be borne, and ye yourselves touch not the burdens with one of your fingers.

Luke 11:46 (KJV)[318]

Disaster struck American medicine in the 1960s when malpractice litigation began a wild and sweeping escalation, endangering the very fabric of our health care delivery system and culminating in 1974 in an almost unbelievable series of crises with doctors on strike, hospital services cut except for emergencies, and acrimoninous and inflammatory confrontations between legislators and doctors making daily newspaper headlines. For the first time in modern memory, there was open warfare between the doctors and the legal profession with verbal blows being exchanged and wounds inflicted which to this day remain unhealed.

It is no exaggeration to say that a state of war exists between malpractice lawyers and the medical profession; the reader can check this by putting on a white coat and sitting around in the staff lounge or cafeteria of any major hospital and listening to the conversation. There is very little prospect for peace without major changes in the law, changes being fought by legislators, many of whom are lawyers with an obvious conflict of interest, blocking reasonable demands for relief made by practicing physicians. How did this come about? Originally, malpractice insurance was designed to provide a mechanism for punishing medical negligence and was based on the concept that the guilty practitioner had performed below the usual standards of care observed in the community and that, as a result of his negligence, the patient had incurred an injury. The doctor, as a member of a

318. Bible: Luke 11:46.

learned and respected profession, was accorded deference and, except for really gross negligence, could seldom be successfully sued for malpractice; but this attitude gradually changed.

Before World War II, malpractice litigation was relatively rare. In 1948, an internist could still carry liability insurance of $5,000 to $15,000 for a premium of $23 every six months. As late as 1959, equivalent coverage cost the internist only $30 every six months. In the next decade, business really began to pick up, premiums began to rise substantially, reflecting an increase in the number of cases and escalating awards. Even the hospitals, initially immune from suits, required increasing amounts of malpractice insurance coverage.

Between 1960 and 1970, annual malpractice premiums, paid by physicians, dentists, and hospitals in the United States, soared from approximately $65 million to over $330 million. This rise impressed the HEW Commission on Medical Malpractice of 1971, but it was small compared to what happened a few years later as the upward spiral continued. By 1974-1975, in New York State *alone,* the annual cost of malpractice premiums had skyrocketed to $224 million, compared with $330 million in 1970 for the *entire nation,* and a prediction was made that by 1978 the annual premiums in New York State alone would rise to $500 million! By 1975, the average annual premium for a physician in New York State was $4,700, with individual payments ranging from $1,763 to $21,584 for orthopedic surgeons, with no end in sight. Doctors were actually quitting practice because of these high premiums, some of the older ones retiring early. Younger doctors, faced with high premiums in certain specialties decided to leave New York State for regions of the country with a better malpractice climate. Or, failing this, some opted for salaried positions that would take them out of the so-called "entrepreneureal" private practice system. The problem was now affecting many aspects of health care delivery, and no one could long escape its impact. Since most of the costs of malpractice insurance were eventually passed through to the consumer and taxpayer, no one was immune.[319]

Hospital malpractice insurance premiums also underwent massive escalation, rising to $1,447 a year per bed in 1975-76, and within

319. McGill, W. J.: Protection of professional life in a litigation-prone society. *Bulletin New York Academy of Medicine, 53:*766-74, Nov. 1977, p. 769.

twelve months becoming almost impossible to obtain at any price, driving many hospitals to "self-insurance."[320]

A cost that hardly existed a generation ago now absorbed 1.7 percent of the $14,200 million spent on health care expenditures in New York State, 1.9 percent of the $5,860 million expenditures on hospitals, and 4.5 percent of the $2,750 million expenditures on physicians' services. Malpractice problems were compounded in 1974 in New York State when Employers of Wausau, a Wisconsin company and for many years the principal insurer of physicians, withdrew from the market because it was unprofitable and was replaced, effective July 1, 1974, by Argonaut, a California-based organization that immediately raised the rates by 93.5 percent and announced in December 1974, a further increase of 196.8 percent effective in January 1975.[321] The medical profession, now thoroughly aroused, could see no reason for the abrupt and massive premium increases and challenged their propriety, demanding an investigation. Suspicions were expressed, and with justification, that Argonaut's need for the increases was due to its investment and stock market losses rather than adverse experience with malpractice claims. Apparently, to avoid a showdown and the thorough investigation this would entail, Argonaut quit the field of malpractice insurance in New York State, effective July 1, 1975, leaving the doctors to fend for themselves.

Physicians sought legislative relief, but they were up against a legislature dominated by lawyers, many of whom were associated with law firms taking malpractice cases. Conversations between legislators and doctors became quite heated, the lawyer-legislators taking the tack that the legal profession had already suffered enough economic deprivation with the passage of no-fault automobile legislation. "We lost automobile litigation and we had to turn to malpractice to make a living." "Why are you doctors so upset, the insurance premium is tax deductible and you can pass the charges along to the patient by increasing your fees."[322] And, indeed, studies made in Michigan and confirmed in other localities indicate unequivocally that firms doing auto-

320. Report of the Special Advisory Panel on Medical Malpractice, State of New York, 1976 ("The McGill Report").

321. *Ibid.*, p. 79.

322. *Medical World News*, Aug. 25, 1975, New York, When a Malpractice Carrier says "Good Bye."

mobile negligence litigation shifted to medical malpractice suits after the passage of no-fault automobile legislation. Clearly, little was to be expected of lawyer-legislators without extraordinary pressure to act in the public interest rather than self-interest.

Racing for the deadline of July 1, 1975, when their existing policies with Argonaut would be terminated, the doctors sought without success to obtain any significant relief from the New York State Legislature. With considerable fanfare, the Act of May 21, 1975, Chapter 109, was passed by the Legislature and publicized as a great contribution to solving the medical malpractice problem. Without going into the details of this Act, it was completely unsatisfactory for the doctors and offered no substantial solution to the malpractice crisis. The Medical Malpractice Insurance Association, set up under Chapter 109 to provide insurance coverage for hospitals and physicians, was poorly conceived and badly organized. On May 24-25, 1975, the House of Delegates of the New York State Medical Society voted overwhelming disapproval of Chapter 109. Realizing that working with the lawyer-dominated legislature was a waste of energy, the doctors seeking to stir up public opinion resorted to reducing services and hospital admissions to emergency requirements. People became aroused and began bombarding their legislators. Doctors' offices became propaganda centers for relief. The hospitals quickly realized that nothing functioned without physicians.

Even these pressures failed to obtain the desired relief in Albany. In fact, efforts were made to place the striking doctors in a very bad light, accusing them of neglect of the Hippocratic oath, lack of idealism, being money-oriented, greedy, avaricious, unethical, and immoral. Sermons in various publications preached this theme almost to the exclusion of a fair appraisal of the needs of doctors and the ultimate harmful impact of the malpractice crisis upon health care delivery to their patients. The arguments against the doctors were of nineteenth century vintage and unrealistic in the 1970s.

A bone was tossed to the doctors by Governor Hugh Carey of New York who appointed a special panel in June 1975, the McGill Commission, to study the malpractice problem and to report back to the Governor and Legislature by January 1976. The doctors were tired of panels and commissions; they wanted action, and a verbal minority wanted to really shut down the hospitals. Fortunately, cooler heads prevailed. The one substantial saving grace that averted a great catastrophe was that the doctors had succeeded by the Spring of 1975, in obtaining permission to establish their own malpractice insurance firm from the State Commissioner of Insurance. Entitled The Medical Liability Mutual Insurance Company, it offered coverage to physicians in New York State at only a 20 percent increase over the Argonaut rates, effective July 1, 1975. This development, without any help from the State legislators, saved the day, at least for a time, and the transition from Argonaut to the doctors' insurance firm was remarkably smooth. Looking back on all of this, the one positive result of the malpractice war in New York State was the creation of a doctor-owned malpractice insurance company that has been very successful and should obviously have been started years ago.

With immediate disaster averted, the doctors looked to the McGill Commission for long-term relief. Having insurance available for purchase was a stop-gap measure. What was needed were substantive changes in the tort law, statute of limitations, informed consent, contingent fees, and numerous other inequities in the adversary tort system of settling malpractice suits. Would the McGill Commission do the job? It did not, unfortunately, for a wide variety of reasons, some of which were beyond its control.

McGill said in his report:

> The problem is that the definition of malpractice, well established in law, has been superseded by subtle changes in the sociological outlook of juries and insurance companies in their handling of claims. In view of such settlement practices, malpractice insurance premiums have continued to grow without relation to negligence; our best physicians and hospitals are being sued, not just the poor practitioners. A new doctrine has developed subtly and without formal articulation. . . . This new doctrine holds in effect, that a person who has suffered an injury through some form of medical accident deserves compensation. In view of the existence of an insurance system offering protection against suits claiming negligence, such compensation can be worked out only through the finding or fault. Thus, juries view the human dimensions of such accidents and ask for awards on the grounds that the injured deserve it and the insurance company can afford it. . . . Transformation of the tort law and insurance system has occurred rapidly dur-

ing the past decade.[323]

The Commission felt:

> clearly, we are facing a prospective breakdown in the system of tort law and malpractice insurance, perhaps not this year, next year, or within five years, but inevitably.

The McGill Commission, after considerable thought and study, felt any insurance system with "friction," or administrative costs and legal fees eating up a major portion of the premiums, leaving only 25 to 40 percent for the injured patient, was grossly inefficient and needed revision. Among its other recommendations were

> limitation of contingency fees, elimination of the *ad damnum* clause in the complaint, itemization of awards, limitation on maximum amount awarded for "pain and suffering," structured awards, and trust arrangements.[324]

The main recommendation attacking the tort-liability insurance system was quickly labeled "no-fault" by the legislators and Senator Dunne of the Commission who wrote a strong dissenting opinion. The concept of no fault has always been anathema for the lawyers-legislators and was rejected by them out of hand. Governor Carey, in April 1976, submitted to the legislature a list of recommendations for malpractice insurance relief, but it was a watered-down version of the McGill report and, even then, much of it was rejected by the legislature. Except for the availability of malpractice insurance made possible largely through the MLMIC without legislative or gubernatorial help and to a lesser degree by the MMIA (Chapter 109), the malpractice relief sought by the doctors and the measures recommended by the McGill Commission were largely ignored by the State Legislature whose reluctant moves to cope with the crisis have been characterized as applying an adhesive bandage to a major wound.

The McGill Commission's warning of disaster ahead and its prediction of an inevitable breakdown of the tort-law/liability system in the near future seems not to have made any appreciable impact on the lawyer-legislators. Only an aggressive campaign by the people at large will bring about any substantive change. While on the subject of the people, they are not without blame in the development of this crisis. McGill and many others have

323. McGill, W. J.: Bulletin New York Academy of Medicine, Nov. 1977, pp. 769-71.
324. *Ibid.*, p. 771.

pointed out that we have become a nation of litigants, looking to the law, the lawyers, and the courts to settle almost any conceivable dispute. McGill ascribes much of this to the development of an adversary society in the United States, and he believes that the mechanism of award that has changed tort law into a compensation system is to be expected in view of this society's adversary nature and its emphasis on the redress of grievances. He places his hope for a solution on the building of "a more harmonious system." In effect, he places his hopes for change on an optimistic appraisal of the capacity of human beings to rise above self-interest and to seek the high ground of public interest.

With eloquence he asserts in the final paragraph of his address:

> We must develop forms of insurance compensation and adjudication of disputes that can extract us from the adversary struggles characteristic of the courts. We must move away from the model of bargaining which is exemplified by labor disputes for settlement of such issues. We must do this if we expect to solve any of our society's larger problems. As we begin to solve the medical malpractice problem. We shall begin to solve many other problems of and equally divisive character. It will probably take longer than a lifetime to conclude such a monumental healing effort because the evil we now confront has been developing for more than four decades.[325]

Well said, but, I am sad to say, hardly an immediate solution for paying that enormous malpractice insurance premium and no solace at all for the innocent, idealistic, hard-working doctor being sued unjustifiably, not because he was negligent but because it is a way for a patient to claim compensation for his illness.

If the appeal to idealism and the plea for people not to sue so freely because it creates disharmony in our society is doomed to failure as I think it is, what is the solution? Where can we turn? Many wise and experienced individuals have given considerable thought to this subject, but no panacea has emerged; there are no easy solutions. Witness the HEW Commission study, "Commission on Medical Malpractice of 1971-1973" which, after sixteen months of deliberation and at least two million dollars spent, had labored mightily and in the opinion of the McGill Commission "brought forth a mouse."[326] Why did this commis-

325. *Ibid.*, p. 774.
326. *Ibid.*, p. 768.

sion fail to achieve a satisfactory goal? Why did it fail to realize that the malpractice problem was of crisis proportions? Why, for example, did it minimize the threat of malpractice lawsuits stating that "there is less than one chance in 100,000 of an incident occurring that will give rise to a medical malpractice suit each time a physician or dentist treats a patient"? Why did the Commission fail to realize that malpractice insurance was becoming difficult to obtain, escalating in cost, and headed for disaster? How close was the Commission to the grass roots, to the physician on the front line, actually delivering health care and maximally exposed to the threat of law suits?

Lest there be any misunderstanding, let us make it very clear that where actual malpractice has occurred, there is every reason to punish the perpetrator and to compensate the injured person quickly, effectively, and fairly. However, it is a matter of record that true medical malpractice is an infrequent occurrence. There are some honest mistakes, significant numbers of unsatisfactory results, but few downright instances of gross malpractice. Remember that 90 percent of all the malpractice suits ever filed in the United States have come since 1964. This phenomenon bears absolutely no relation to the quality of medicine being practiced that is better than any in the world. In fact, it is our best doctors and best institutions, those caring for the sickest patients and undertaking the greatest risks, that are being sued, not the minority of poorer ones. The explanation is not to be found in a decline in the standards of medical care or in the professional performance of the doctors. It lies elsewhere.

Where else in the world is litigation so openly invited as it is in the United States? Although it is not supposed to be mentioned in court, every litigant knows that doctors carry malpractice insurance, and it is common knowledge in New York City that hospitals require that their attending staff be covered in the amount of $1 million for one occurrence and $3 million for multiple claims. We have a society eager to gamble; witness the proliferation of legal and illegal games of chance, the give-away television shows and lotteries. Why work when you can get rich overnight be wagering a small sum or depending on the luck of the draw? With all that money sitting out there, with the press publicizing million dollar and multimillion dollar awards, such as the recent one for a misplaced belly button, with hungry, aggressive negligence lawyers, some of them called ambulance chasers in the old days, available like bounty hunters for a price, the cards are stacked so that it takes a truly magnanimous person to resist the temptation to blame the doctor for a real or imagined wrong and to seek financial retribution. The temptation is especially severe because the patient stands to risk or lose absolutely nothing by instituting the suit. No other major country in the world permits an individual to sue without requiring that he post collateral and be responsible for court and defense costs in the event that he should lose the case. Only in America can this happen! No wonder there seems to be no end to litigation, especially medical malpractice law suits.

The magnitude of the problem was grossly underestimated by the HEW Commission of 1973, due in part to the fact that it limited the study to claims closed in 1970, reflecting conditions in the 1960s when the problem was of smaller dimensions. In 1970, medical malpractice claims were filed in the U. S. against 26,500 physicians and other health care providers. By 1975, it was estimated that the number of claims filed would expand to 40,000 and the Insurance Services Organization (ISO) projected a 12 percent annual increase, predicting, if the escalation continued, by 1980 medical malpractice claims would reach 82,000 or more. In 1969, one out of every 23 doctors (4.3%) covered by the St. Paul Fire and Marine Insurance Company was involved in a malpractice claim and, by 1974, one out of ten (10%) was being sued for alleged malpractice. And this was with a company that does not sell insurance in such hardhit states as New York and California where the rise in cases has been of astronomical proportions. In Maryland, one out of every three orthopedic surgeons and one of every four obstetrician-gynecologists and anesthesiologists were involved in malpractice litigation in 1974. In California it is even worse, one estimate being that the average Los Angeles physician is sued once every seven years. Reliable estimates indicate that by 1980, the number of malpractice actions per 100 M.D.s will reach 35 to 40 in California and 18.4 in New York, with no end in sight.[327] Is it any wonder

327. AMA Source Document, prepared by the Editors of *PRISM*. Malpractice in Focus. Chicago, American Medical Association, 1975.

that a hot-selling automobile bumper sticker being used by friends and relatives of doctors reads: "Support a lawyer. Send your son to medical school."

The Contingent Fee: An Invitation To Barratry and Champerty

Many other topics were discussed in the HEW Commission's Report, but the segment of it that riveted my attention was the one on legal aspects of malpractice, the so-called Westat report. I happen to be one of the physicians who feels very strongly that a major factor in the medical malpractice problem is the contingent fee and its accompanying evil, the fee split or kickback. Despite the reams of opinions, essays and statements written on this topic, I have seen nothing to dissuade me from my belief that this is at the bottom of our problem with malpractice.[328]

Doctors Can't Split Fees—Why Should Lawyers?

If the contingent fee and the fee split or kickback to the referring lawyer and payoffs to runners and case finders were outlawed, I predict that the number of malpractice claims would plummet with immediate and dramatic relief from the current crisis. What is the evidence or argument to support this thesis, one that is strongly opposed by, guess who, the trial lawyers? These "heroes" on white horses argue that without the contingent fee, the poor would lose their "key to the courthouse." How else can the poor man sue his doctor or the hospital, they ask. My answer is that lawyers should try to emulate the doctors by giving their services without fee to their clients who cannot afford them.

Medicine, in compliance with its Hippocratic oath, has been doing this for years in its wards, clinics, and in private offices. What have the lawyers been doing? How many free clinics for legal aid are there? Is there any form of widespread Blue Cross-Blue Shield coverage for those seeking legal aid? Why is legal aid for the poor so minimal in this country? Why isn't it expanded? How does a middle-class worker get legal advice for reasonable fees? How much, or how little, *pro bono publico* work is done by the prestigious and very wealthy established law firms? How sincere are the malpractice lawyers when they

328. Westat Report: Appendix to Report of Secretary's Commission on Medical Malpractice. DHEW Publ. No. (OS) 73-89, Jan. 16, 1973.

speak of their concern over the little fellow who cannot afford to sue his doctor? How can one believe there is any real concern when it is a matter of record that malpractice lawyers reject claims under $10,000 to $20,000 because there isn't enough financial incentive? Let's face it, all too often the sole concern of the malpractice lawyer is to make money and to win his case, letting the chips of the reputations he attacks fall where they may.

The contingent fee, like poker, is essentially an American invention, the United States being the only major nation, with the sole exception of six provinces in Canada, which permits it to stand. This arrangement gives legality to the lawyer to gamble on getting nothing if he loses but one-third to one-half of the court award if he should win. The lawyer's share is right off the top, before other bills are paid, and the lawyer may get more out of a successful suit than the injured plaintiff. In addition, lawyers are allowed to kickback or split fees with a lawyer who refers the client to them, the amount being in the range of one-third of the lawyer's fee. Most of the time the "feeder" lawyer does nothing except exact his pound of flesh and provides no legal services to the client whom he refers. Oftentimes, the client is unaware that a major portion of the award will be kicked back to the referring lawyer who may act as if he were doing him a favor. Contingent fees and fee splitting and kickbacks are illegal in medicine, and they should be abolished in all of the professions, especially the law. If you need any further support for my argument against contingent fees and fee-splitting, look at the malpractice premiums paid by British doctors in their country where the contingent fee is illegal, $58.25 per annum, as compared with the astronomical figures of their American colleagues.[329]

But money, although important, is only part of the problem. Think of the anxiety, the frustration, the anger of the doctor being sued, most of the time without valid proof or reason. His reputation is assailed, and no matter whether he wins or loses he is hurt both professionally and in his community. The time expended in a defense is almost incredible. The attack upon the doctor, his character, and his reputation, conducted in open court under the rules of adversary conflict, is an assault upon every principle a good doctor holds dear. No doctor emerges from such

329. *Medical World News*, April 21, 1975.

an encounter quite the same. He distrusts the attacking lawyers, has nothing but contempt for their methods of operation, and has grave reservations about the entire judicial system that places him at such a disadvantage. Accustomed to scientific inquiry by rational thinking, he soon finds that the legal adversary system and its proponents are seldom interested in what is scientifically true. They are interested in winning at any cost, and whether the defendant doctor has done the right or wrong thing has little to do with their basic motivation. The trial lawyer's stock in trade is to make an ass out of the defendant doctor, using tactics often remote from those the true physician has been brought up with. The truth is not the issue, it is a staged performance in an arena the trial lawyer relishes and the good doctor abhors.

Anyone who has ever witnessed the selection of a jury for a trial wonders how the system works as well as it does. If the prospective juror is well educated and well informed, all too often the opposing lawyers will disqualify him. Rather than a true cross-section of the people, the jury ends up representing lawyers' preferences geared to winning their cases. Under the existing rules of adversarial confrontation, how can a jury of average people possibly learn enough to express valid opinions on highly technical medical problems? Is it any wonder that Chief Justice Warren Burger has come out for eliminating juries in civil cases that are too long, too complicated, or too technical for the average layman? This is a reform in our legal system long overdue, especially in medical malpractice.

Once a doctor has been sued for malpractice, it is bound to influence his approach to other patients. Much has been said about defensive medicine, the ordering of tests and consultations primarily to protect the doctor against a malpractice action. This is a costly development in medicine, but it is only a small part of the real problem. There are many times and instances when doctors refuse to see a patient because of fear of becoming involved in litigation. With the current vogue for a so-called "vacuum-cleaner" approach to law suits, anyone called to see a patient may be involved in a suit that is aimed at one principal who may, or may not, be at fault. Even the most peripherally involved physician may be subpoenaed and subjected to interrogation, deposition, court appearance and, in the event of a bad outcome, even the completely innocent may be punished and assessed damages. The dimension of this problem is difficult to identify, but it is of major proportions. Physicians or surgeons asked to perform a risky operation or procedure may hesitate to intervene and risk a malpractice suit in the event of failure or a poor result.

The point I wish to make is that the introduction of the malpractice threat into the doctor-patient relationship is one of the worst developments I have witnessed in American medicine during my fifty years in it. To this day, the issue of the contingent fee remains unresolved, an embarrassment to the elite of the bar and the battle cry of the trial lawyers. I doubt that it will ever be settled, certainly not as long as the sole arbiters are lawyers who judge themselves, make the laws, adjudicate and administer them. As recently as February 15, 1978, the *New York Times* headlined "Lawyers Shun Curbs on Suing Physicians–Plan to Reduce Cost of Medical Malpractice Litigation Turned Down at Bar Parley." The report describes the response of the House of Delegates of the American Bar Association to the recommendations of its own ABA Commission on Malpractice which, after several years of study, advocated several mild reforms, all of which were flatly rejected.

Once again, the legal profession has demonstrated its intransigence and its inability to rise above self-interest. Fortunately, the doctors are no longer alone. The general public is becoming increasingly hostile to lawyers and is in a mood to take aggressive action, not in the vein of Shakespeare's revolutionaries in *Henry VI,* Part II, "The first thing we do, let's kill all the lawyers," but to subject the legal profession to the public scrutiny and accountability that it has for so long evaded for itself and sought to impose upon medicine.

A distinguished professor of law at Harvard University, Lawrence H. Tribe, has joined the fray in an article appearing in the *Atlantic Monthly,* July 1979, entitled "Too Much Law, Too Little Justice–An Argument for Delegalizing America." He says:

> The United States now has three times as many lawyers per capita as England and twenty times as many as Japan. . . . In this century, the number of American lawyers has grown twice as fast as the population as a whole, and the profession is expanding more rapidly than ever. Over 126,000 students enrolled in law school in 1978–

> more than twice the enrollment fifteen years ago. In the same brief period, the number of lawyers has increased by more than 50 percent from 300,000 to 460,000. Multiplying even more quickly than lawyers are laws and lawsuits. . . . Clearly, something is awry. . . .This intoxication with law costs us dearly. Legal fees have soared to more than 25 billion a year. Because much of that expense is tax-deductible, the tax system in effect finances the litigious society.[330]

As a physician, I was really amazed to find that the prestigious HEW Commission on Malpractice was unable to tell us how many lawyers there are in the United States because there is no official central registry of lawyers. It had to base its analyses on the unofficial Martindale-Hubbell Law Directory, and "estimates" supplied by the American Bar Association which ranged in the neighborhood of 272,000 lawyers in private practice in 1972. *Time* magazine, in its issue of April 10, 1978, estimated that the number of lawyers in this country had within fifteen years increased from 296,000 to 462,000, a major discrepancy between its figures and those of the HEW Commission, even if due allowance were made for those lawyers not in private practice.

Without an official registry of lawyers with their specialty qualifications, the HEW Commission had to pick its sample of malpractice lawyers on hearsay with the help of the three trial lawyers on the Commission who named those familiar to them. What a primitive way to design a federally mandated, nationwide, well-financed study! Lawyers rather than trained survey investigators were recruited to interview lawyers, the argument being that they would be more comfortable with their own breed. My feeling is that they were all too comfortable and too cozy. Participation of those interviewed was on a voluntary basis, and in New York City of the twenty-one "potential subjects" identified by the HEW Commission as malpractice lawyers, only four participated. The interviews, such as they were, required no documentation and were essentially anecdotal—a naive way to interview a trial lawyer! All in all, the study is a prime example of how not to conduct an investigation of anything—especially trial lawyers—and I can find no excuse for its failings.

Again we witness the futility of permitting lawyers to investi-

330. Tribe, Lawrence H.: Too much law, too little justice—an argument for delegalizing America. *The Atlantic Monthly*, July 1979, pp. 25-30.

gate or regulate lawyers. And this is the very profession that is spearheading the drive to subject doctors to more and more regulation by bureaucrats and lay persons! Let the lawyers look at themselves. Why, for example, isn't there an official registry of all lawyers in the United States? Why aren't lawyers required to take special examinations for certification as specialists? How does the average layman know whether his lawyer has any competence in the problem being brought to him? Is he a tax specialist, a specialist in corporate law, a trial lawyer, a criminal lawyer, a real estate expert, or a divorce specialist, to mention only a few? Where is the blue book that the profession owes to the public as tangible evidence of its willingness to identify its practitioners and to safeguard the public from misrepresentation and fraud? When Warren Burger, Chief Justice of the United States Supreme Court, lashes out in public against the majority of trial lawyers whom he describes as grossly incompetent, he has ample reason for doing so and there are many, within and outside the profession, who agree with him. For example, in November 1973, Chief Justice Burger told an audience of New York lawyers, "We are more casual about qualifying the people we allow to act as advocates in the courtroom than we are about licensing electricians."[331] He has continued to pursue this line and as recently as 1978 caused consternation in the ranks of the legal profession by repeating his assertions and refusing to retract despite threats of retaliation and demands for an apology.

It is high time the legal profession has imposed upon it many of the regulations and restraints it has imposed, or seeks to impose, on others. No profession should be a law unto itself. I submit that the legal profession has failed miserably to regulate itself in the public interest. Its professional code of ethics is flagrantly disregarded by its members and poorly enforced. The voices for reform have gone unheard for years. With Watergate, Koreagate, and other evidence of gross malfeasance, lack of integrity and faulty ethics and morality, the public is now aroused to a degree that it has lost confidence in its legislators, regulators and representatives of government, many of whom are lawyers who make, interpret, adjudicate, and enforce the law. To name a few, witness the recent spate of books and articles on this sub-

331. Goldstein, Tom. *The New York Times*, Feb. 19, 1978.

ject: (A) Unequal Justice, (B) The Trouble with Lawyers, (C) Crisis at the Bar, (D) Why Crooked Lawyers Go Free, (E) A Plague of Lawyers, (F) The Finest Judges Money Can Buy, (G) Woe Unto You, Lawyers, (H) The Million Dollar Lawyers, (I) Lawyers on Trial.*

The time has come for the legal profession to put its house in order and to submit to outside regulation so that the reform it has so vigorously rejected may be instituted in the public interest.

In closing this chapter on the disaster visited upon American medicine by the malpractice crisis, I address myself again to the role of lawyers in promoting and abetting this conflict primarily for their self-interest and clearly against the public interest. They must take a major portion of the blame for the existence of the crisis. It is true that the general public is also guilty, the plaintiffs all too often seeking the pot of gold at the end of the rainbow by filing claims that even their own lawyers admit are at least two-thirds of the time without any merit. Add to this, juries who are overly sympathetic to the plaintiff and hostile to "rich" doctors and insurance companies, judges who may seek to solve social problems through acquiescing to awards for injuries having nothing to do with malpractice but designed for rehabilitation or reimbursement of individuals from the easiest available financial source. Finally, a population of people becoming more and more litigious every day, egged on by underemployed, avaricious, self-seeking lawyers with little regard for ethics or the public interest. How else can one assess their role in pushing the medical profession and the hospitals to the very wall, completely indifferent to the holocaust it has and is perpetrating on the American

* (A) *Unequal Justice.* Jerold S. Auerbach. New York, Oxford University Press, 1976.
(B) *The Trouble with Lawyers.* Murray Bloom. New York, Simon & Schuster, 1968.
(C) *Crisis at the Bar.* Jethro K. Lieberman. New York, W. W. Norton & Co., 1978.
(D) Why Crooked Lawyers Go Free. James N. Miller. *Reader's Digest,* Sep. 1979, pp. 47-54.
(E) A Plague of Lawyers. Jerold S. Auerbach. *Harper's,* Oct. 1976, pp. 37-44.
(F) *The Finest Judges Money Can Buy.* Charles R. Ashman. Los Angeles, Nash Publishing, 1973.
(G) *Woe Unto You, Lawyers.* Fred Rodell. New York, Berkley Edition, Berkley Publishing Corp., 1980.
(H) *The Million Dollar Lawyers.* Joseph C. Goulden. New York, G. P. Putnam's Sons, 1978.
(I) *Lawyers on Trial.* Philip M. Stern. New York, Times Books, 1980.

people?

Ethics and morality need to be introduced, debated and implemented in the law schools of the country before it is too late. Where is the voice of the deans of the schools? Why have they merely stood by as did many of the Germans in Nazi Germany while the profession of medicine and our hospitals were being attacked by self-seeking trial lawyers whose chief interest it was to get rich? Why does a young Harvard Law graduate cry out to no avail as a voice in the wilderness for the teaching of ethics in his prestigious law school?[333] The papers are full of criticism of the legal profession. Who among the lawyers will lead them out of the wilderness or barrenness they have created? When will the law schools be subjected to a Flexner-type investigation to close the poor ones, the part-time road to the court house, the night school avenue to legal opportunity? We are already inundated by lawyers; why produce 50,000 more each year? Let us shut down the bad schools and elevate the standards of the good ones.

In conclusion, I endorse with pleasure Chancellor Allen Wallis' commencement address of 1974 at the University of Rochester School of Medicine, entitled "Doctors and Lawyers."

Doctors and Lawyers

> You who are receiving degrees in medicine or in the sciences related to medicine undoubtedly realize that throughout the country at this season thousands of others are receiving similar degrees in token of their preparation, like yours, for devoting the best parts of their lives to improving the health of their fellow men.
>
> Most of you are vaguely aware, also, that all over the country even larger numbers are emerging from professional schools of another sort, namely schools of law. Probably few of you realize, however, that before your careers have run their courses those lawyers may have more influence than you have over what you do, how you do it, and how you are rewarded.
>
> You may find lawyers defining the range of treatments that you are allowed to use in specified circumstances. Lawyers may prescribe the criteria by which you are to choose among the allowable treatments. Lawyers may specify the priorities you must assign to different patients. Lawyers may require you to keep detailed records to establish at all times that you are in full compliance. Lawyers

333. Israels, M. J.: A dissenting opinion on Harvard law. *The New York Times*, June 12, 1975.

may punish you unless you can refute beyond a reasonable doubt their presumption that your failures result from not following all of their rules, regulations, and requirements. And lawyers may decide what incomes you deserve.

Should you have the temerity to differ with the lawyers, you will be backed by the authority of your knowledge, your science, your skill, your art, your experience, your judgment, your dedication, and your conscience. Which is to say that in the eyes of the law you will have precious little backing; for knowledge, science, skill, art, experience, judgment, dedication, and conscience—whatever else their merits—do not constitute due process of law.

This control of health care by lawyers will come about through a process in which many of you, and most of your contemporaries, believe unquestioningly. That is the process of turning to the government to solve all problems, real or imagined, large or small, widespread or confined. . . .

Scarcely anyone has confidence in any branch of government (except, ominously, the military), so we create new government agencies to monitor the old ones. Increasingly, confidence in private institutions and professions also is eroding, and the accepted solution is to regulate them through government, even though government is respected and trusted even less than the institutions it is charged with regulating.

It is this process of putting the least trusted of all institutions, government, in charge of less distrusted institutions and professions which may result in lawyers acquiring a far larger measure of control over health care and research than they have today. For what we call "government" is, after all, made up of people, and not necessarily superior people, much less perfect people. While not all people in government are lawyers, lawyers usually participate in writing rules, regulations, orders, guidelines, and directives, and the adjudicators and enforcers almost invariably are lawyers. So we can expect the work of those now receiving degrees in health to be closely regulated by those now receiving degrees in law.

. . . The lawyers have you outnumbered, but on the average they are no match for you in intelligence, industry, or dedication. Just don't let them ambush you while you are absorbed in caring for the sick.[334]

---

334. Wallis, W. A.: *An Over-Governed Society*. New York, The Free Press, Macmillan Publ., 1976, pp. 71-73.

Chapter 29
ACADEMIC MEDICAL CENTERS

In the early 1930's, as a medical student and house staff member and later as attending physician, I had the pleasure of making rounds with Dr. William S. McCann, the Dewey Professor of Medicine at Rochester, New York; Dr. Frederic M. Hanes, Chairman of Medicine at Duke University; Dr. John P. Peters, John Slade Ely, Professor of Medicine at Yale; Dr. Francis G. Blake, Sterling Professor of Medicine at Yale; Dr. Walter W. Palmer; Dr. Robert F. Loeb; and Dr. Dickinson W. Richards at Columbia-Presbyterian Medical Center in New York, as well as with other distinguished members of their staffs. These men were very different individuals with varying life-styles, but they had many qualities in common. Among these were brilliance, high competence as clinicians and teachers and investigators, leadership, widom, charisma, and incomparable standards and dedication to their patients and students. Over and above all of these were integrity and intellectual honesty with a deep commitment to respect for the identity of each individual patient.

These great teachers set the tone for the house staff in a way no textbook could possibly have done. The poorest and most undesirable patient was accorded the respect owed to his being ill. No patient, whether he was on the ward or in the most expensive private room, was addressed by his first name by his physician unless he was a personal friend. Decorum and dignity were preserved for all. On teaching rounds, as the teachers moved from private rooms to the wards, they wore the same clothes, exhibited the same manners, conducted the same dialogues irrespective of the social class or economic status of the patient, serving as superb role models for the junior staff. By their own example, in the eyes of their students, caring for the patient became just as important as curing the disease. Who will ever forget having witnessed the aristocratic and fastidious Hugh Auchincloss, Sr., Professor of Surgery at Columbia-Presbyterian, clearing a patient's "intestinal obstruction" on rounds by rolling up his gold cluff-linked shirtsleeves and digging out by hand, a large fecal impaction! Or what student will ever fail to remember the classmate who blurted out on Doctor Loeb's ward rounds that the patient being examined had cancer in a day when that word was not used at the bedside. Loeb's reaction was to order the student out of the hospital, to banish him from the medical school. The next day, the penitent student, seeking reinstatement, visited the professor and was taken back into the fold. "I just wanted you to know what it is like to have someone pronounce a death sentence on you," said Loeb.

In those days, the outpatient clinic was not neglected. House staff took regular turns in the various clinics and were assigned patients whom they would follow for the duration of their tenure. Every effort was made in the major university outpatient clinics where I worked to see that each patient had his or her "own doctor" so that patients would not wander about like lost souls. Medical students served regular tours in the outpatient department where they gained experience in primary care and office-type medicine under the vigilant supervision of assigned preceptors with wide experience in clinical practice. The attending staff, because of its long tenure and relative stability, provided the ambulatory clinic patient with continuity of care and direction. The senior professors also worked in the clinics side by side with the house staff and junior attending staff, giving the entire atmosphere of ambulatory care the dignity and purpose it deserved. Above all, it was a great feeling to know that the poor were getting as good advice as the wealthy, and that is why we were showing up day after day in that busy, teeming clinic. Which profession other than medicine can say this? Has anyone ever seen a courthouse surrounded by free legal aid clinics for the poor? This is the way it was with the Vanderbilt Clinic and other university outpatient clinics before World War II, but something went awry. With the passage of time, erosion and decay of the urban centers, and the flight of the middle class and their doctors to the suburbs, the neglect of the Samaritan role of medicine for its technology, the massive expansion in full-time positions, the trend to avoid primary care, this position could not be sustained, and undersirable changes became manifest.

Why did the profession of medicine, riding high on a crest of popular admiration and respect, its members returning from service in World War II to the well-earned plaudits of the people, witness a shift in position? It was soon to be placed on the defensive by a consumer-oriented nation of people, suspicious and critical of its doctors, demanding more comprehensive health care delivery and insisting that medical care be a right available to all on demand with no out-of-pocket payment.

In a recently published superb essay entitled: *The Academic Medical Center–A Stressed American Institution,* David E. Rogers, President of the Robert Wood Johnson Foundation, has put his finger on some of the things that went wrong.

> During the past decade, an unusual symbiotic relation that has linked the government and academic medical centers in a highly productive venture has begun to come apart. The special partnership, which gradually evolved in the years immediately after World War II, reached full flower during the mid-1960s. The relation developed because both parties shared concerns about medical matters and each had something to offer the other. Mutual interests included a desire to increase the national capacity to conduct biomedical research of high quality, to improve and upgrade the knowledge base and skills of new physicians, to strengthen the training of medical specialists, to regionalize better the sophisticated high-technology services in tertiary-care hospitals and to give services of higher quality to those unable to pay for private medical care.[335]

This arrangement was mutually beneficial, the government gaining from the input and cooperation of the academic medical centers as evidenced by improved staffing of the Veterans Administration Hospitals, the production of well-trained specialists for work in community hospitals as well as academic centers, and the development of neighborhood health centers in ghetto areas. The

---

335. Rogers, David E. and Blendon, R. J.: The academic medical center: a stressed American institution. *New Engl J Med, 298/17:*940-50, Apr. 27, 1978, p. 940.

academic centers gained as they were enabled

> to move to build a strong biomedical research capacity, a broader range of high-quality specialty training programs of international distinction, and to strengthen medical education greatly in the process. Through the back door of government research funding, teaching medical centers were also able to increase their medical services to low-income people, particularly those with serious complex illnesses in which their high-technology services excelled—to the benefit of all concerned. But now things are going awry, and the interaction is increasingly confrontational. From the federal point of view, academic medical centers, formerly believed to be a part of the solution, are now being regarded as the cause of the problem. Medical school deans who used to be asked to Washington for advice are now called there to be lectured on how unresponsive their institutions are to national concerns.[336]

Some blame this on a rising tide of antiintellectualism across the nation and in Congress, but this seems at best a simplistic explanation. Whatever the cause, the adversarial confrontation is becoming steadily worse, with the federal government seeking to use its control of the purse strings to impose upon academic medical centers innumerable restraints, regulations galore, and bureaucratic red tape and controls. Instead of containing health care costs, government policies have actually encouraged their escalation, the cost to hospitals of PSRO's alone being $300,000,000 in one year with little or no evidence of any cost benefits except to the insurance companies who have reaped a bonanza through shortened hospital stays with no discernible improvement in the standards of health care. Beyond this, academic freedom is being menaced by the government's clumsy approaches to the delicate problems of curriculum content, admissions quotas, failure to train primary physicians, and the maldistribution of physicians in practice. How and why did a marriage and partnership that seemed so right go sour?

In his analysis of what went wrong, David Rogers focusses largely on what he calls external pressures exerted upon the academic medical centers. He records that "of the 120 centers, 31—or more than one quarter, including some of the most prestigious ones—sit squarely in the midst of the largest, most troubled, decaying inner cities. Indeed over half—61—are in the 40 largest cities. Herein lies a problem"[337] When these academic centers

336. *Ibid.*, p. 940.
337. *Ibid.*, p. 941.

were first built, they were in areas of greatest need, surrounded by pockets of poverty in a middle-class environment with a balanced demographic mix of people. With the steady decay of this inner city, the middle class fled to the suburbs, leaving the city to the indigent, various types of misfits and losers, a predominance of poorly educated southern blacks who had migrated north in steadily increasing numbers and great numbers of illegal aliens. With the flight of the middle class, there went enterprises, job opportunities, and economic stability, and it was not long before the medical profession chose to follow the trend to the suburbs.

Except for a few characters like "The Last Angry Man," doctors could no longer be found in the central city or ghetto, and few young physicians would elect to establish conventional practices in these areas.[338] With the disappearance of private practitioners, there was no choice for the people of these neighborhoods except to go to emergency rooms of the existing hospitals. Some of these institutions, responding to economic pressures, were also abandoning their innercity locations and relocating in the suburbs. The academic centers, almost alone, held the fort, stayed put and became more and more the major resource for health care of the decaying neighborhoods. Their emergency rooms, designed for small volume, were soon overwhelmed, and financial demands upon the institutions would head them toward bankruptcy for services rendered largely without reimbursement. The highly sophisticated tertiary care academic center, designed as the court of last resort, was poorly prepared for these developments and was plagued with problems for which its staff, its policies, its goals, and its orientation were grossly inadequate and often inappropriate. Confronted with overwhelming problems of alcoholism, drug abuse, a decaying physical environment with unbelievably primitive housing and sanitary conditions, criminal activity on a scale seldom seen, and a breakdown in the criminal justice system, the academic center was now almost the only source of stability in these communities and was asked to perform functions for which it had little or no commitment or preparation. In addition, these institutions became a main source of employment and were, in the process, pressured into hiring more and more semiskilled

338. Green, Gerald: *The Last Angry Man*. New York, Charles Scribner's Sons, 1956.

local residents of limited educational background who, in turn, would soon, through group efforts, union activity, and community boards, attempt to control policy and governance of the medical centers. With the advent of Medicare and Medicaid and the dramatic expansion of Welfare Aid, increasing loads would be placed on the centers, already heavily burdened, and soon the trend would be to mass produce egalitarian medical care rather than to concentrate on high quality tertiary medical care for a smaller number of individuals, the role for which the academic centers had originally been designed.

Additional external pressures were placed upon the academic medical centers by "medicalization" of social problems, says David Rogers,[339] invoking a theme originally developed by Renée Rox:[340]

> Last on our list of powerful external forces creating problems for academic medical centers is the interesting shift in national perceptions about what constitutes a "medical" problem. During the last decade, many conditions that seem to have emerged as unfortunate responses to the stresses, strains and shortfalls of modern society have been moved into the purview of medicine. The overuse of alcohol, addiction to mind-altering drugs, problems of violence or of child abuse, problems previously labeled "behavioral," marital incompatibilities, sexual identity problems, certain behavior long considered criminal, compulsive overeating, and even gambling —these and many other problems—have now been "medicalized."

The impact upon the professional staff of academic medical centers was devastating, especially for those who had elected to pursue the scholar's life, isolated and shielded from the mundane struggles and petty annoyances of the world outside the ivory tower. Even those committed to clinical medicine found their scientific education inadequate for dealing with societal ills and their middle-class background a handicap in coping with the problems of the ghetto and in understanding the language and mores of the gutter. Many resented the medicalization of societal problems. and felt that physicians were being asked to step in where the courts, the family, the church, society as a whole and the government at large had abdicated and had failed to maintain control. Government, seeking a scapegoat for its own deficiencies

339. Rogers and Blendon, *New Engl J Med*, p. 946.

340. Fox, Renee C.: The medicalization and demedicalization of American society, *Daedalus* (Proc. Am. Acad. Arts & Sci.), *106/1*:9-22, 1977.

and a mechanism for solving the very problems it had failed, quite miserably, to resolve through its own efforts, looked to the academic medical centers to perform miracles among the assorted alcoholics, drug addicts, psychopaths, perverts, and other dropouts from civilized society who were crowding into their clinics, often displacing the more deserving poor and the worried well. This was a role for which academicians were poorly suited and ill-prepared by selection, precept, and commitment and one that a good many resented. To understand why this was so, we need to examine not only the external pressures on the academic centers but also what was happening within these centers. It is all well and good to blame "them," the outside world, for what went wrong, but something also happened inside the academic centers that contributed to the problem rather than to the solution.

Internal Problems in Academic Medical Centers

Some of the blame has to be ascribed to compliant obeisance to the Flexner full-time system pressed upon the academic medical centers by its ardent advocates. We have seen how this accelerated after World War II and really exploded when large governmental funds became available. Whereas in 1950, federal research fund allocations amounted to $73 million, by 1973 they had risen almost fortyfold to $2.8 billion, leading Rogers to say,

> These large infusions of research monies led to a dramatic change in both the size and the character of academic medical centers. No longer were they to be simply places to teach medical students and the hospital of last resort to care for those with complex and life-threatening illnesses. They also became the centers for new biologic science. Faculties were rapidly expanded, and most of those recruited were selected for their research backgrounds and potential. Indeed, these new faculty members were recruited primarily for work in the laboratory not patient care. The funds to support them were public dollars, while clinical work and, to a lesser extent, teaching were actively discouraged. The number of full-time faculty grew by 300 percent–from 13,681 to 39,300–between 1962 and 1976.[341]

Empires sprang up in academic centers, directed by faculty owing little or no obligation to the broader goals of the university, or to community needs, and concerned chiefly with the furtherance of their own research projects. With salaries, equip-

341. Rogers and Blendon, *New Engl J Med,* p. 943.

ment, and budget provided by government funds and large allowances for overhead, these research-oriented entrepreneurs were often in a position to dictate terms to the deans of their schools and to enjoy freedom from any supervision or overall control. All too often, policy was set by individuals having large grants but with limited perspectives of the general goals, aims, and purposes of the academic centers. There was little or no awareness of or concern for problems in the community and the need for change in meeting the demands for health care delivery. The medicine of tomorrow took over while the problems of today were neglected. The faculty and faculty committees were predominantly controlled by the basic science and research group. Curriculum and admissions policy were set by the same people whose teaching obligations were not very heavy, leaving ample time for committee meetings and prolonged luncheon discussions. The talkers and planners took over, while the doers involved in day-to-day patient care were less available and relegated purposefully or through their apathy or default to lesser roles in critical decision making. Where were the deans of the medical schools while this was going on? Outnumbered and vulnerable, oftentimes poorly trained and ill-equipped for the new demands of the position, struggling for survival, their half-lives reduced to three or four years by sometimes vicious infighting, compromising instead of leading the way, powerless to set and determine broad policy —in effect, figureheads, with a few exceptions.[342]

Full time had taken over in a massive way but radically different from the system that Flexner had originally imposed upon Hopkins where the clinician was expected to see patients and the surgeon to continue to operate but to do this without monetary consideration while continuing to teach, investigate, and direct large clinics. The new fulltimer was primarily a researcher who avoided patient care like the plague and often sought every excuse to escape from teaching medical students and house staff.

Dr. Dickinson W. Richards, Nobel laureate in medicine, superb clinician and teacher, a stimulating writer on medical history and education, addressed himself to this theme when he raised the question: "Are Our Medical School Faculties Qualified to Teach

342. Glaser, R. J.: Medical care, education and research. *New Engl J Med, 271/27:* 1398-1403, Dec. 31, 1964.

Medicine?" In this essay, he questioned some of the post-Flexner developments in the academic medical centers, especially those having to do with part-time teacher practitioners, and concluded—

> The effects [of the Flexner scheme] on the practicing clinicians who serve as teachers, insofar as these survive, are severe. They are truly second-class citizens. Their counsel is tolerated but not accepted, while the resident reigns supreme. They themselves become discouraged, and often fall further behind. We still do have clinicians, actually practicing clinicians, who are doing top-quality research; but their path is not easy, their academic recognition is held back, and their numbers are diminishing. Clinical investigation, as such, is receiving relatively less attention, at a time when it is increasingly needed, and when it must become more rigorous. Correspondingly, the full and comprehensive and continuing care of the patient, especially in relation to his family and community, is given low priority.[343]

343. Richards, D. W.: *Resident and Staff Physician*, October 1971, pp. 76-88.

Chapter 30
OPEN-HEART SURGERY

The July 8, 1980 issue of *The Washington Post Magazine* features staff writer Nicholas Lemann's story, "The Lives in the Day of Dr. Lefrak," replete with three full-page color photographs of the doctor at work under a subtitle, "Money Just Doesn't Interest Me . . . I Love Heart Surgery. I Just Love It."[344]

Dr. Edward Lefrak, thirty-seven years of age, a 1969 graduate of the Indiana University School of Medicine, only three years in private practice after spending eight years in residency training in cardiovascular surgery, specializes in open-heart surgery. He will perform 500 such operations this year, 400 of them coronary artery bypass procedures. From these he will gross upwards of a $1.5 million in fees, making him, in Lemann's judgment, one of the highest paid people in Washington and, I would add, probably one of the hardest working. Lefrak operates in a nonuniversity community hospital and does little or no teaching. The story of his meteoric rise to affluence and prestige tells us a great deal about current trends in medical economics, practice, and education.

The crux of this story is the introduction in 1967 and the subsequent success of coronary artery surgery utilizing vein grafts obtained from the patient's legs for bypassing obstructions in diseased coronary arteries with resulting improvement in the circulation to the heart muscle. This operation, done with the trappings and all of the drama of open-heart surgery, had enormous appeal for those afflicted with angina, was relatively simple to perform for an experienced cardiac surgeon assisted by a good pump team, and could be done with very low mortality in substantial volume. The group of patients in need of such surgery—male, middle-aged, employed, responsible, and possessing

344. Lemann, Nicholas: The lives in the day of Dr. Lefrak. *The Washington Post Magazine,* July 8, 1980.

excellent health insurance coverage—was an answer to the prayers of hospital adminstrators seeking to fill beds and increase hospital income and prestige. Lemann described the operation more crassly as a "good money-generator for doctors and hospitals."

Initially promoted as prolonging the life of patients with coronary artery disease, the operation is now accepted as effective treatment for angina pectoris, improving the quality of life without statistical evidence of life extension except in obstruction of the left main coronary artery or in triple coronary artery obstruction where it may be life-saving. Lefrak performs his surgery in Fairfax Hospital, Fairfax, Virginia, whose trustees decided in 1977 to start an open-heart surgery program and imported Doctor Lefrak, fresh from a training program in Houston and Portland, Oregon, to become its director.

What motivated Fairfax Hospital, a nonuniversity, nonteaching community hospital, drawing its patients from the Washington, D. C. area, to embark on an ambitious open-heart program? Almost certainly, economic factors played an important, perhaps the decisive, role. A successful program would fill beds with middle-class, well-heeled, and well-insured patients, important considerations in a period of declining bed occupancy and diminishing hospital revenue. The patients would all pass PSRO and Utilization Committee review. Third-party payors would ensure that most of the hospital bill would be paid through insurance, only a fraction of it to come from the pockets of the patient. Of a $23,00 hospital and doctor's bill, only $1,075 would be out of pocket. Public relations aspects of the program were important; its success would attract favorable attention of the general public and generate interest in fund raising and other activities of the hospital. Other considerations played a role in the trustees' decision, not the least of which probably was the weakness and low volume of the open-heart programs of the three university medical schools in Washington, D. C., where vested interests obstructed innovation and the importation of new blood. An additional stimulus to the trustees may have been the striking success achieved by another nonuniversity community hospital, Washington Hospital Center, whose open-heart program was initiated in 1974 under the direction of Dr. Jorge Garcia, one of its surgical trainees who had been recalled from the Cleveland

Clinic.

By stepping into the void created by weakness in the university medical school programs these two community hospitals soon became responsible for the overwhelming majority of open-heart operations performed in the Washington, D. C. area.

In the fall of 1979, says Lemann,

> a task force of local heart surgery experts issued a report on the state of the art locally that pronounced the programs at Georgetown University, George Washington University and Howard University "unacceptable" for their low volume of cases and high mortality rates. The report showed Lefrak with the lowest death rate in the area for bypass operations in 1978, 1.7 percent; Garcia's team at the Washington Hospital Center with 3.2 percent, second lowest; and Hufnagel (at Georgetown University) with a rate of 11.8 percent, more than double anyone else's. The report was well publicized and had the effect of officially enthroning Lefrak and Garcia as the area's premier heart surgeons. The staffs of the university hospitals were outraged. . . .

Clearly, these two young men and their community hospitals had stolen a march on the university centers, a position they have not relinquished as their programs have continued to flourish.

> Garcia now has two other heart surgeons working with him, and together they will do about 900 operations this year. Lefrak just hired a second surgeon and will do about 500 cases this year on his own. Garcia's mortality rate for bypasses last year was 0.8 percent. Lefrak's last death on a bypass case was last October. . . .
>
> Lefrak admits that he makes a great deal of money and does not spend any of it because he works all the time. He is described by Lemann as being positively hostile to money and describes its acquisition as an anti-goal; but he continues to accept the money and to deposit it in a zooming 5 ½ percent savings account. . . .
>
> Garcia, the son of a farmer in the Philippines, lives in a house in Potomac with a private tennis court and seems more interested in the finer things in life. Asked what he likes best about America, he grins and says, in slightly tortured English, "Free Enterprise! You can do anything you want. It doesn't matter who you are that is my favorite thing."

The story of the Washington, D.C., open-heart programs has a message and raises several questions. First, and perhaps foremost, is the failure of three major university medical schools and their hospitals to meet the challenge of open-heart surgery and in the process neglect to bring to the people of that area the benefits of modern cardiovascular surgery. Why did it fall upon the trustees of two lower echelon community hospitals without university standing to bring Washington, D. C., into the modern era of open-heart surgery? Granted that their motives may have been suspect, predominantly economic or financial, at least change for the better was brought about.

This accomplishment calls to mind Dr. David Rogers' comment that changing course for a large academic medical center has become as complicated as reversing course of a large modern battleship compared to earlier days when institutions were smaller and could be turned around quickly and easily, like a canoe. Therein lies a lesson. Have medicine and its leading institutions become so big and unwieldy that they have lost flexibility and maneuverability in an era of turbulence and change calling for quick and innovative decision-making? At a time when being bigger is equated with being better, can being smaller be more efficient, higher in quality, and more productive? Are academic, university-controlled medical centers so large and unwieldy that they may be headed, like the dinosaur, for extinction? Is it not time for decentralization rather than merger? Is the bloom off the rose of the university as the dominant force in controlling and setting policy for medical education, training, and health care delivery? Let the Washington, D. C., experience speak for itself.

On the short haul, the superiority of the programs at the two community hospitals is being judged primarily by their low mortality rates. On the long pull, other considerations must be given emphasis. Coronary artery bypass, as is true of many other therapeutic measures, does not cure heart disease; it palliates and, in some instances, extends life, but the underlying disease process remains untouched. How many of Lefrak's or Garcia's patients really needed the operation? How carefully were they selected? Were medical measures given an adequate trial? How are the patients being followed? In a university academic medical center, one would hope that experience with this group of patients would be shared in education, training, teaching, and research, with a large population of medical students, nursing staff, technicians, house staff, attending staff, and research scientists focussing on the prevention of heart disease and on long-term care of the patient. Virtuosity and skill in performing an operation, no matter how advanced, should not be the sole or dominant factors in judging the success of a program. The real solution is to introduce highly skilled surgeons into the academic programs, keep them reasonably happy, and expect and demand that they collaborate with cardiologists and that they train others to acquire equally high surgical skills. They should be part of a team, not the whole show.

Other questions are raised by the Washington story. Is it equitable that a young surgeon, only three years in private practice, gross in excess of $1.5 million a year in fees while the insurance plans providing these rewards squeeze every dollar they can from the payments made to physicians in less glamorous fields who seldom gross one-tenth as much as the surgeons? While the open-heart surgeon, with minimal overhead (most of it provided by his hospital), is rewarded for his efforts at the rate of $1000 an hour, who decides that a physician in his office, with substantial overhead out of his pocket, be reimbursed less than twenty dollars for a Medicare visit and a fraction of this for Medicaid? Is it fair that a young doctor, just starting practice fresh out of a residency, be able to establish a higher profile for Medicare fees and end up being far more generously reimbursed for his services than the old established practitioner whose profile and fee schedule designed for harder times were much lower? These inequities have led to considerable dissatisfaction and unhappiness. Is it then any great surprise that some physicians resort to five-minute visits, hustling, pingponging patients, performing unnecessary tests, x-ray studies and electrocardiograms all for the purpose of expanding their income? The remarkable thing is that only a minority of physicians resort to these unethical practices while the majority remain steadfast to the high traditions of their profession. By working longer hours and longer days, they cope with the demands of higher and higher overhead, increasing malpractice premiums, soaring inflation and inadequate insurance reimbursement allowances.

It is all well and good to demand that the physician lavish time, effort and personal, individualized attention on each patient and extend every effort toward preventive medicine and ambulatory care and on keeping the patient out of the hospital. Still we have a system of payment that favors inpatient hospital care, technical procedures, and tests, all of which are reimbursable while outpatient ambulatory care is often not paid for by insurance and even when it is reimbursable it is at niggardly rates. The overhead expenses of the physician in private practice receive scant attention when reimbursement formulas are calculated by insurers, or at least it seems that way. The impact of soaring malpractice premiums has been virtually ignored. All too often, the effects of inflation have to be absorbed by the doctor, who is admonished by the AMA to keep his fees down to avoid adverse publicity. Disgruntled patients and insurance companies with powerful legal resources at their fingertips can complain to grievance committees of the County Medical Society or the State of alleged overcharging by doctors. In such a conflict, the doctor is usually at a substantial disadvantage.

Professional office rent in New York City has soared out of sight with levels of thirty dollars or more per square foot prevailing. Doctors who started practice in New York in the 1930s paid less rent per month for a two-room office than they now pay for *one square foot* of office space—more than a 100-fold increase in rent alone. To top it off, the latest gambit is to attempt to force a long-established physician to purchase at highly inflated prices the office he had been leasing for years and to add to this an extraordinarily high monthly maintenance charge for services seldom rendered to him. Add to this the salaries and fringe benefits, special taxes, pension plan, and other outlays required for the myriad of personnel and ancillary services needed to cope with modern medical practice. These may include nurses, technicians, secretaries, receptionists, bookkeepers, accountant, lawyer, malpractice insurance premiums, answering service, cleaning service, utilities, garage rent, telephone bills, etc. Of a gross income of $150,000, it is not unusual for more than half to be consumed by overhead expenses.

Is it any wonder that many physicians are eschewing solo practice, taking institutional salaried positions, forming groups, or staying in academic medicine, leaving the field to an assortment of gynecologists, plastic surgeons, radiologists, proctologists, and others who can generate large incomes. Doctors are notoriously underpaid for thinking, talking, listening and reassuring, and they have difficulty in paying their bills at present rates of third-party reimbursement for these aspects of their work without cutting corners and shortening the length of their encounters with their patients. A visit is a visit and is paid for at the same level whether it takes one hour or ten minutes; whether it takes the skin off the doctor's back to survive the episode; or whether the doctor is a star, brilliant, dedicated, accurate and compassionate; or mediocre, unscrupulous, incompetent, callous, stupid, or venal.

It should be emphasized that the amount of time the doctor actually spends with a given patient may be only a fraction of that spent in reviewing x-ray films, laboratory tests, and the literature or in just plain worrying and wrestling with the problem. This is the kind of work lawyers charge for by the hour but is not rewarded by health insurers. In this respect, medicine should take a leaf from the legal profession. All insurance and reimbursement formulas favor getting *things* done as opposed to thinking and decision making, the real essence of good medical care. Witness the substantially higher incomes of radiologists, endoscopists, clinical pathologists, and surgeons as opposed to family practitioners, internists, and pediatricians.

The system of paying doctors for their work must be redesigned if people wish to have doctors who will spend time with them to perform the acts of reassurance and comforting that are all that are needed for 75 percent of the complaints for which patients consult doctors. This applies no matter who pays the bill —private funds, government, insurance, or whatever. While on this topic, the unconscionably high incomes of some hospital-based specialists, who receive a percentage of the gross take, are sources of much dissatisfaction within the profession and are serving to severely overinflate medical costs. I have in mind the incomes of hospital-based radiologists, anesthesiologists, and so-called clinical pathologists. They have a monopoly and serve a captive audience, the hospital patient, who has no freedom of choice and must accept the person assigned. The clinical pathologist never sees the patient and still he may derive an enormous income from allegedly being responsible for the laboratory that does thousands of tests. Recently it was disclosed that a clinical pathologist in a small 145-bed hospital in Elkton, Maryland, was paid nearly $500,000 in salary in 1975. This is not an isolated example. I regard it as an abuse of a monopoly, and I feel that it has to be corrected by our own profession before someone else does it for us.[345]

A recent expose, published in *The Daily News* of New York on November 23, 1980, entitled, "The Medical Perk Barrel—or—How Doctors Get Rich," contains allegations that, if proven to be true, are nauseatingly offensive to the rank and file of the medical profession. Among the accusations are these:

> . . . that in hospitals here and elsewhere in the country, doctors are given not only handsome salaries but also a long list of perks (fringe benefits) that include chauffeur driven cars (in one instance a Jaguar), college expenses for their children, free office space, mortgages at low interest rates, gourmet meals, country club fees, liberal travel expenses, and lucrative private practice deals. Ultimately, the millions of dollars in costs are paid by taxpayers through higher Medicaid, Medicare, and Blue Cross bills.

The matter is now under investigation by a New York State Senate Task Force on Financially Troubled Hospitals whose chairman, State Senator Thomas Bartosiewicz (D., Brooklyn), describes the "multi-million dollar perks for doctors as a modern day version of Robin Hood in reverse—rob from the poor to give to the rich." Some might question the source and sincerity of this accusation originating as it does in the New York State Senate whose predatory raids on the public till for its own "perks" have aroused public outrage in the past.

345. *American Medical Association News,* Nov. 1, 1976, p. 15. Re: clinical pathologist, hospital, Elkton, Md.

Chapter 31
COSTS OF HEALTH CARE

Grave fears have been expressed about the enormous sums being spent by Americans on health care, the most recent estimate being $165 billion in 1978, roughly 9 percent of the Gross National Product (GNP).

My reaction is this. Why not stress the good accomplished rather than focus attention on an artificial ratio of expenditures thought to be appropriate in relationship to other priorities in our lives? Why not publicize statistics such as those prepared by the U. S. Department of Commerce showing that Americans paid out more for their automobiles in 1975 than they spent on their total health care, the actual figures being $112.5 billion for autos, as compared with $86.4 billions for health care, leading one editor to comment "and the American public shelled out about $26 billion more a year on the care and feeding of autos than on its personal medical care."?[346] And this was well before galloping inflation, the energy crisis and soaring gasoline bills.

Even more titillating are these facts. In 1976, Americans spent as much or more on their lawyers as they did on their doctors. In 1977, they spent $28.2 billion on alcohol, $25 billion on legal fees, $50 billion on gambling (almost certainly a gross understatement), $16.5 billion on tobacco, $11.5 billion on toilet articles and cosmetics, $2 to $3 billion on cat and dog food and, by one estimate, $175 billion on leisure activities in 1978.[347] Is it not time to question priorities on the expenditure of the Gross National Product rather than to focus the criticism on health care expenditures? And, while we look at medical expenses, let us not forget that in 1977, in New York County alone, "the largest number of patients, over 13,000 using up the largest

346. *Medical Economics*, Dec. 15, 1976, p. 240.

347. American Medical Association Research Information Center, H. M. Enos to author, Nov. 13, 1978.

number of patient days, over 136,000, and accounting for the largest single expenditure of 20.4 million dollars, were patients admitted to hospitals for alcoholism and drug abuse."[348] Even this is known to be the tip of the iceberg, excluding alcohol-related admissions covered by one or another euphemism or camouflage.

Many proposals have been advanced to reduce health care expenditures, some by the very same politicians who have never been known for cutting costs for anything they touch. For those in government who, in the guise of reducing health care costs, inflict ever more costly government regulations upon this "industry," I say, end the charade. PSROs alone added $300 million to the health care bill last year with absolutely no evidence that health care standards were improved. During 1978 alone, in New York State forty dollars was added to the daily cost of each hospital bed by regulations imposed upon the hospitals by government agencies, again having nothing to do with the quality of health care.[349] Similar restraints and costs have been inflicted upon industry and ultimately the consumer by over-regulation in the hands of a proliferating federal bureaucracy. My answer to this is a plague on government regulations and its bureaucrats. Rather than to place a cap on hospital costs, let us put it on government spending. Cut the budget. Allow the government so much money for its annual budget except for bona fide emergencies and demand that there be no overruns. Let the government live within its means. Let no one make the excuse that the spawning bureaucracy serves to employ more people. I would rather place a pick and shovel in the hands of those who need this kind of "made" work.

Having taken this position on overregulation of our hospitals by government and its bureaucracy, it is not suggested that hospitals are without blame. They have their own bureaucracy, built-in flaws and featherbedding. It is common knowledge that the productivity of hospital workers is well below that of employees in other segments of our industrial system, and major efforts must be made to improve performance. Of course, a hospital cannot

348. Goessel, E. A., Med. Director, New York County Health Services Review Organization. *NYCHSRO News*, Winter 1978, p. 2.

349. Crandall, R.: Is government regulation crippling business? *Saturday Review*, Jan. 20, 1979, pp. 31-41.

be run along the lines of a shoe factory. Like a fire department, it must be staffed around the clock, twenty-four hours every day, to be ready for any emergency. At any given moment during the twenty-four hours there will be surplus personnel with little or nothing to do. This is the price one must pay for adequate coverage to cope with emergencies. Granted this, there is one aspect of hospital performance that merits close examination. This is the custom of closing down important segments of the hospital on weekends, especially on three-day holiday weekends now so popular, providing only emergency services with a skeleton crew. My position is that the cost of maintaining our hospitals (over $300 a day in New York City) is so high that hospitals and the people they serve can no longer afford the luxury of a five-day week. Hospitals should be geared to render full service seven days a week, and the sooner they get around to do this the better. The current system is wasteful and fails to derive optimal and efficient utilization from our multimillion dollar hospital plants. It is in this area that productivity can be increased, but it will take a significant revolution in work habits of doctors, nurses, and lay personnel, including administrators, to achieve these goals.

The average man is misled by the charts and statistics showing enormous increases in spending for health care, for he is led to believe that the services being rendered today are the same as they were years ago and that they simply cost more and more and that the doctors and the hospitals are ripping off people. What he may fail to realize is that whenever we medicalize a societal ill, we charge the bill to medicine and not the jails, the social institutions, the government, the churches, and the organizations that in the past have dealt with the same problems. As we go from sin to crime to sickness and medicalization in our management of societal ills, we inflict the costs upon the health care system, and the very people responsible for this trend make newspaper headlines, protesting rising health care costs and demanding more and more regulation and governmental controls. Couple the expenditures for our automobiles with the $45 billion being spent by Americans each year on alcohol and cigarettes, add to it the enormous sums being spent on junk foods, pornography, compulsive gambling, divorces, abortions, drugs, and the like, and one may wonder how much of the GNP is left. Add to this mélange the medicalization of many other assorted societal ills, and is it any wonder those costs attributed to "health care" are skyrocketing with no end in sight? There will never be enough money to provide for all of these, and maybe we should be grateful for this. Priorities and values will have to be established, not only for the good of the individual but for society in general. To look to the government to make these personal decisions for us is to court disaster. Each one of us must take a position and express it, not leave the final decisions to the dropouts and failures in our society.

Medicalization of Old Age

A major cause of soaring health care costs is the medicalization of old age in America, which has brought with it many abuses, enormous expense, nursing home scandals and ripoffs, undesirable abandonment of the elderly by their families, and institutionalization and "warehousing" of people who, with some help, might be able to fend for themselves in their own homes. Services originally rendered under social service agencies or religious auspices are now part of the medical bill that is eating up the GNP. Families are encouraged by the legal system to abandon elderly parents, to dissipate or hide resources, and to turn parents over to governmental agencies for support. The recently published story of the old man who was divorcing his sick wife of over forty years in order to obtain Medicaid for her in a nursing home is tragic and almost beyond belief.

Getting old in America can be a very sad experience when it should be a golden era in the life of a human being, a time devoted to leisure, enjoyment of freedom from competition and stresses of modern life, and opportunity to enjoy the fruits of one's labor, preferably in the midst of familiar surroundings and loved ones. To deal with aging as a predominantly medical problem requiring institutional or custodial care is a travesty abandoning most of the goals to which the elderly aspire and are entitled. The nursing home is no place for most of our senior citizens. It is not the solution and, in fact, has become part of the problem. A society that has made possible the successful exploration of space should not and cannot allow itself to flounder helplessly in solving this problem. The medical establishment, focussing most of its energy, personnel, and resources on technology, acute care, intensive care units, and dramatic surgical procedures needs to be reminded and prodded to focus more of its efforts on what McKeown has called its Samaritan or pastoral role, one that has been grossly neglected in the hustle and bustle of modern day medical practice. McKeown defines this role in the following terms:

> Under the Samaritan or pastoral role (of medicine), I include all services, other than investigation and treatment, which are needed during acute illness, during convalsence and for prolonged periods, in some cases for the rest of their lives, by chronically ill or handicapped people.[350]

So long as the institutions for the mentally retarded and chronically ill remain physically and geographically separate from acute care hospitals, there will be no dramatic improvement in nursing home, custodial, and long-term institutional care. I agree with McKeown that the time is ripe for medicine to assume greater responsibility for and direction of this neglected aspect of the care of human beings. Perhaps a leaf can be taken from the experience in Canada where beds declared underutilized in acute general care hospitals are simply transferred to long-term purposes and are so listed. In New York City, where surplus acute-care beds exist, entire hospitals have been closed and left to rot rather than modified or adapted to long-term care for which there is great need.

Similarly, when an acute-care hospital in New York City has a low occupancy rate on certain floors, for example obstetrics or pediatrics, these beds and floors are simply eliminated and closed down rather than assigned, as in Canada, to long-term care. These trends are wasteful, inefficient, costly, and clearly not in the best interests of the community and its people; they serve to add to the problems of the long-term care of the elderly. It would seem to make more sense to have flexible regulations for hospital bed occupancy rather than a rigid formula that recognizes only one aspect of the problem. Bringing the chronically ill under one roof with those acutely ill might stimulate house staff, nursing staff, attending staff, and administration to commit themselves

350. McKeown, Thomas: *The Role of Medicine: Dream, Mirage or Nemesis.* Princeton, Princeton University Press, 1979, p. 135.

more fully to their Samaritan or pastoral role.

Having said this, it remains to stress again that old age should not be and never should have been medicalized. Social agencies, government, religious organizations, and the people at large should address themselves to the broad problem of what is to be done for the elderly, the majority of whom are not sick and do not require constant day-to-day medical assistance. The answer may lie in providing the elderly with safe, specially designed, minimal maintenance and low cost housing, opportunities for supervised activities and utilization of leisure, communal eating facilities for those who wish, and accessibility to medical assistance if and when it is needed. Instead of merely complaining about soaring medical costs, let us attack the problem at its source by making certain that medical care is applied to medical problems and not primarily to correct social and societal ills.

RESPONSIBILITY OF THE INDIVIDUAL FOR HIS OWN HEALTH

Any discussion of the costs of health care would be incomplete without referring to the responsibility of the individual for maintaining his own health. In America, we have been witnessing a decline in morals and ethics and aberrant life-styles of a substantial segment of our population, inviting major hazards to their health. Gifted leaders are crying out for change and some of the most eloquent are in the medical profession, seeking to attack illness and disease at the source. The late Dr. John Knowles expressed with vigor, frankness, and clear insight the opinion that the great advances of the future in medicine will come not primarily from research laboratories but from a movement that will insist that each individual not only have the right to good health but, more importantly, be made personally responsible for it.[351] Why should society as a whole be punished by higher health insurance premiums and taxes because an individual chooses to drink himself to cirrhosis of the liver, the seventh leading cause of death in America?[352] Why should the cost of health care of those who persist in smoking be placed on the bill for all of us? Why should sexual promiscuity with its harvest of venereal disease, illegitimate pregnancy, and 1.1 million abortions per year be

351. Knowles, John H.: *Doing Better and Feeling Worse.* New York, W. W. Norton and Co., 1977, pp. 57-80.

352. *Ibid.*, p. 40.

subsidized out of the pockets of more responsible members of the community? Knowles was of the opinion, and I agree, that "control of the present major health problems in the United States depends directly on modification of the individual's behavior and habits of living." However,

> the knowledge required to persuade the individual to change his habits is far more complex, far less dramatic in its results, far more difficult to organize and convey—in short, far less appealing and compelling than the need for immunization, getting rid of sewage, and drinking safe water.[353]

The final paragraph of his essay makes the real point,

> When all is said and done, let us not forget that he who hates sin, hates humanity. Life is meant to be enjoyed, and each one of us in the end is still able in our own country to steer his vessel to his own port of desire. But the costs of individual irresponsibility in health have now become prohibitive. The choice is individual responsibility or social failure. Responsibility and duty must gain some degree of parity with right and freedom.[354]

If one accepts Peter Sedgwick's viewpoint that "the future belongs to illness . . . we are going to get more and more diseases, since our expectations of health are going to become more expansive and sophisticated,"[355] there seems no end in sight for expenditures on so-called health care. Is it any wonder that Ivan Illich in his controversial "Medical Nemesis" castigates the medical profession, saying "The medical establishment has become a threat to health," pointing to iatrogenic ailments and blaming the medical profession for medicalizing societal ills and in the process depriving man of his innate power to cope with illness and death by making him excessively dependent upon specialized professional health care. In the process, Illich seems to forget the great advances we have made in medicine and seems to be asking us to return to the dark ages. He seems to forget that people are themselves responsible for many of these trends. Why focus the blame upon the doctors?

Were Illich the sole voice against medicalization, one might dismiss his comments as those of an extremist, but there are others raising their voices on this theme, one of the most respected

353. *Ibid.*, p. 61.
354. *Ibid.*, p. 80.
355. Sedgwick, Peter: Illness—mental and otherwise. *The Hastings Center Studies, 1:* 1973, p. 37.

being Dr. Lewis Thomas, President of Sloan-Kettering Cancer Center, and a highly regarded physician, educator, researcher, and administrator. Recently Thomas warned,

> If people are educated to believe that they are fundamentally fragile, always on the verge of mortal disease, perpetually in need of support by health-care professionals . . . there can be no limit to the number of doctors' offices, clinics and hospitals required to meet the demand. In the end we would all become doctors, spending our days screening each other for disease.[356]

In another gemlike short essay, Thomas had this to say about illness and medical care:

> The great secret known to internists and learned early in marriage by internists' wives, but still hidden from the general public, is that most things get better by themselves. Most things, in fact, are better by morning. It is conceivable that we might be able to provide good medical care for everyone needing it, in a new system designed to assure equity, provided we can restrain ourselves, or our computers, from designing a system in which all 200 million of us are assumed to be in constant peril of failed health every day of our lives. In the same sense that our judicial system presumes us to be innocent until proved guilty, a medical-care system may work best if it starts with the presumption that most people are healthy.[357]

This is an ingenious concept, perhaps an ingenuous one, but hardly one acceptable to most politicians, poverticians, activists, and those believing in the efficacy and need for preventive medicine. Between the extremes of medicalization of all of our ills and the benign neglect of most minor and self-limited ailments, there has to be a middle ground where the battles for health maintenance and better health care can be fought without placing ruinous demands upon our financial resources.

---

356. Thomas, Lewis: *The Medusa and the Snail.* New York, Viking, 1979, p. 49.
357. Thomas, Lewis: *The Lives of a Cell: Notes of a Biology Watcher.* New York, Viking, 1974, pp. 85-86.

Chapter 32
TOO MANY DOCTORS OR TOO FEW?

Is there no balm in Gilead? Is there no physician there?
–Jeremiah 8:22[358]

At 11:16 P.M. on Friday, January 27, 1979, a distraught young woman dialed 911 for emergency assistance for a seventy-year-old man who had collapsed of an apparent heart attack at 13 West 54th Street in New York City. First on the scene, a five-story town house, were two policemen from the Midtown North Precinct, Anthony Graffeo and George Frangos, who said they had received the call from the 911 dispatcher at 11:18 P.M. , and arrived shortly thereafter to find the victim unconscious, lying supine on the floor of the sitting room. "He was still warm," said Officer Frangos. "His face was reddish, not kind of polka-dot blotches or bluish, the way they get a little later. He wasn't at that stage yet. We started CPR [cardiopulmonary resuscitation] and called to rush the ambulance. . . . The secretary was trying to give him artificial respiration," Officer Frangos said. "We took over, looked for pulse or breathing. I didn't hold onto his arm for a long time, but I didn't feel any pulse. I started pressing on his chest. We took turns pressing on his chest. By then–maybe two minutes–the ambulance crew arrived." Quoting directly from Robert D. McFadden's *New York Times* report of January 29, 1979:

> The first medical team on the scene were members of a Roosevelt Hospital ambulance crew, Jim Paturas and Randy Huff. Their log showed a departure time of 11:18 and arrival at 13 West 54th Street at 11:22 P.M. Four minutes later, they radioed for a two-man St. Clare's Hospital paramedic team, which arrived at 11:37, according to its logs.
>
> . . . The St. Clare's team quickly hooked up a portable heart monitor, and a motionless green horizontal line appeared on its

358. Bible: Old Testament. Jeremiah 8:22.

screen, indicating that the heart was not pumping blood.

One of the medics asked if a relative was present. No one responded. He asked if anyone knew of the patient's recent medical history. Again no one responded. He asked if any one was present when the heart attack occurred. Again no one responded.

Mr. McCabe inserted a plastic endotracheal tube down Mr. Rockefeller's throat and into the lungs, and he attached an oxygen supply. A 5 percent dextrose solution in water was fed through intravenous tubes in both of Mr. Rockefeller's arms.

Sodium bicarbonate to counteract acidosis that develops when breathing stops was administered at 10-minute intervals.

Epinephrine, a hormone that stimulates the heart, was given.

Abnormal Heart Rhythm

After Mr. Rockefeller was worked on for five or six minutes, the motionless electrocardiogram line developed into a small wave, indicating ventricular fibrillation, an abnormal heart rhythm that is just above the level of clinical death.

The paramedics repeated the drug dose and added 500 milligrams of calcium chloride, described by Mr. Rodgers as a "heavy duty" heart stimulant.

Mr. McCabe, speaking by radio to St. Clare's asked for instructions. A doctor suggested a dose of dopamine, which is used to raise blood pressure. They tried it, but to no effect.

Standing nearby, Mr. Hoffman, who was still holding an intravenous tube in one hand, had a phone and a walkie-talkie in another and was making arrangements to have Mr. Rockefeller taken to Lenox Hill Hospital, at 100 East 77th Street, between Park and Lexington Avenues, where the Rockefeller family doctor was standing by. Dr. Esakof would not say who had called him and it could not be learned who had placed the call.

When Mr. McCabe overheard him, he broke in to say that procedure required that they take the patient to the nearest hospital, St. Clare's, at 51st Street and Eighth Avenue.

"You don't understand," Mr. Hoffman said, telling the attendants that the patient was Nelson Rockefeller.

Mr. McCabe was stunned. He explained later that he and his partner were so intent on their work that they had not paid attention to the patient's identity.

The ambulance arrived at Lenox Hill at 12:06 A.M.

It was Dr. Esakof's decision to move Mr. Rockefeller to Lenox Hill, where he is a member of the staff and it was he who pronounced the patient dead at 12:20 A.M. after further attempts to revive him proved futile.[359]

My purpose in describing this episode in some detail is to il-

359. *The New York Times*, January 29, 1979.

lustrate that our system of emergency care in the borough of Manhattan, densely populated by physicians and hospitals with large house staffs, failed to bring a qualified M.D. to the side of a mortally stricken man when he needed one the most. If it happened to a Rockefeller, what happens to John Doe, and why?

We boast of great advances in medical technology and Emergency care and millions are expended on these each year, but the fact remains that ambulances that in the good old days used to carry M.D.s to the scene now arrive with non-M.D.s called technicians and some with paramedics who have been trained to render advanced life support. The excuse is that doctors are in short supply and needed at the hospital and cannot be spared for ambulance-riding duty. Some even claim that paramedics are better at this sort of work than doctors. Maybe they are, but ideally a doctor should be at the scene of any serious emergency. In the days when our hospitals had only one-fifth of the house staff they now possess, we somehow managed to send doctors out on emergency ambulance calls. Now we send "technicians" to perform duties that a physician should be performing. The system needs revision and a resetting of priorities in the commitment, assignment, and deployment of house staff. Emergency care is much too vital to be placed entirely in the hands of non-M.D.s. Ask any family whose loved ones have been stricken and left to the devices of the first available ambulance. For the patient and his family there is no substitute for the presence of a doctor in these moments of crisis. A system that provides for anything less has failed to meet its obligation to the care of the patient and invites criticism and dissatisfaction from the public it serves.

Granted that many ambulance calls may be unnecessary and more efficiently answered by non-M.D.s; there should be another mechanism for getting a doctor to the scene of a serious emergency. At St. Vincent's Hospital and Medical Center of New York, this need had been fulfilled in part by the establishment of a mobile coronary care unit that responded to emergency calls for patients suspected of having a heart attack. This ambulance carried a doctor and paramedics and was equipped to institute advanced life support with electrocardiographic monitoring. Unfortunately, because of the alleged shortage of house staff, a physician no longer accompanies the ambulance, a giant step backwards in my opinion. In communities where there is no hospital, the solution has been to equip ambulances with audio-visual communication systems that convey to a doctor in a regional hospital details of the emergency for which he or she may give advice and instruction to non-M.D. personnel.

LACK OF AVAILABILITY OF DOCTORS

Handling of emergencies is not the only source of complaints about doctors and their work. It has become next to impossible to locate a doctor after office hours, on the weekend, or on Wednesdays or Thursdays, known in the suburbs as "doctor's day off." Many patients complain that they have little or no chance to get on the golf course at the country club on those days because of the doctors and they resent this, for they believe that doctors should be dedicated people with little or no free time for these activities. I have some strong medicine to offer to alleviate or cure these complaints. The quickest cure for unavailability of physicians is to produce enough of them so that their virtual monopoly will be eliminated. In New York City, during the Great Depression, there was no problem with lack of availability of a doctor. If he happened to be playing golf, driving a yacht around the island, socializing when he should be working, and away more than present, the answer was quite simple—he lost his patients to someone who was more readily available. This may sound pretty rough, but those who cry out for rugged individualism and the free enterprise system should be prepared to take it or leave it.

The large yachts tied up at marinas and owned by doctors have done the image of our profession untold harm and form the topic for much adverse cocktail party chatter and cartoons. In a similar vein is the publicity accorded the large Cadillacs and Continentals owned and driven by doctors and their families, many of whom are now indulging in ownership of sleeker and ever-more expensive cars of foreign make—Mercedes, Ferrari, Rolls Royce, Porsche, Jaguar, *et cetera* almost *ad nauseum.* I suppose one might question why people resent and envy these evidences of affluence on the part of doctors while they admire them in their lay neighbors. The fact remains that people do resent ostentation and the trappings of affluence in doctors. One answer to this problem is to educate and train more doctors, getting away from a monopoly and encouraging bona fide competition in the hope that in a free market doctors' incomes will not reach excessively high levels in comparison with those of their neighbors. This brings us to the question: Do we have too many doctors or too few? The answer is moot, the facts inadequate, and the opinions and judgements based largely on individual bias and prejudice rather than scientific proof.

My personal belief is that we need more doctors by a considerable margin over the 16,000 graduating from our medical schools each year, and I shall present my reasons for this opinion. The issue of a doctor shortage has been clouded during the past decade by the importation of alien FMGs (Foreign Medical Graduates) in vast numbers, the yearly equivalent of the entire output of American medical schools. True, the latest health manpower bill stipulates that the admission to the U.S.A. of FMGs of alien birth be cut back sharply, but I suspect that those fearing a surplus of doctors are anticipating a rear-guard action, lobbying, and political moves to delay the implementation of this embargo. The fact of the matter is that without FMGs there will be a significant doctor shortage for some years to come unless remedial action is undertaken. This will be felt by institutions with unattractive programs having little or no appeal for American graduates. The prediction of the Congress that there would be a surplus of native-born physicians by 1980 is clearly in error and again illustrates the folly of predictions based on faulty data. Perhaps it was the only way Congress could get out of the predicament in which it was placed in 1965 when the Department of Labor declared there was a shortage of physicians in America and opened up the flood gates for virtually unrestricted admission of many thousands of alien FMGs. In a similar vein, I express skepticism of current predictions of a surplus of doctors by a federal administration (Carter) whose main goal was to cut its budget by eliminating capitation grants to medical schools and seeking every conceivable justification for this ill-advised action.

Barring a postponement of the implementation of the restrictive new policy on FMGs, for the first time in a decade we shall need to be more aggressive about facing up to a shortage of doctors to meet the needs of the people. With universal health insurance coverage, demand will undergo major increase, in compliance with Wildavsky's law that patients seek medical care up to the level of their insurance. If there is little or nothing out of their own pockets, the sky (or the insurance level) will be the limit. All I can see is the prospect of increasing demand for doctor services calling for more medical graduates well beyond the current projections.[361]

Emphasis on disease prevention, the battle cry of the current crop of government leaders setting health care policy, will create additional pressures upon the system and will require more doctors. Continuing medicalization of societal ills will stress the system even more. Abortion, drug abuse, and alcoholism, previously treated as crimes, have been medicalized and condoned and included in society's bill for health care rather than crime control. As these trends proliferate, ensuing demands on the health care system will be of major proportions, upsetting the old-style ratios that were designed to fit the values and mores of the 1920s and 1930s rather than the 1970s or 1980s.

THE WORK ETHIC

Doctors do not want to work as hard as their predecessors. Osler's claim that the master-word in medicine is WORK is being challenged by a new generation who finds difficulty in accepting it as a way of life. Physicians emerging from internships, fellowships, and residencies that stress time off-call rather than on, with less and less night work or weekends on duty, functioning essentially on a 9 to 5 weekday schedule, find difficulty in adjusting to around-the-clock demands of private practice. Many fail to adjust to this new way of life and seek to escape it by practicing in groups, by committee, partnership, or in institutions. Irrespective of their motivation, the facts of life are that most of the current crop of doctors and their immediate families simply will not accept the heavy work schedules and long hours of their predecessors. As a result, substantially more doctors will be needed merely to equal the performance of the same number of physicians of an older generation.

361. Knowles, J. H: *Doing Better and Feeling Worse.* Chapter on political pathology of health policy, by A. Wildavsky. New York, Norton, 1977, p. 108.

WOMEN IN MEDICINE

The major influx of women into medicine, averaging 30 percent of each medical school class, is one of the great advances of this century, making up for the losses to medicine occasioned by discrimination and bias. The change is relatively recent, and insufficient time has elapsed for evaluating its long-term impact on physician performance. There are some data available, but they need updating and need to be viewed without the bias and sometimes rancor of either male chauvinists or excessively ardent feminists. Over three-fourths of women physicians are married (over half of them to other physicians), and those who marry have averaged three children, slightly more than reported for other married women in their socioeconomic class. Given the heavy and intimate demands of motherhood and family life and the increasing scarcity and cost of domestic help, over the long pull I predict that the average woman physician will not be able to keep pace with her male peer in the delivery of health care. My estimate is that, over a thirty-year span, it could take four women physicians to equal the work performance of three male physicians in the practice of medicine. Having said this, I brace myself for the expected barrage from those who differ. Evidence supporting me has been presented by Lopate in her monograph on women in medicine.

> A comparison of the practice patterns of men and women physicians graduating between 1931 and 1956, showed that almost 9 percent of the women were inactive, in contrast to less than one percent of the men. In addition, only 54.5 percent of the women worked full time, while 88.8 percent of the men had full-time practices. Although many women, particularly if not married, devote 60-80 hours a week to their profession, women physicians on the whole do not put in the same long schedules as men. Nor do they see as many patients per hour as the men do, since they generally spend a longer time with each one.[362]

For those feminists who challenge my prediction, my answer is to express my admiration for those women who have succeeded so well in combining the roles of wife, mother, and physician. So what if we need four women physicians to equal the practice performance of three men. Medicine has gained in the process!

---

362. Lopate, Carol: *Women in Medicine.* Baltimore, The Johns Hopkins Press, 1968. p. 145.

EARLY RETIREMENT

Additional pressures, tending to reduce the physician work force, are mandatory retirement from institutions, industry, partnerships, group practice, government, and academic positions. The relatively recent availability to physicians of Social Security and liberalized pension plans have made retirement more feasible for physicians, who in the past kept working until they dropped dead. Excessive paper work and overregulation and demands for recertification, relicensure, and continuing medical education have already influenced some doctors to retire early. Last but not least, that cancer on the clinical practice of medicine, the malpractice crisis with its ever-growing substantial premiums is making it difficult for doctors to taper off practice or to take part-time positions as they grow older. It is all or none, and many are opting for the latter. Escalating costs of maintaining an office practice with no end in sight, coupled with government and third-party insurers' efforts to regulate, i.e. limit, doctors' income, are driving some physicians out of practice, and I predict an acceleration of this trend. The attrition rate for doctors is certain to rise in the future as more and more quit practice early. Uncorrected, this will be a major factor in contributing to a doctor shortage. Any projection of the numbers of doctors needed to supply the needs and demands of the people of the United States must make adequate allowance for these relatively recent developments. The old doctor-patient ratios are out of date and need revision to meet modern trends.

"SUBSTITUTES" FOR DOCTORS

Another thing that has gone wrong in medicine is a serious misconception regarding the role of physician assistants, nurse practitioners, midwives, and other "substitutes" for doctors. This is an extremely popular concept that is spreading like wildfire across the country with, I believe, a half-baked appreciation of what the role should be. Busy practicing physicians have always employed extenders and assistants, some to a greater degree than others. No doctor worth his salt would try to practice medicine today without a good nurse, a competent secretary, a good accountant and bookkeeper, and other technical help, to name only a few members of the team assisting him and freeing up valuable time for optimal utilization of his medical skills. There is nothing new about so-called health extenders. What is different today is that aggressive attempts are being made to *replace* the doctor rather than to *extend* his activities. The extenders, especially the nurse practitioners and the physician's assistants, seek to function independently by practicing medicine on a fee-for-service basis, without any sort of supervision or direction by an M.D. This is a very undesirable trend in America and in the long run will serve to give some of our people fifth-class medical care as a substitute for the services of a bona fide physician. Without going into detail, my reaction to these ill-adviced demands of nurse practitioners and physician's assistants is that if they want to practice medicine independently, let them go to medical school for the superb education designed by the leaders of our profession to prepare men and women for a lifetime of service to the American people. There are no shortcuts. Anything short of this is settling for incompetence. Let us call a halt to the current trend to permit people to practice medicine without going to medical school.

WHERE HAVE ALL THE NURSES GONE?

Before leaving the topic of nurse practitioners and the like, a few comments must be directed to the current severe shortage of registered nurses, a situation that has reached the stage of a national scandal despite ample warning signals sent out by hospitals and physicians for a number of years. In my publication of 1977, under the auspicies of the Committee on Medical Education of the New York Academy of Medicine, entitled, *Nursing Education: Status or Service Oriented?* I predict dire results if nursing's hierarchy should succeed in their campaign to close the hospital diploma nursing schools that were then producing the majority of registered nurses in America. I blame a great deal of the current shortage of nurses on this error in direction and policy, and I recommend that the leaders in the nursing field who were responsible for this fiasco be publicly identified and censured.

To what purpose do we direct nursing education to higher and higher academic achievement and increasingly sophisticated levels of university degree acquisition, stressing new roles for nurses and in some instances seeking not only to extend the physician but to replace him, when the infantry soldier of nursing, the bedside nurse, has become a scarcity. No army can consist solely of high ranking officers. Where have all the privates gone? When the leaders of a great profession through their misguided efforts impose upon the sick and helpless of this nation a serious shortage in nursing personnel, especially of those who should be laying hands on patients and rendering bedside care, the time has come for drastic remedial action and repudiation of those responsible for this disaster.

Chapter 33
TOO MANY SPECIALISTS?

Not only do I believe that more physicians are needed, but there is ample evidence that the kinds of doctors and their distribution must undergo change. There is general agreement that we are producing too many specialists and not enough generalists. The causes for this are not simply money, selfishness, and creature comfort, although these are important considerations given the mercenary and self-centered society from which many of the new doctors are coming. The explosion of medical knowledge and technology has been so massive that young men and women of integrity, high purpose, and idealism, the very ones we need most, express anxiety and uncertainty over their ability to function as generalists. They are so bright and talented that they cannot reconcile themselves to practicing medicine with a superficial knowledge of many fields and no in-depth command of any. I have talked with a number of these young people who are seeking specialty training because they see in the demands of general practice weaknesses in themselves and in their preparation that will plague them for the rest of their lives. These same individuals have little faith and less patience with the "moulting" process through which specialists used to rise through the ranks of general practice, self-educated and to a great degree self-made. Now the new people demand to have it all in one sequence, residency training followed by subspecialty training and emergence, not as a general physician but as a narrow subspecialist. Prodding them in this direction are the role models seen in most academic institutions, virtually all of them subspecialists. Those who cannot make it in these academic surroundings as subspecialists are the second-class citizens called general internists—or at least this is how the students and house staff see it—given the present rather low esteem in which the general internist is held.

American Board Certification

Undesirable trends have also appeared in the various boards that serve to regulate the certification of specialists and subspecialists. The American Board of Internal Medicine, for one, must share the blame for the proliferation of subspecialists and the decline of the general internist leading to the lopsided overproduction of subspecialists of the past decade. I single out this Board because it deals with the largest segment of specialists, and it happens to represent my own area of special interest. I am certain that the other Boards have similarly erred. What went wrong? In a hard-hitting discussion of this problem, in September 1978, Dr. Robert G. Petersdorf, then Chairman-Elect of the American Board of Internal Medicine, had this to say:

> Before 1970, the Board (Internal Medicine) required four years of training in general internal medicine, plus two years of training in a subspecialty, or two years of practice, before a candidate was eligible to take the written examination in general internal medicine. If he passed the written, he then took an oral examination, usually within the ensuing twelve months. The entire certification process took at least seven years after the candidate received the M.D. degree and, in many instances, much longer. Only a very few successful certificants, less than 200 a year in the aggregate, took the established board examinations in cardiology, pulmonary disease, gastroenterology, allergy and immunology, and the end product of the examination process for 95 per cent of the candidates was certification in internal medicine. In the late 1960s and early 1970s, the Board made several decisions that greatly accelerated subspecialization. It abolished the oral examination, did away with the practice requirement, and shortened the entry requirement to the certifying examination to only three years of general internal medicine, or to two years of medicine plus the first year of a two-year training period in a subspecialty—the short track.[363]

The elimination of the oral examination was, in my opinion, an unmitigated disaster. The actual testing of the candidate in his personal approach to the patient should never have been abandoned. This is the ultimate test of the competence of the candidate to practice clinical medicine. All that "book larnin" may mean very little if it is not applied effectively at the bedside and on the physician-patient encounter that is the essence of medical practice. The excuses given that there were not enough

363. Petersdorf, R. G.: The doctors' dilemma. *N Engl J Med, 299/12:*628-34, Sept. 21, 1978.

examiners and that the oral examinations were uneven, subject to individual bias, and imposed excessive tensions on the candidates are really for the birds. Plenty of well-qualified examiners were available for the job if one went out of academe to seek them. Why were more of the practicing internists not enrolled as examiners? I submit a major factor was the bias of the Board toward academic full-time medical educators as their chief examiners. Above all, the elimination of the oral examination served to reduce the art of physical examination, history taking, and decision making to a very low position in the training and testing of the clinician. Candidates were bound to feel that these aspects of medical practice were unimportant, and nothing could be further from the truth. The oral examination should be reinstated. When it is, I predict there will be a dramatic upsurge of interest in history taking and physical examination on the part of medical students and house staff.

Petersdorf goes on to criticize the massive proliferation in subspecialties authorized by the American Board of Internal Medicine and the enormous number of applicants it encouraged.

> As a consequence, in the 1975-76 examination cycle more than 5,000 candidates took these subspecialty examinations (this number does not include allergy or nuclear medicine). Nor has the pace slowed; 2,453 candidates took the five examinations that were given in June 1978. The largest number of candidates took the examination in pulmonary disease, 755, and the lowest, 309, the infectious disease examination. Even with my great personal loyalties to infectious disease, I cannot conceive a need for 309 more infectious-disease experts unless they spend their time culturing each other.[364]

Petersdorf continues, pointing out that even the figures he quotes "do not include cardiology and gastroenterology, traditionally the two best populated examinations or oncology, the most rapidly growing." He predicts that the candidates in the 1978-1979 subspecialty examination cycle will exceed 6,000 with no end in sight. Petersdorf blames the shortening of the training requirements for the explosion in the subspecialties to the neglect of general internal medicine, and I couldn't agree more.

Those of us on the firing line in medicine witnessed the cheap-

---

364. *Ibid.*

ening of the value of a specialty and subspecialty certificate with large numbers of individuals certified as specialists and subspecialists with limited clinical experience or expertise. The process was too fast and too superficial to produce the kind of specialist we struggled so hard to produce in the past. Many of these candidates emerged as neither fish nor fowl. Most should have been guided to general internal medicine.

Despite its protestations of innocence, the American Board of Internal Medicine must accept the blame for over production of splinter specialists and a denigration of clinical practice inherent in its elimination of the oral examination and the practice requirement of prior days. To correct these errors will not be easy, but it is not impossible. Petersdorf makes a number of suggestions, some of which may be acceptable while others are not. In any event, as the upcoming Chairman of the American Board of Internal Medicine, he may have an opportunity to test his beliefs. Mistakes have been made, and the way to certification in internal medicine and the subspecialties is much too easy.

Every medical educator worth his salt has his own proposals for improving programs in his specialty, and I am no exception. When I first established the Upjohn Fellowships in Gastroenterology in 1962, they were for one year, and it was not until nearly ten years later that we were forced by changing ground rules of the American Board of Internal Medicine and pressure from the competition of NIH training programs to extend the tenure to two years. My trainees who completed the one-year fellowships were every bit as competent in clinical gastroenterology as those taking two years, and their subsequent careers have shown no differences between the two groups. The hallmark of my fellows has always been their sound clinical training in internal medicine, their commitment to service to patients, and their availability for rendering comprehensive and primary care. I know from personal experience that in a one-year fellowship I can educate and train a bright young doctor to acquire the skills, the language, the grasp of literature, and the clinical approach to sound decision making in gastroenterology. Basically, these graduates are excellent internists with a hobby* and special skills in gastro-

* Any favorite pursuit, topic, or object; that which a person persistently pursues with zeal or delight. *Webster.*

enterology. I feel this is an excellent foundation for future growth and development.

My proposal is that we develop programs in internal medicine requiring three years in general medicine, including ambulatory and primary care as well as in-hospital care, and to cap the program with one year in a subspecialty, be it gastroenterology, cardiology, oncology, hematology, renology, endocrinology, metabolic diseases, infectious diseases, or any of the other major areas. Shorter rotations through these subspecialties have not been satisfactory, in my opinion, and do not serve the purpose I seek to achieve. For some who desire it, the fourth year could be in administrative medicine as a chief resident. On completion of the four years, the candidates will qualify for the certifying examination in internal medicine.

For those who wish to go into subspecialties, I would demand three to five years of clinical practice before allowing admission to the subspecialty board examinations. For those who see as a weakness in my proposal the neglect of future academicians and research workers, my answer is to set up a minority of special programs for such individuals and to stop trying to make a research scientist of every fellow in gastroenterology, cardiology, or whatever and desist from trying to make a clinician out of every laboratory scientist. The trend toward neglect of clinical medicine and service to patients has already gone too far.

My proposal will serve to nudge some into the practice of general internal medicine where many will remain, serving the people who need them so much. Those who emerge from this with the drive to enter a subspecialty will have been tested in combat and will be better subspecialists for the clinical experience they have gained. Some will drop out, and with overproduction already upon us, it would be a blessing. Were this quickly implemented, a major and important trend would be instituted to return general internal medicine to the position it once held as the most basic of all the specialties and the most needed. Then we could begin to really talk about giving the public a keen, well-trained, available internist as the modern replacement for the old-style family practitioner, who is really an anachronism in today's world of medicine.

Finally, should we not take a hard look at the American Board of Internal Medicine and the other specialty boards, seeking to find out how they went astray and lost contact with the needs of the American people to the point that Congressional action appears imminent on the question of overproduction of specialists and subspecialists? Academic distinction alone should not be the sole or determining factor in the selection of members for these boards. In the public interest, there must be a major input by distinguished practicing clinicians.

Chapter 34
FAMILY MEDICINE:

Here Today, Gone Tomorrow

Role models are extremely important in guiding student career choices and unless the general internist is accorded the recognition he deserves and is more visible and respected in his teaching hospitals, no amount of legislation or regulation will serve to divert medical students into careers as general physicians. I do not believe that the establishment of divisions and residencies in family practice or primary practice is the answer to this need, although they do represent efforts toward change. I am skeptical about the academic viability of programs in family medicine. In the first place, I see the family as an endangered species and agree with some others that unless steps are taken, we may well run out of families before we run out of energy.

Any physician who practices in a large city knows that the so-called nuclear family has been steadily undergoing erosion. Of the 56 million families estimated to exist in the United States, only 16.3 percent are of the traditional nuclear type with "breadwinning fathers, homemaking mothers and resident children," and even these appear to be headed for dissolution and change.[365] Whole families no longer live under one roof for any great length of time. Children are off to school, college, or their own pads. Grandparents either live in their own apartments or house or are sent into nursing homes or are committed to institutions. The family, such as it is, does not receive its medical care from a single physician. The wife, or mother, has her gynecologist, the husband may receive his care from the company doctor, the children have their pediatrician, the adolescent and teenager have their own urologist and gynecologist, and the poor seek care in the nearest available clinic or Medicaid mill. The truth of the matter is that family medical care has, by and large, become greatly fragmented.

365. Howard, J.: *Families.* New York, Simon and Schuster, 1978.

Add to all of this, the trend for people to go to a headache specialist for their headaches, a gastroenterologist for their stomach ailments, a cardiologist for cardiac complaints, a diabetes specialist for diabetes, and one must ask what is family medicine and is it a realistic concept in this day and age? In some quarters, the solution has been to set up family practice units in the hope that its graduates will seek careers in providing the family with comprehensive health care. What seems to have been overlooked is that families are themselves fragmented, and they may not really want to place their lives and health in the hands of any single individual.

I seriously question the policy of selling family medicine as a future to our bright young physicians, especially in the face of the decline in the nuclear family. I have the feeling that some of the proponents of this movement are being influenced more by nostalgia, sloganeering, a desire to do the popular thing, and a yearning to return to the good old days than by the facts of life. My own impression is that the nearest and perhaps closest approach to the ideal person to render personal health care is a physician well trained in general internal medicine with some knowledge of pediatrics and easily accessible and willing to serve his people. To achieve this goal, what we really need to do is to adapt and improve the medical school curriculum and residency programs in internal medicine and pediatrics to make them more responsive to the needs of patients for general medical, primary, ambulatory, and comprehensive medical care. Having watched physicians moult and make career and specialty changes with the passage of years, I have serious doubts as to how permanent the commitment of our current graduates will be to family and community practice. My prediction is that after a few years many will decide to seek further training in specialties or may choose to take the path of self-education in training for a specialty, abandoning family practice. There must be another way to approach this.

The Hidden System for Primary Care

I believe that the specialties and subspecialties are here to stay and will continue to proliferate. Not only do the medical students flock to them, the general public, despite the clamor of a few for the old-style general practitioner, demands specialty care.

Even in rural areas, the farmer's wife wants an obstetrician to deliver her children, her husband wants an orthopedist when he fractures a bone, and both of them demand a well-trained surgeon if they need an operation. When this is true in rural areas, you may well imagine what it is like in large cities. Granted the viability and proliferation of specialties, how do we meet the demands for primary care? I believe that it rests with the recognition and encouragement of what David Rogers calls the "hidden system" of general medical care, which he describes in these terms:

> It is perfectly clear that the largely specialist-oriented private sector of medicine now handles the primary-care needs of most of the population. This system has two very real problems: it is hidden, and it requires a special ticket for entry (e.g., a surgeon may handle the primary-care needs of a patient who originally came to him for surgery, but not as a first-contact physician for a patient with undifferentiated problems). . . . Some figures have been published suggesting that certain "specialists," notably pediatricians, internists, and obstetricians, do much more general practice than they are generally willing to admit. Eighty per cent of the disease processes most frequently managed by pediatricians and internists are the same as those handled by general practitioners.366

There are many advantages in this hidden system, which is good for the patient as well as the doctor. In the first place, it forces the specialist or subspecialist to try to stay abreast of trends in general medicine as well as in his subspecialty. Instead of depending on a general practitioner for referrals, the specialist has direct and primary access to patients and has the opportunity to apply his skills at earlier stages of illness when the prospect of effective therapy may be more promising. Having gained his patient via this route, the specialist is ethically entitled to continue to treat him, and the problem of noncompliance in therapy is minimized. Nothing can be more frustrating to a consultant-specialist than to make recommendations that neither the patient nor the referring doctor choose to follow. Having to rely on the referring doctor to transmit the consultant's opinion to the patient may lead to misunderstanding and, on occasion, to misrepresentation. The hidden system, which is largely controlled by satisfied patients and their families who refer them-

366. Knowles, J. H: *Doing Better and Feeling Worse.* Chapter by David E. Rogers, The Challenge of Primary Care. New York, W. W. Norton and Co., 1977. p. 100.

selves and others into the system, has the advantage that at least someone was satisfied with the doctor's work and is expressing it by referring others. This is in the best spirit of the free enterprise system and should be encouraged rather than blocked. How often have I wished that a patient had been referred to a consultant earlier in his illness, perhaps in time for more effective therapy. How often have I praised the system of free choice that has led the patient to make a change in his doctor for the better.

IMPROVING THE CURRICULUM AND TRAINING PROGRAMS IN INTERNAL MEDICINE

Rogers' closing comments on the hidden system strike at the very core of the problem. Noting that specialists provide a great deal of primary care, he feels that redesigning their training may better prepare them for "what they in fact will be doing anyway [and] might decrease the criticism of specialty-oriented programs, while improving the availability and quality of general care."[367]

A step in this direction has been taken by Dr. Lawrence E. Young, the highly respected Dewey Professor and Chairman of Medicine at the University of Rochester School of Medicine, who "retired" five years early in 1974 to become Alumni Distinguished Professor of Medicine in charge of a new program in Rochester focussing on primary care delivered by internists. This program, the Associated Hospitals Program in Internal Medicine, with a heavy emphasis on outpatient ambulatory medicine has been very popular and oversubscribed. It is designed to provide the resident with a nicely balanced educational experience, time spent in ambulatory settings alternating with assignments to ward service in major teaching hospitals. This is a good start, but it may well be only touching the tip of an iceberg for numerically it can provide only a relatively small number of disciples. Furthermore, how many Larry Youngs are there available to direct such programs? What is really needed is to modify existing residencies in medicine to provide adequate and appropriate exposure to personal, continuing, and comprehensive care of patients within the limitations of the time frame of three or four years of medical residency. I must confess that when I was in my internship and residency at Duke and a fellowship at Yale, outpatient experience

367. *Ibid.*, p. 100.

was woven into the fabric of the general medical residency effectively and impressively. But something happened with the passage of time, and there was an erosion of status of the outpatient service as an integral part of the medical residency. I blame this in a large measure on the takeover of the teaching of medicine in university centers by full-time salaried faculty who regarded outpatient work as, at best, a necessary evil.

The decline of prestige of the part-time teacher who brought so much to the medical students from his experience in the community and in private practice had a great deal to do with the weakness that developed in all of the teaching programs overemphasizing the acutely and severely ill and neglecting the "walking wounded" and the worried well. Things became very lopsided and patient care suffered. While programs such as Doctor Young's at Rochester are sorely needed and offer a glimmer of hope for reform, the nuts and bolts work should be performed by all medical educators, especially in internal medicine, who must seek to return to the medical residency emphasis on caring for the patient as well as curing him. For this, there is no better teacher than the part-time instructor whose main occupation is in the day-to-day practice of medicine with all of its trials, tribulations, and problems, not to mention its emoluments. If the medical student sees these men and women at work as highly respected members of the teaching staff and not as second-class citizens, he will not fail to be favorably impressed by their roles and may be inspired to emulate them. At least the student will have exposure to a real choice in career decisions and not be confined to the full-time academic model that is not only unrealistic but, for the majority, unattainable and undesirable.

My plea then is for a return to power and influence of the greatest asset a medical school and hospital may have, the practicing clinician who volunteers committed time for teaching and training. For those in this category who have special talent and skills in teaching and administration and are subject to heavy demands, I believe that a modest base salary should be provided with opportunity to develop private practice. If you have the right person, there need be no limitation on private practice. If you have the wrong person, no restrictions will prevent abuse. The real answer lies in careful selection and by the highest standards being set by those in charge.

Having said so much in praise and defense of part-time teachers, I must stress that I expect these individuals to exhibit the highest ideals, integrity, compassion, skill, and commitment to patient care and to be all of these without thinking primarily of the financial reward. The true rewards should be in the enormous satisfaction that accrues to the physician-teacher, who by training and educating his students, house staff, and colleagues is able to extend his gifts of healing and wisdom far beyond the relatively few patients he can reach in person or at any given moment in time. The part-time volunteer clinician-teacher I am speaking of is, in the Oslerian tradition, admittedly an exception in today's society, but these are the men and women I speak of when I extoll the virtues of the part-time teachers of medicine and argue for their return to power.

Chapter 35
WHY FLEXNER'S FULL-TIME SYSTEM FAILED

As a matter of fact, the rank and file of doctors are no more scientific than their tailors. . . . Doctoring is an art, not a science.
—*George Bernard Shaw (1913)*[368]

Doctor Eugene A. Stead, Jr., of Duke University, is a brilliant physician and medical educator, Emeritus Chairman of the Department of Medicine and an individual of exceptional perspicacity, with a knack for terse, witty, pungent, and accurate expression. In a biography entitled, *E. A. Stead, Jr.—What This Patient Needs is a Doctor,* he makes these comments.

> I am also less impressed with the benefits of putting all doctors on a salary and reducing the fee-for-service aspect of medicine. Some patients need more medical attention than the doctor believes they need. He gives this service willingly for a fee. He gives it grudgingly if he is on salary. The patient isn't always wrong. . . . Dr. Wilburt Davison commented many years ago on the distribution of senior faculty giving care to patients in the Duke Medical Center after 5:00 P.M. on weekdays and on Saturday afternoons or Sunday. He found that salaried doctors were not in the patient care areas but the fee-for-service doctors were. A recent check shows that Dr. Davison was a good observer. The distinction in the patient care areas of the Duke Medical Center of doctors on salary and those on fee-for-service on Saturday afternoons is similar to that observed 25 years ago.[369]

Full time has been acclaimed by many educators as the greatest advance of the century in medical education, and few dispute this insofar as the *preclinical* departments are concerned. It is in applying this concept to the clinical divisions that controversy and debate have arisen. In the preclinical departments, defined as those preceding the clinical years in medical school, e.g. anat-

368. Shaw, George B.: *The Doctor's Dilemma.* Baltimore, Penguin Books, Inc., 1954, p. 25.

369. Stead, E. A., Jr.: *What This Patient Needs Is a Doctor.* Ed. by Wagner, G. S., Cebe, B., and Rozear, M. P. Durham, Carolina Academic Press, 1978, p. 88.

omy, physiology, biochemistry, pathology, microbiology, and pharmacology, the commitment of the "whole time" and full energy of the faculty to their medical school duties of teaching, training, and research was a salutary change and without any question served to revolutionize the education of medical students. Although Abraham Flexner actively promoted full time in the preclinical chairs, he cannot be credited with this innovation, which had already been introduced into a number of medical schools then in existence, including Johns Hopkins, long before he appeared on the scene. Every physician in America is deeply indebted to the full-time system of medical education in the basic or preclinical departments for the sound foundation he possesses in the scientific aspects of medicine. Those of us who have been through this experience will never forget it. Here the principles of rational scientific thinking and reasoning, observation, self-disclipline, rigor, integrity, inquisitiveness, skepticism, and scholarship are inculcated by teachers and role models who represent some of the most brilliant, dedicated, and talented minds in America. To this relatively small cadre of teachers we owe the tone and character of the mode of introduction of raw college recruits into the mysteries and challenges of modern scientific medicine.

The system of medical teaching in America is geared to one-to-one personal contact between teacher and pupil. Oftentimes, the first reaction of a freshman to medical school is surprise at finding the classes to be small with the faculty outnumbering the students, a far cry from undergraduate education. It is a system that emphasizes individual instruction, and it does not lend itself to mass production and hopefully it never will. This is the stage of the medical student's career when he should develop what we hope will be lifelong habits of study, contemplation, and devotion to the comprehension of basic mechanisms of health and disease. In anatomy he learns structure; in physiology, function; in biochemistry, mechanisms; in microbiology, causes or etiology; in pathology, what went wrong; and in pharmacology, how to treat. Under no circumstances should this learning process be diluted or diminished. For most medical students there will never again be another opportunity for daily and intensive exposure to the basic sciences and scientists who determine to a major degree whether a physician will be scientifically competent. Although some students will, after clinical training, return during fellowships to pursue basic scientific endeavors, for most, the period of this intensive exposure is limited to the first two years of medical school.

It is for this reason that every effort must be made to preserve and to intensify this experience in this era of expanding basic scientific information rather than to dilute it by introducing extraneous and often irrelevant material into the curriculum.

The debt of every doctor to his preclinical teachers is seldom given the wide publicity and recognition it deserves; without these men and women, physicians might be no better informed than well-educated laymen, competent in the art but sadly lacking in scientific preparation for medical practice. For the general public, the role of the full-time basic scientists in our medical schools needs publicity, support, and adequate recognition. From this relatively small group of scientists have come many major advances in the diagnosis, understanding, treatment, and management of disease, and with these have come international acclaim and a substantial share of Nobel prizes.

Abraham Flexner, carried away by the impressive accomplishments of preclinical teachers under the full-time system, leaped at the opportunity to impose the same system on clinical teachers. Here he made a number of serious mistakes, many of which have been described in the preceding pages. I have presented detailed and verbatim statements by some of the greatest clinicians America has ever seen, who opposed strict full time and refused to stay with it. The public statements and the private records, divulged by confidential memoranda on the conflict, reveal an almost Machiavellian approach by Flexner and a small coterie of medical friends, chiefly nonclinicians, designed to force their beliefs upon individuals and institutions using as leverage large sums of Rockefeller money to achieve their goals. The evidence is clear that Flexner placed the Rockefeller Boards in the unsavory position of dictating institutional policy as a condition for contributing large funds. Years would go by before the dissenting voices of outstanding laymen, outraged by these tactics, would be heeded in the councils of the Rockefeller Boards and result in the rescinding of all conditions imposed upon their grants. Flexner was never gracious about his defeat on this issue and continued, even after retirement, to make life miserable for any dean or medical school deviating one iota from his utopian and unworkable scheme.

We have seen numerous and valid objections to strict full time presented by experienced and idealistic doctors who tried to make it work and failed. First and foremost, it imposed restrictions on the clinical professors in the medical school that were never placed upon other professors in the university, implying that clinical professors could not be trusted to regulate themselves. Flexner's overemphasis on medicine as a science was unrealistic; the practice of medicine is not a science but an art, and physicians are not intended to be primarily scientists. The art of medicine soon declines if the physician or surgeon fails to practice it in daily personal contact with his patients. Surgical skills atrophy from disuse. Diagnostic and decision-making skills diminish when underutilized. Flexner, the academician, seeing only flaws in the clinician, had little or no understanding of the role these factors play in the making of a great clinician and teacher. Flexner's lack of interest in the community and his concept of the medical school as an ivory tower—or citadel of excellence—led us to disaster in coping with the increasing demands and needs of people in the community for health care. What Flexner failed to appreciate was that strict full time, by his definition, never envisioned service around the clock but really meant 9:00 A.M. to 5:00 P.M. on weekdays with no one except house staff available at night, on weekends, in emergencies, vacations, during long absences on site visits, national society meetings, grant reviewing and NIH activities, etc. Flexnerian full time was science-centered, not service-oriented. Neither had Flexner foreseen the massive proliferation of committee assignments, administrative demands, and nonprofessional activities eating up much of the day for the full-time staff, leaving very little time for teaching, scholarly pursuits, contemplation, and research, his real *raison d'être* for full time. The full-time professor was, in truth, a part-time clinician, while the part-time teacher was a full-time physician.

In addition, Flexner, by demeaning the participation of the university professor in private practice, was cutting off the lifeline of financial support for the medical center from the surrounding community. This was an especially grave error that Flexner as a nonphysician failed to appreciate. Philanthropists like to give money to hospitals and institutions where their own doctors work. Witness the major gifts of the Harkness family to the Columbia-Presbyterian Medical Center, where their personal physicians were on staff, among them Dr. Albert R. Lamb and Dr. Fordyce B. St. John. Recall the major fund-raising activities of Frank Billings at the University of Chicago based upon his warm personal relationship with his private patients. And high on any list is the performance of Dr. William S. McCann of the University of Rochester, who raised over twenty million dollars from his private patients for the medical school, assuring his department of medicine of an endowment that is the envy of many schools.[370] Every major voluntary hospital or school has similar tales to tell. If the doctors had not been in the personal private practice of medicine, who knows where all of that money might have gone. This potential for fund raising was completely ignored by Flexner, who failed to appreciate that a warm doctor-patient relationship established by following Peabody's precepts could do more for fund raising in medicine than a thousand slick brochures and eloquent letters.

Finally, Flexner was unaware that the strict full-time role model was a very poor example for the majority of medical students, most of whom were destined to enter private practice. The system was much too solicitous and protective of the comforts of the full-time teacher, with little thought given to the patients assigned to his care. Who would see the patient in an emergency, after hours, or on the weekend? Who would teach primary care or family care? Who would make the house calls? Is it any wonder that students sought to emulate their teachers, looking for salaried jobs with regular working hours, no night duty, and no weekend work? Is it any wonder that poor work habits and an overweening desire for leisure and recreation should engulf the medical profession?

How can the modern day medical internship or residency, which heavily stresses time "off call," ever produce the physician who will be available around the clock for his patients once he

370. Romano, John, (Ed.): *To Each His Farthest Star.* Fifthieth Anniversary, University of Rochester Medical Center, Rochester, University of Rochester, 1975, p. 483.

leaves the protection of his hospital or ivory tower? Doctors of the current medical house staff are classified as "full-timers" despite the fact that they are on duty from 9:00A.M. to 5:00 P.M. on weekdays, with only every third night on duty and every third weekend on call. No wonder we need, in a major teaching hospital, 245 house staff doctors to take care of the same patient load that only thirty years ago was handled by forty-five interns and residents. Not only is this financially wasteful, it is a dreadful way to train and prepare young doctors for a profession of service to the public. I submit that we should take a hard look at these trends among house staff and institute remedial measures to make better clinical practitioners of them and to instill in their way of life the concept of rendering service, something the full-time system has failed to do.

In exposing the weaknesses of the full-time system in the clinical departments, it is not intended to deny that there are some positive features and strengths in the plan. There are distinct advantages in having on the premises of the hospital or medical school a cadre of highly respected, skilled clinical teachers, administrators, and investigators on full-time salary. Objections arise when the system calls for all, or the majority, of clinical teachers to be on full time. Even more criticism arises if the full-time faculty is seldom visible to the students and patients, is away more then present, shirks clinical teaching assignments, and prefers to isolate itself from the community served by the hospital and medical school. Major objections arise when, as is so often the case, individuals with little or no experience in the personal practice of medicine are selected to become department heads, the choice seldom being based on proved clinical competence but largely on research publications and on the hope that somehow clinical competence will emerge. Demonstrated clinical competence and experience should be a major factor and not a minor one in the selection of those who are to direct clinical departments. In the rush to recognize scientific achievement and administrative talent, professional clinical competence has been grossly neglected, and we have paid a price for this in the decline in the clinical capabilities of the average medical school graduate who all too often emerges from four years of medical school lacking the basic skills to be a physician. For those who point to brilliant exceptions, to these criticisms found on every faculty, the answer is that the emergence of such individuals is more a tribute to their own ingenuity and excellence than to the full-time system under which they work.

Chapter 36
NEW MEDICAL SCHOOLS NEEDED:

Not the Post-Flexner Dinosaur Model

Returning to the doctor shortage, which I believe exists and on which point I find myself in disagreement with some authorities, what remedies do I propose?

Undeniably, we need more new medical schools. The tragedy we must terminate is the turning away at the gates of our own medical schools, some 25,000 per year of our highly qualified young people despite their excellent records, high intelligence, exceptional ideals and motivation, simply because there are not enough places.

We need more medical schools quite different from the existing ones. Before describing the kind of new schools we need, I shall lay the groundwork for my argument by clearing out some of the underbrush that has proliferated about the Flexnerian legend. First, let us consider Flexner's view that a medical school had to be an integral part of the university, physically as well as conceptually. He quoted the German university model as the ideal of ideals, but on close inspection it is quite clear that Flexner was mistaken about the workings of the German universities and their *Kliniken.* His concept that the professor of Sanskrit should be paid the same salary as the professor of medicine or surgery in the medical school completely overlooks the real facts of life.

This topic was thoroughly aired by Dr. Robert H. Ebert of Harvard Medical School in a recent sparkling essay, "Medical Education in the United States," in which he examined the hospital phase of medical education in Germany in Flexner's time and compared it with modern-day practices in America.[371] Ebert pointed out that although the German teaching hospitals

371. Knowles, J. H.: *Doing Better and Feeling Worse.* Chapter by R. H. Ebert, Medical Education in the United States, New York, W. W. Norton and Co., 1977, pp. 171-184.

were under the university umbrella, the German university was highly decentralized and "little more than a loose federation of autonomous departments" called *Kliniken*. There was almost no communication among the various *Kliniken*, even those within the same university, and the teaching of medical students was largely didactic, by lecture, and with little or no direct exposure to patients. Ebert felt it was a "successful model in terms of research and advanced training in scientific medicine. But it was a poor model for the education of medical students, and it produced a large number of rather badly trained general practitioners and a relatively small number of very well trained specialists." He then stated that the German model could not be adopted in America for a number of reasons and proceeded to identify them; he stressed the differences in organization of the American and German universities and the vastly different hospital structure in the two countries, the German hospital being government owned, whereas the American ones were in the main privately owned and controlled. Imposing the German system upon American medical schools and hospitals seemed out of the question in actual practice, but this did not appear to deter Flexner who embarked on his quest with considerable vigor. One of his serious mistakes was to underestimate the service function of the teaching hospital, in fact, Flexner repeatedly ignored service for science.

Ebert, in commenting on the developments of the past seventy years' since Flexner, asked these questions:

> But had the teaching hospital in fact become a part of the university? There were many who would note the predominance of full-time faculty, the high quality of research, and the commitment to teaching, and would say "yes." They would claim that clinical departments—or at least some clinical departments—were every bit as academic as the basic-science departments. And there would be some truth to these claims. But do any or all of these claims make the teaching hospital an integral part of the university? Not necessarily, for a fundamental difference between the teaching hospital and the rest of the university always remains. The hospital must provide a service—namely, the care of the sick—which is unrelated to the primary role of the university, and it must provide that service day in and day out, year in and year out, whatever the requirements may be for teaching and research. . . . Unlike the university, the patients served—not the students—represent the primary constitutency of the hospital. . . . The teaching hospital is certainly

> academic, but it represents the part of the educational system devoted to the training of the physicians. It works with the university, but it is not an integral part of it.[372]

Returning to Abraham Flexner and his dream that the university should dominate the medical school and its hospitals, his notions regarding financial rewards for clinicians versus academicians were unrealistic chiefly because he did not appreciate the importance of the service aspects of a doctor's existence. Teaching medical students and house staff and directing research is only part of the clinical professor's work, much of his time being devoted to rendering or supervising the rendition of service to patients in the university hospital and clinics. This service obligation runs around the clock, 365 days of the year. Contrast this with the usual obligations of a university professor who has to teach a few hours in the year, has most of the time at his own disposal for scholarly pursuits, and has virtually no service obligations and few requiring the intensity of physical and mental commitment demanded of the clinical professor.

In real life, physicians in private practice earn more money than undergraduate teachers who are in the main dependent upon university salaries that never seem adequate. The practicing physician has several other options, engaging in private practice, going on full-time salary, or a variety of combinations of the two, while the undergraduate teacher seldom has these options. Holders of Ph.D. degrees are numerous and in surplus supply, while the M.D. is in short supply and in high demand. These considerations influence the salary scale for the two groups. Medical schools have to pay higher salary to their faculty than the undergraduate school does to its own teachers. One would think that, in this day and age, these facts should be well known to university faculty and their leaders, but the issue remains acrimonious and divisive, the undergraduate faculty openly or covertly resenting the larger incomes of the clinical faculty.

Physical proximity of the university to the medical school by no means assures an amicable and effective relationship between the two. I have seldom seen any great input of undergraduate faculty of the university into the teaching activity of a school of medicine. This is not to say there should not be, but

372. *Ibid.*, pp. 177-78.

my point is that there is none. Even in the medical school itself, seldom do we see a professor of biochemistry or physiology making rounds with the clinicians, and there is much room for improvement in the relationships between preclinical and clinical professors despite the fact that their offices may be only a few doors away from each other.

Flexner's belief that the entire clinical staff should be on a full-time salaried basis has been discussed in detail in earlier chapters and demonstrated to be a misguided, unworkable, uneconomic, and impractical venture, totally out of touch with the care of the patient and the needs of the community.

Knowing these facts to be true, the Flexnerians who have planned most of the new medical schools have continued to seek this "unattainable ideal" and have required that university and medical school and its hospital be built together, sometimes under one roof, and usually *de novo*. Instead of building a new medical school around an established and vigorous hospital with a sound track record and loyal clientele, the Flexnerians have all too often elected to build a new university hospital in the desert or in some isolated community usually after they have built the medical school, and sometimes even the university, on an attractive but relatively inaccessible site far from the people it is designed to serve. The initial cost of these centers is prohibitive and their maintenance even more so. No wonder the experience is that it generally takes ten years from the birth of the concept to the admission of the first medical student to these medical schools. When federal funds seemed unlimited, they were spent like water. No wonder the money has run out.

With most of the existing medical schools conforming to the Flexnerian dinosaur type, the time is ripe for innovation and trial of new models emphasizing low initial cost, low maintenance, and efficient and dedicated commitment to the principal mission of a medical school, the education and training of physicians for the practice of medicine.

Instead of building a $100 million university hospital in the desert, let us start with an existing, highly regarded hospital with a good staff and excellent trustees in a community able and willing to give substantial support. The staff of the hospital can be strengthened by a small cadre of full-time salaried clinician-teachers, experienced in rendering patient care on a one-to-one basis, and committed to encouraging growth and development by providing sympathetic and innovative direction and leadership to a largely part-time voluntary staff and to a smaller geographic full-time staff interested and competent in teaching, rendering service, and undertaking clinical research. This staff should be in the main self-supporting through its own efforts and not require an enormous budget. Such a staff will be respected in the community, will have its roots in the neighborhood, and will serve it well. It will be more apt to stay put and not be as freely mobile as one without private practice ties facilitating movement from one better paying position to another, like a rolling stone.

Where will the preclinical or basic science faculty come from? One approach is to affiliate the medical school with a suitable university in a loose network, the basic sciences being taught at the university, the clinical subjects at the hospital. Another alternative, which I prefer, is to select a basic science faculty specifically for this kind of medical school, demanding that its chief purpose not be limited to basic laboratory research but to the teaching of physiology, anatomy, pharmacology, and biochemistry to students who are for the most part going to be practitioners of medicine. This is not to say that these departments are to be second-class. They need to be so oriented that teaching medical students is their number one priority. This is not to forbid any research. It is to stress teaching activity and to reward this appropriately. Instead of finding the institution crawling with Ph.D. candidates, who in the current era sometimes outnumber the medical students in the basic sciences, the medical school will really be turned back to the medical students, and most of the Ph.D.s will be diverted to the university setting where they really belong.

This kind of medical school would represent an American version of the British Hospital schools in London, which have for many many generations produced 90 percent of the physicians and surgeons of Great Britain. Clinically, these schools have consistently turned out an excellent product. Schools developed along these lines could be started up almost overnight if the leadership were vigorous and energetic. They would not require enormous capital funds and massive endowment. They could be set up in almost any community of 50,000 or more people and distributed across the country where they are needed most. Their graduates would be more apt to settle where they have studied. The university hospital's commitment to patient care and community health care would be sincere and documented by its past performance.

These concepts are by no means original, but for years they have been minority opinions while Flexnerian theories have held sway. In a recent monograph, *Medical Education Since 1960: Marching to a Different Drummer,* the evolution of "Community-Based Medical Schools" is thoroughly aired.[373] The movement has much in its favor and incorporates some of the suggestions presented in the preceding discussion. There is the fear in some quarters that the emphasis of these schools on service may lead to dilution of their commitment to scientific medicine. We need both in a well-balanced relationship to each other. The important and key point is that alternatives to the Flexnerian approach to medical education are undergoing study and experimentation and they need to be supported and encouraged.

ADMISSION TO MEDICAL SCHOOL

For years, most of those involved in medical education have been critical of existing methods of selecting students for admission. At a time when we have been leaning more and more on grades to the degree that some medical schools have set a 3.6 out of 4 average as the cutoff point for interviews, we find considerable evidence that grades do not mean as much as they did. They have undergone dilution, and we have been warned by our deans of this trend. For example, Duke University Medical School recently warned its interviewers of the altered significance of college grades. The dean cited the example of an applicant from a prestigious university for whom his professor of organic chemistry had written a letter of recommendation stating in part that the applicant stood 176th in a class of 316 and received an "A."

Even more disturbing is the trend to more and more aggressive

373. Hunt, Andrew D. and Weeks, Lewis E., Ed.: *Medical Education Since 1960: Marching to a Different Drummer.* Battle Creek, The Michigan State University Foundation with the cooperation and support of the W. K. Kellogg Foundation, 1980.

grade grubbing and vicious competition among premedical students. Reports of cheating, vandalism and destruction by some premedical students of their competitors' experimental material and data are especially serious, and, while known to their peers, seldom reported or punished. Would grade grubbing be less severe if less emphasis were placed upon the 3.6 or above level? I know there are plenty of candidates with 3.0 averages who would make excellent physicians, and I believe the emphasis should be on other aspects of the candidate's qualifications. Cheating and other unethical and antisocial activities are especially serious in those seeking to enter the medical profession and should be detected and punished early rather than accepted as normal or acceptable practice in today's world.

The MCATs (Medical College Admisstion Tests) have not provided much help in the selection process. The most that can be said for them is that individuals with high MCAT scores will almost certainly get through the first two years of medical school, but they fail to predict performance in the clinical years. Dissatisfaction with the MCATs has been so great as to lead to the development of a new type of MCAT examination designed in part to better measure noncognitive as well as cognitive skills. The first new MCATs were administered in 1977, the scientific problem section being the only really new part, and it is much too early to gauge their value, but I have an uncomfortable feeling that they may not tell us much more than the old ones. The search for methods of predicting clinical performance is being actively pursued but they remain elusive.

One stimulus for this quest is the criticism that medical schools have been overproducing specialists and subspecialists and neglecting the generalists who are in short supply and considerable demand. Faculty role models, predominantly specialists, have been blamed for this trend. While they must accept much of this responsibility, there are many who feel that part of the difficulty stems back to the kinds of students selected for admission to medical school. The emphasis has been overwhelmingly on scientific training and competence almost to the exclusion of other qualities that may be much more important in the makeup of a physician.

Should we not take a close look at the composition of medical school admissions committees? How many are dominated by basic scientists with limited comprehension of what it takes to make a good doctor? How strongly are the clinical services represented? Are there practicing clinicians on the committee? Should some thought be given to having well-informed laymen as well as doctors among its membership? How can we spot and measure noncognitive traits in applicants for medical school? How do we measure character, integrity, leadership, decision making, morality, ethics, compassion, caring, empathy, ability to communicate, ability to work as part of a team, capacity for giving more than taking, staying power, and steadiness under fire? These are important traits we treasure as those of the ideal physician and we must find ways to identify them. With evidence accumulating that the Myers-Briggs psychological tests for personality type may yield objective data identifying traits of the student who is likely to head for primary care medicine rather than subspecialties, why don't we use them?[374]

Finally, for those who argue that we shall be faced with a surplus of doctors during this decade and that no new medical schools are needed, my reply is to question the statistical basis for this belief and to express this caveat. Why, of all of the learned professions, should medicine be singled out to practice birth control on its progeny? Is there any precedent for this in America in the legal profession, engineering, teaching, or the ministry? Why should we deny any competent and dedicated young man or woman, perhaps your own children, the opportunity to study medicine? If this policy should lead to an oversupply, let the rules of free enterprise resolve the issue. If doctors are making too much money, why not break up the monopoly by producing more of them and introducing competition for patients into their everyday lives?

374. Myers, Isabel B.: *Introduction to Type,* 2nd Ed. Center for Applications of Psychological Type. Gainesville, FL., 1976.

Chapter 37
L'ENVOI

Le Cri de Coeur

Live pure, speak true, right wrong, follow the King–
Else, wherefore born?

The Round Table
Gareth and Lynette
Alfred, Lord Tennyson[375]

The list of things that went wrong in the making of the American doctor is far from complete, but at least a number have been identified. This is not to infer that everything that happened was bad, for many wonderful advances were made, contributing substantially to the better education and training of the doctor, placing in his hands a formidable array of diagnostic and therapeutic weapons of almost incredible sophistication for the fight against disease. I have chosen to concentrate on what we might call negative factors rather than positive ones. I have elected to stress what I perceive to be failures and undesirable trends in the education and training of physicians for rendering service to people rather than to emphasize the major discoveries and great scientific achievements of the past helf century that have made American medicine the envy of the world. My reason for this is that despite the major advances in medical technology of the past fifty years, and perhaps to some degree as a result of them, the general public is now more critical of the American physician than it has ever been. Through its politicians, and a minority of M.D.s, it seeks to impose upon the medical profession at large well nigh overwhelming bureaucratic control and over-regulation at the very time in our history when the record of medical achievement and the health status of the nation have never been better.

Having devoted much time and effort to identifying what went

375. Tennyson, Alfred, Lord: *The Poetical Works of Tennyson.* Cambridge Edition, G. Robert Stangle (Ed.). Boston, Houghton Mifflin Co., 1974.

wrong, I would betray my professional instincts were I not to seize this opportunity to recommend therapy to cure or prevent the ailments I have diagnosed. Are the conditions I have described beyond remedy? Is it already too late? Is not the central theme of *The Last Angry Man* as relevant today as it was in 1956? Written by Gerald Green (currently a celebrity for *Holocaust*) about his uncle, Samuel Greenberg, M.D. (1886-1952), a general practitioner who continued to practice in his deteriorating Brooklyn neighborhood long after his colleagues and better patients had fled, it describes the conversion of a TV executive who came to "con" the old doctor into participating in a "This is your life" type program and staying to admire him in death, if not before.

> There aren't enough people left who get mad, plain mad (said the TV producer). Not mad for a cause or a purpose, but just generally mad at all the bitchery and fraud we take for granted. We accept it. We like it. We want to be had. That's where he was different. He knew he was being cheated and he didn't like it one tiny bit, whether it was some old biddy doing him out of his two dollars or a corporation telling him they made better cathartics. He was the last angry man.[376]

Sam Abelman (Dr. Samuel Greenberg) was not the last angry man, nor was he even next to the last. There are many others in the profession of medicine who share his kind of anger toward some trends in our society, our institutions, our profession, and ourselves. I, for one, simply refuse to stand by, mute, accepting as inevitable the undesirable developments and moral decay of the past several decades. A society that allows permissiveness, promiscuity, and irresponsibility to run amok; adultery to become a way of life; teenage sex the rule rather than the exception, venereal disease to run rampant; with the breakdown of family life, with over one million abortions during the past year (almost half that number of "unwanted" teenage pregnancies), drug abuse and alcoholism almost beyond belief, charging these and more to the health care bill and then objecting to the escalating costs of these irresponsible activities and demanding that government and tax subsidy pay for them, that society has to be regarded as a sick organization.

---

376. Green, Gerald: *The Last Angry Man*. New York, Scribner's Sons, 1956, pp. 486-90.

I raise my voice against attempts by government and its spokesmen to control our great profession and their efforts to label it a trade and to treat it as such.

I decry the performance of some academic leaders of American medicine who lost sight of personal and primary care of the patient and what McKeown has called the Samaritan role of medicine and focussed to an excessive degree on basic research and the medicine of tomorrow to the neglect of the problems of health care delivery of today. I am unhappy that many of our learned societies and specialty organizations that should be providing leadership have become kudos-awarding associations dominated and led by individuals who appear to have lost touch with the man in the street and with the actual practice of medicine. I blame the overproduction of subspecialists on our specialty boards whose makeup is excessively dominated by academicians, some of whom have never really experienced the trials of personal medical practice and many of whom have lost touch with the personal health requirements of our people.

I decry the overemphasis on technology, testing, and procedures dominating American medicine. I object to a system of health care that inappropriately rewards doing things to people to the neglect of thinking, communicating, and caring for the patient.

I am appalled that prominent academicians engaged in medical research have cheated, fudged data, and plagiarized in order to advance their careers. Can the man in the street be blamed for losing faith in scientists? When *The New York Times* headlines on its front page, "Columbia Medical Chief Resigns; Ex-Associate's Data Fraud at Issue,"[377] where will it end? Have we not reached a stage when decaying moral and ethical standards, even among the elite, cry out for reform in our profession, our society, our legal system, and in our day-to-day life and activities? Who among us will rise up to carry the torch of reform to lead us out of the current morass?

I blame the profession of medicine for permitting self-interest, greed, avarice and, on occasion, dishonesty to impair its image. So long as Medicaid mills, Medicare fraud, fee-splitting, kickbacks,

377. *The New York Times,* August 9, 1980, front page.

unnecessary operations, "no show" jobs and the like exist, there will be no peace for the medical profession. When doctors seek what is in it for themselves and act in self-interest rather than the public good, medicine as a whole will suffer, and the majority of doctors will have to pay the price for the misdeeds of a few. I blame the medical profession for emphasizing its own creature comforts tothe exclusion of concern for the sick. The virtual disappearance of the house call and the lack of availability of doctors after office hours, on the weekend, or on "doctor's day off" have reached the proportions of a national scandal. Medicine, in its finest sense, cannot be practiced as a trade confined to "business hours." Committees and groups of doctors are inadequate substitutes for one's own physician. Every patient is entitled to have his or her own doctor.

I object to the selection process for admission to medical school for overemphasizing grades and neglecting to seek out and to identify the traits those of us on the front line know to be essential in a man or woman seeking to become a physician. I decry the current climate of excessive competition for grades in the sciences that have set apart "premed" students in the universities and led to their being regarded as pariahs by their nonmedical peers. Even more do I decry the cheating and dishonesty alleged to be common in the struggle for high grades and wonder why the malefactors are not identified and kicked out of college. I object to the narrowness of current premedical education and its failure to provide individuals with a broad base of knowledge and strengths in the humanities as well as the sciences. While I would not go so far as Lewis Thomas in advocating a return to the study of Greek in the premedical curriculum, I urge that the study of modern languages be reinstalled.

I cry out against a system that turns away 25,000 of our best young people each year at the gates to medical school, not because they are incompetent but because there are not enough places. And then, to compound this evil as we have for years, imports from foreign countries, chiefly in Asia, the equivalent of the total annual output of our own medical schools, are depriving the country of origin of their own graduates and utilizing the resources of poor and so-called developing nations to provide doctors for the richest nation in the world. I, for one, cannot understand why we do not have more medical schools in America and am unwilling to accept the excuses. I deplore newspaper headlines like the one in the *Washington Post* of October 25, 1978, announcing "U.S. Won't Help Start More Medical Schools," the chief protagonist then being Health, Education and Welfare Secretary, Joseph A. Califano, Jr., who said we have reached the point of creating a doctor surplus. A "surplus," if it exists or will appear, produced in my opinion by the senseless U. S. policy of importing foreign medical graduates, chiefly from Asia, in enormous numbers, during the past decade or more. Remedial legislation has been passed to plug the loophole, but evasive tactics are being employed by several groups and I predict it will be some years before the flood will be cut to a trickle. From what I see of the medical education scene, perhaps it is high time for the U. S. Government to step aside as the *major* arbiter of where and when new medical schools should be built. The record of the past seems conclusive to me that private voluntary sources have done a better job in developing new medical schools than big government. We need more medical schools, preferably not of the Flexnerian dinosaur model. Taking a leaf from the auto industry, we need compact models with better fuel mileage.

I believe, despite the protestations of many, that we do not have enough medical schools in America to produce the doctors needed for all of our people. I have no fear of overproduction if we cease to import foreign medical graduates to cope with the demand. If doctors want to preserve the free enterprise system they hold so dear, let us produce enough of them so that the law of supply and demand will be operative in a free market providing solely that the product be a superior one, highly qualified and morally and ethically committed to the highest possible standards. Nothing would make me happier than to see the individuals who enter medicine primarily to make money disappear from the scene to pursue other areas of endeavor. I believe the doctor who seeks only to take on the "easy cases" that do not take very much out of him is a misfit in the profession. Perhaps the economic necessity may drive him to accept the bad as well as the good, and in the process perform a great public service. The individual who seeks a life of ease and luxury is out of place in medicine as I see it, and society would be better off without him.

To our philanthropists and philanthropoids, I urge recommitment to those goals so brilliantly pursued and embraced by the Rockefellers, Harkness, Eastman, Duke, et al. To the church, irrespective of creed or sect, I urge return to committed involvement in the field of health care. Let us do the job ourselves and not depend upon government and bureaucracy to do it for us or to us.

Franz Ingelfinger has said,

> The paradox identified by Thomas, Cooper and Wildavsky is born of the fact that society, although it itself has abandoned the old-fashioned virtues, still demands to find them in the sons of Hippocrates. Physicians, indeed, are expected to be chimera-like creatures who, on one hand, should be expert in the fabulous knowledge and skills of the scientific century, but on the other, should simultaneously display the humanity, compassion, and devotion attributed to "the good old doc!"[378]

Ingelfinger continues, pointing out that society in general has become depersonalized, urbanized and homogenized. He asks, "Should doctors, who en masse are ordinary if specially educated folk, be expected to seek different objectives and to observe a different ethos." My answer is a loud and resounding *yes, of course*! In fact, my position is that those aspiring to a career in medicine must be held to the highest possible standards of morality, ethics, sincerity, and compassion toward their fellowman. I set standards for those entering the profession far above the median for the rest of our society. The doctor should be different, above reproach, and subjected to standards reserved for no other profession except perhaps the ministry. If this is too much to expect or demand, then look for medicine to plunge in public esteem rather than to rise higher. Look for medicine to retreat from its high ground to the level of the trade our enemies are seeking to push us into. I don't believe it is asking too much; I believe it is a practical goal. We have thousands of eager, idealistic, bright, and dedicated young people seeking each year to enter medicine. Let us not sell them short. They will respond to good leadership. Set the standards high and select only the best!

378. Ingelfinger, F. J.: Medicine: meritorious or Meritricious? *Science, 200/4344:*942-46, May 26, 1978.

Clearly, the time is ripe for change and improvement and more than anything else for the restoration to medicine of some of its old virtues and qualities that in recent years have worn rather thin. Other voices have been raised on this front; one of the most respected that of Sir George Pickering, who said in his Schroeder Lecture at Dartmouth College in 1976:

> I believe that the profession of medicine is now facing a dilemma which may destroy it unless the nature of the choice is seen clearly and faced with insight, courage, and resolution. The dilemma is similar in Britain and in the United States. Should medicine behave as a learned profession or as a technical trades union? . . .
>
> Fifty years ago when I first visited this country, medicine was at its best deeply respected as a learned profession. The great doctors were learned and the less great would have liked to be and respected those who were. Professional standards were high; service to the sick and integrity were the watchwords. Professional bodies sought to maintain and enhance standards and discourage those who erred or who sought to err. Now medicine seems to be in danger of ceasing to value or respect learning. What would have been regarded as unprofessional behaviour is not only tolerated but encouraged by the larger organisations of both senior and junior doctors. This is what I mean by medicine on the brink. In my more realistic and more pessimistic moods, I suspect that we are no longer pausing at the riverbank but that we have already crossed. Yet medicine increasingly attracts the best of our young. If they can detach themselves from the myopic selfishness of their predecessors and resist the stupidity of some of their leaders and some bureaucrats and politicians, I am sure there is still hope. The tide of battle may have set against the idealists, but it is not yet finally lost.[379]

I agree with Sir George that time is running out for us, and the optimist in me says we still have a chance. The question is how to fight this battle, how to reverse these undesirable trends in our society, and how to recruit the troops we need to turn the tide.

> For those who have already lost, or may be in the process of losing, faith in the importance of individual effort in achieving high goals, and look only to the government and large organizations to achieve progress, my message and my hope is that they may return to the battlefield refreshed and inspired by the magnificent record of past achievement in medicine compiled by individual men and women of high spirit and courage who, paraphrasing St. Ignatius Loyola, gave and did not count the cost, fought and did not heed the

379. Pickering, Sir George: Medicine on the brink: The dilemma of a learned profession. *Perspectives in Biology and Medicine*, Summer 1978, p. 551.

> wounds, toiled and did not seek rest, labored and asked for no reward.[380]

The great medical institutions that have sprung up across the country did not arise *de novo* from the soil or by spontaneous generation. Each one is the product of inspired, dedicated individuals who sought to advance medicine and to better the quality of life of his fellowman. To name the Rockefellers, Senior and Junior, Carnegie, Johns Hopkins, Vanderbilt, Payne Whitney, Morgan, Harkness, Brookings, Eastman, and Duke is to make only a partial list of the great benefactors. Add to these the names of Frederick T. Gates, Abraham Flexner, Henry S. Pritchett, Charles W. Eliot, Daniel Coit Gilman, Wallace Buttrick, James H. Kirkland, Rush Rhees, W. P. Few, laymen who saw the vision of the benefactors and translated them into reality.

Topping it off, the truly great leaders of the revolution in American medical education: William H. Welch, Osler, Halsted, Mall, Cushing, Howland, Abel, Howell, Simon Flexner, Edsall, Billings, to name a few followed by their illustrious students, George H. Whipple, Wilburt C. Davison, Milton Winternitz, William G. MacCallum, Walter B. Cannon, G. Canby Robinson, Barker, Thayer, Wilder Penfield, Alan Gregg, Francis, W. Peabody, Robert F. Loeb, Walter W. Palmer, Thomas Rivers, Francis G. Blake, Frederic M. Hanes, John P. Peters, Warfield Longcope, Dickinson Richards, George W. Corner, Wallace O. Fenn, Edward F. Adolph, William S. McCann, Stanhope Bayne-Jones, George R. Minot, William B. Castle, Florence Sabin, and the like. Each of these individuals deserves a vignette and more, but space does not permit it.

For this specific discussion, my point is that American medicine owes to each a tremendous debt for individual activity in advancing scientific medicine to the high pinnacle it has reached. The going was seldom easy and many obstacles had to be overcome. Success was not gained without enormous effort, sacrifice, and dedication. Witness George Whipple foregoing the temptation of a year in Europe to stay home in Rochester to oversee in person every foot of construction in the new medical school he was building in Rochester, cutting expenses wherever possible,

380. Loyola, St. Ignatius (1491-1556): Prayer for Generosity (1548). *Bartlett's Familiar Quotations*, 14th Ed. Boston, Little, Brown & Co., 1968, p. 180b.

conserving his endowment for scholarly use, not dissipating it on bricks, mortar, or marble. The calmness, fairness, and integrity of a Walter W. Palmer in cooling off the angry antagonistic Abraham Flexner, in the classic confrontation that saved the Columbia-Presbyterian Medical Center from going down the drain by persuading the General Education Board and Flexner not to rescind the Rockefeller gifts because of the failure of an attempt at full-time staffing. The wisdom and financial sagacity of Wilburt C. Davison in committing Duke University Medical School to geographic full time and group practice when these innovations were regarded as anathema by Flexner and his board. These were individual actions and deeds, some of them fraught with danger. If ever there was a time in American medicine when the word crisis could be spelled as do the Chinese, with two characters, one–danger, the other–opportunity, this was it. Most importantly, these individual leaders had the competence, the courage, and the staying power to succeed in achieving their goals. America will forever be in their debt, and America must never forget them.

Let us return to Jacques Barzun and his message for the professions, "that their one hope of survival with anything like their present freedoms is the recovery of mental and moral force."[381] In medicine, I believe the so-called mental force that I take to be scientific and technological competence of the average physician has never been higher. I have no quarrel with this. We choose the best students, we hope, and subject them to a grueling, demanding pace that turns out a first-rate scientific product, among the best in the world. It is in the area of what Barzun calls the moral force that some deficiencies have appeared and have led to much of the difficulty the profession is experiencing with the public. Unless this moral force is strengthened and improved, medicine will continue to lose ground despite its enormous technological and scientific advances. Can a society that seems to be rivaling ancient Rome in its failings be asked to produce sons and daughters who will rise above the mediocrity and lead the way to decency, morality,compassion, and genuine concern for each and everyone? I not only believe it can, I happen to feel

381. Barzun, Jacques: The professions under siege: private practice versus public need. *Harper's, 257/1541:*61-68, Oct. 1978, p. 68.

that it must if it seeks to survive. The guide lines for our society were laid down centuries ago in the ageless Ten Commandments and amplified by Christ (Mark 12:30-31):

> Thou shalt love the Lord thy God with all thy heart and with all thy soul, and with all thy mind. This is the first and great commandment. The second is like unto it. Thou shalt love thy neighbor as thyself. On these two commandments hang all the Law and the Prophets.[382]

When a great medical educator, Robert F. Loeb, placed first in his list of Laws for Treatment, the Golden Rule, we know that the passage of centuries has not dimmed the luster of this basic tenet of human behavior. Yet, think of the many instances where these rules and admonitions have been ignored and flaunted. Is it any wonder that society appears to be lost and floundering?

Perhaps one of the great weaknesses in our method of educating people for the profession of medicine is that we have emphasized scientific competence to the neglect of morality, integrity, compassion, and plain everyday kindness. Medicine started in the Church, its early schools being church controlled and its earliest practitioners priests of the church. The hospitals originated as church related units and were in the main charitable institutions. Witness in New York City alone the profusion of church related teaching hospitals: Presbyterian, St. Luke's, St. Vincent's, Mt. Sinai, to name only a few and with no intent to slight the others. Early on, the evidence of a religious presence was for most of these institutions a fact of life. It set them apart. With the passage of years, the intervention of big business methods, the control by third-party payers (including the government), secularization of the institutions has become a way of life. With this development, I submit that we have lost something very real that may account for the reaction of the public who feel that our hospitals have become impersonal, cold, remote, insensitive, unsympathetic, and money oriented.

Granted that the physician is the key to the hospital, its core, its essence. I place upon him the responsibility for maintaining the morale, compassion, concern, kindness, and the concept of service to the people entering its doors. By his life-style, his dress, his competence, his language, his self-discipline, his cleanliness,

382. The Bible: New Testament. Mark 12:30-31.

his kindness, his understanding, his willingness to serve others with pleasure, the doctor will influence untold numbers of people with whom he comes into contact. The doctor is always on stage no matter whether he is on an elevator, in a corridor, in a coffee shop, an office, or in the emergency room, or operating theatre. If he conducts himself as a good human being as well as a highly trained one, the effect on those nearby can be inspirational. From this stems the reputation of the hospital. If the doctors set the standard, the rest will follow for better or for worse. Is this asking too much of the doctor? I, for one, do not believe it is. I think it is essential and, indeed, mandatory for doctors to conduct their lives in this way. I believe doctors must somehow find the motivation, the integrity, and the decency to pursue this way of life as a member of a profession devoted to healing and helping others. There are those who will take issue with my position and maintain that doctors should come down from their pedestals, eschew their role of exceptional beings, and become as one with the common man. I have the impression that if we seek to reduce the physician in our society to a mediocre role, the general public will lose more in the process than it will gain. The human being who places his life in the hands of his physician needs to feel that his physician is above reproach, has superior skills, and is by no means a common person.

As President Hoover said in his essay, "The Uncommon Man":

> In my opinion there has been too much talk about the Common Man. . . . Thus we are in danger of developing a cult of the Common Man which means a cult of mediocrity. Let us remember that the great human advances have not been brought about by mediocre men and women. They were brought about by distinctly uncommon people with vital sparks of leadership. . . . *It is a curious fact that when you get sick, you want an uncommon doctor;* if your car breaks down, you want an uncommonly good mechanic; when we get into war, we want dreadfully an uncommon admiral and an uncommon general. . . . For the future of America rests not in mediocrity, but in the constant renewal of leadership in every phase of our national life.[383] (Italics inserted by Doctor Lepore.)

I believe that most of the criticism physicians are faced with today has little to do with their technical competence, and I have identified some of the major areas of controversy in previous

383. Hoover, Herbert C. Essay: The uncommon man, in book entitled, *On Growing Up*. New York, William Morrow & Co., 1962, pp. 153-54.

chapters.

I believe it is not too late to institute remedial measures for the cure of the things that have gone wrong. The patient is not moribund, but he is getting weaker and therapy cannot be too long delayed. Any good practitioner knows that if the patient is doing poorly, someone else will be called to change the therapy. Let the medical profession initiate its own reforms before its detractors and the bureaucrats take over.

What remedies do I propose? I believe the practice of medicine is not a science but an art based upon scientific principles with its major purpose to provide service to people. By failing to emphasize service to the people and the community, Flexner's strict full-time scheme directed American medical education away from health care delivery and the personal care of the sick, and we are paying the price for this now. My proposal for change is to have the medical schools revert to Dr. Walter W. Palmer's position that their clinical teaching staffs be made up of a small cadre of full-time men and women joined with sympathetic and cooperative physicians on geographic full time and a substantial group of part-time voluntary staff based in the community. All would be committed to providing full service to the university, their hospitals, their patients, and the community regardless of the number of hours involved. The service funtion of medicine would not only be of a high technological order but would be given with compassion, dignity and, above all, with strict adherence to the Golden Rule.

I believe with Peabody that "the secret of the care of the patient is in caring for the patient." No physician of any experience can fail to appreciate this beautiful passage in Peabody's great essay.

> The good physician knows his patients through and through and his knowledge is bought dearly. Time, sympathy, and understanding must be lavishly dispensed, but the reward is to be found in that personal bond which forms the greatest satisfaction of the practice of medicine.[384]

It is this personal bond and the joy that derives from it, for physician and patient alike, that we hear so little about in medical training today. Blame this on the lack of good role models. The

384. Peabody, Francis W.: The care of the patient. *JAMA, 88:*877-82, Mar, 19, 1927.

satisfaction that the true physician derives from long-term association with his patients, their families, and their communities is a rich reward for hours, months, and even years of sweat, blood, and tears expended in the care of the sick.

With so much of medical education centered in hospitals and clinics, there is little or no opportunity for the student or house officer to appreciate what the personal practice of medicine entails and what satisfaction there is for the good doctor in the relationships he develops with his patients. I feel sorry for those who have never been exposed to these emotional experiences. They have been cheated out of one of life's greatest and most enduring sources of contentment. I believe more vigorous efforts should be made to bring into the teaching staff of all institutions more role models of physicians in personal private practice whose joy in their daily work and their frustrations too can be transmitted effectively to the students, house staff, and juniors. Instead of irrelevant electives in the fourth year of medical school, why not revive the preceptorship assignments to physicians in practice and modify them to correspond with the needs of the 1980s?

Seeing in the current crisis in medicine opportunity as well as danger, I appeal to medicine to seize the initiative. Our society is in a state of confusion, its values warped, its goals unsure, its direction unclear. The role of the clergy, the teacher, the wise counselor has become less and less important in a society where hedonism, irresponsibility, and lack of restraint have taken over. The great religions appear to have lost control of the people; the teaching profession is under intense criticism, and rightly so; the legal profession, always unpopular with the masses, is enjoying the lowest ebb of its prestige and is under almost daily attack in the press. The medical profession, while also under attack, is of all the professions still among the highly respected. People are coming to their doctors with problems that in the past were reserved for the clergy. Is the average doctor up to the demands of the crisis? I believe he should be and that his education should be designed to improve his effectiveness in this role. Many feel that among the greatest advances to come in medicine will be the role the doctors may play in altering the lifestyle of their patients. This is hard work but it can be done. This is where individual effort, time, and commitment may succeed where other approaches have failed. Every doctor should be a teacher, and every patient should have his own doctor. Therein lies the secret, the opportunity, only if the doctor will seize it and use it maximally and effectively. Here the greatest blows may be struck for preventing personal irresponsibility from progressing to drug addiction and overmedication, alcohol abuse, cigarette consumption, adultery, infidelity, venereal disease, compulsive gambling, dissolution of family life, compulsive overeating, and psychopathic behavior, to name a few.

Let us grasp the opportunity and make the most of it. Each physician has an important role to play in this crusade; if he works hard at it, there is no end to the potential for benefiting his patients and mankind.

For those who seek a panacea in national health insurance or socialized medicine, I offer a warning. Look around at other government controlled institutions. Do we want Veterans Administration type medicine across the board? God forbid! Does any doctor in his right mind want to surrender the freedom of his great profession to the bureaucrats who are already threatening to overwhelm us? Wasn't once enought for Watergate, Koreagate, Amtrak, the Postal Service, poverticians, the energy crisis, five-percenters, the GSA, ABSCAM, and other assorted disasters?

If the doctors treasure their freedom, let them work harder and recommit themselves to the service of their patients, reach the high ground of the priesthood of medicine by the greatest possible effort, and meritably enlist the support of the vast majority of our people who would like to continue to respect, love, and admire their doctors.

As I reach the end of this voyage, I must ask myself this critical question. Am I demanding too much of our doctors in this day and age? My reply is that the message is appropriate for any age, in the past, the present, or the future. Perhaps what I have been trying to communicate to and for our profession and those who seek admission to it was never so well said as in the beautiful timeless letter of St. Paul to the Corinthians speaking of spiritual gifts, chapter 12, verses 4 to 11:

> There are varieties of gifts, but the same Spirit. There are varieties of service, but the same Lord. There are many forms of work, but

> all of them, in all men, are the work of the same God. In each of us the Spirit is manifested in one particular way, for some useful purpose. One man through the Spirit, has the gift of wise speech, while another, by the power of the same Spirit, can put the deepest knowledge into words. Another, by the same Spirit, is granted faith; another, by the one Spirit, gifts of healing, and another miraculous powers; another has the gift of prophecy, and another ability to distinguish true spirits from false; yet another has the gift of ecstatic utterance of different kinds, and another the ability to interpret it. But all these gifts are the work of one and the same Spirit, distributing them separately to each individual at will.[385]

When the spiritual gifts of healing are bestowed and acquired by the physician, he is a man apart from his fellows, obligated to conduct his life in a manner beyond reproach, always remembering St. Paul's admonition that over and beyond the spiritual gifts "are three things that last forever: faith, hope and love, but the greatest of them all is love."[386] My word to those of our profession and those preparing to enter into it is to cherish and guard the God-given gift of healing and constantly seek to live by the rules of St. Paul.

As I reach the end of my story of the past fifty years in medical education and practice, I can think of no finer way to close than by quoting from Daniel Drake's *Essay Number One on Medical Education,* published in 1832.

> With these remarks I close this branch of our subject. If I have spoken freely, it has been as a friend, not an enemy of the profession. I have not written from the recesses of the cloister, but in the midst of society. Observation and personal experience have dictated every sentence, and have afforded me satisfactory evidence of its truth. For this, moreover, I might appeal to all my enlightened brethren in the United States. Not one of them could venture to gainsay, what has been asserted, nor commend the apathy which connives at the errors and abuses, which have been exposed. Let *them* begin the good work of reformation, and society will come quickly to their aid.[387]

385. The Bible. I Corinthians 12:4-11 (New English Translation).
386. *Ibid.*, I Corinthians 13:13 (New English Translation).
387. Drake, Daniel: *Practical Essays on Medical Education and the Medical Profession in the United States, XX.* Baltimore, The Johns Hopkins Press, 1952, pp. 18-19.

NAME INDEX

A

B

C

H

I

J

K

L

M

SUBJECT INDEX

G

H

J

L

M

T